Allergic and Respiratory Disease in Sports Medicine

CLINICAL ALLERGY AND IMMUNOLOGY

Series Editor

MICHAEL A. KALINER, M.D.

Medical Director
Institute for Asthma and Allergy
Washington, D.C.

1. Sinusitis: Pathophysiology and Treatment, *edited by Howard M. Druce*
2. Eosinophils in Allergy and Inflammation, *edited by Gerald J. Gleich and A. Barry Kay*
3. Molecular and Cellular Biology of the Allergic Response, *edited by Arnold I. Levinson and Yvonne Paterson*
4. Neuropeptides in Respiratory Medicine, *edited by Michael A. Kaliner, Peter J. Barnes, Gert H. H. Kunkel, and James N. Baraniuk*
5. Provocation Testing in Clinical Practice, *edited by Sheldon L. Spector*
6. Mast Cell Proteases in Immunology and Biology, *edited by George H. Caughey*
7. Histamine and H_1-Receptor Antagonists in Allergic Disease, *edited by F. Estelle R. Simons*
8. Immunopharmacology of Allergic Diseases, *edited by Robert G. Townley and Devendra K. Agrawal*
9. Indoor Air Pollution and Health, *edited by Emil J. Bardana, Jr., and Anthony Montanaro*
10. Genetics of Allergy and Asthma: Methods for Investigative Studies, *edited by Malcolm N. Blumenthal and Bengt Björkstén*
11. Allergic and Respiratory Disease in Sports Medicine, *edited by John M. Weiler*

ADDITIONAL VOLUMES IN PREPARATION

Allergic and Respiratory Disease in Sports Medicine

edited by

John M. Weiler

University of Iowa
Iowa City, Iowa

MARCEL DEKKER

DEKKER

MARCEL DEKKER, INC. NEW YORK • BASEL • HONG KONG

Library of Congress Cataloging-in-Publication Data

Allergic and respiratory disease in sports medicine / edited by John M. Weiler.
p. cm. — (Clinical allergy and immunology; 11)
Includes index.
ISBN 0-8247-9890-2 (hardcover: alk. paper)
1. Respiratory organs—Pathophysiology. 2. Exercise—Physiological aspects. 3. Asthma. 4. Sports medicine.
I. Weiler, J. M. II. Series.
[DNLM: 1. Asthma, Exercise-Induced. 2. Respiratory Tract Diseases. 3. Sports Medicine. W1 CL652 v.11 1997 / WF 553 A433 1997]
RC732.A42 1997
616.2—dc21
DNLM/DLC
for Library of Congress

97-5181
CIP

Please note: Drugs and dosages presented in this text are intended to provide information but are not guaranteed to be accurate. Before prescribing any of the drugs suggested here, the prescriber should be familiar with the medication(s) and should check package label instructions.

The publisher offers discounts on this book when ordered in bulk quantities. For more information, write to Special Sales/Professional Marketing at the address below.

This book is printed on acid-free paper.

MARCEL DEKKER, INC.
270 Madison Avenue, New York, New York 10016
http://www.dekker.com

Current printing (last digit):
10 9 8 7 6 5 4 3 2 1

PRINTED IN THE UNITED STATES OF AMERICA

To
Kay, Rebecca, and Jamie
and to
the Comets

Preface

Studies and reports presented over the past two decades provide the basis for recognizing the importance of the disorders described in this text. The landmarks in sports medicine are well described in this book and include: 1) testing for drug doping beginning in the 1960s; 2) the 1972 disqualification of an American Olympic swimmer for using a banned substance, and the loss of his gold medal; 3) a report in 1976 by Bierman et al. suggesting that 90% of chronic asthmatic subjects and 40% of those with allergic rhinitis have exercise-induced asthma; and 4) the report that United States athletes who participated in the 1984 Summer Olympic Games in Los Angeles had an 11% prevalence of exercise-induced asthma. Sports medicine is now recognized as a subspecialty, and practitioners are able to take an examination that may lead to certification in sports medicine. Consequently, it is timely and appropriate to present now the first book dedicated entirely to allergic and respiratory disease in sports medicine.

This book is divided into logical sections. Chapters 1 and 2 present a background for the effects of exercise on the respiratory system and describe the mechanics of performing exercise challenges. Chapters 3 and 4 review the history and prevalence of exercise-induced asthma and indicate clearly that we now recognize this disorder in about one in five athletes. Chapters 5–7 propose mechanisms for exercise-induced asthma, focusing on the role of respiratory water loss and mediator release. If mediators play a dominant role in this disorder, then many of the newer anti-mediator agents might be expected to be efficacious in the treatment of asthma that occurs with exercise. Similarly, if a late phase occurs after exercise (Chapter 7), then its treatment might require medications designed to treat chronic asthma.

Chapter 8 describes the treatment of exercise-induced asthma with β-agonists and Chapter 9 addresses the myriad of other medications that have been examined for efficacy in this setting. A remarkably large number of medications, ranging from antihistamines to calcium channel–blocking agents to inhaled heparin to steroids, have proven efficacious. Indeed, new anti-asthma medications are often examined in early clinical trials for efficacy in preventing exercise-induced asthma as proof that the drug may be useful in treating chronic asthma. Chapter 10 examines the role of a nonpharmacological intervention—conditioning and training—in patients with exercise-induced asthma.

Chapters 11–13 are devoted to the upper airway. This section describes the effects of exercise on rhinitis, the recognition and treatment of sinusitis, and upper airway conditions masquerading as exercise-induced asthma.

Chapters 14 and 15 compare and contrast exercise-induced urticaria, exercise-induced angioedema, and exercise-induced anaphylaxis, and provide a basis for the recognition and treatment of these disorders.

Chapters 16 and 17 examine the effects of environment on the respiratory system. High altitude may benefit athletes during training but may also impair their performance, particularly at higher elevations. Similarly, air pollution may produce significant impairment in performance, particularly in athletes who have asthma.

Chapters 18–20 explore selected sporting activities that give rise to special concerns, including scuba diving, football, and winter activities, Scuba diving is particularly important because physicians are being asked with increasing frequency to evaluate whether it is safe for asthmatic patients to dive. These physicians need to know the risks of scuba diving, which are described in detail in Chapter 18.

Chapters 21–24 focus on elite athletes. Chapter 21 describes the role of an athletic trainer in recognizing exercise-induced respiratory disease. This chapter also presents examples of successful athletes with significant respiratory disease, including the case of Amy Van Dyken, who won four gold medals in the 1996 Summer Olympic Games. Chapters 22–24 review drug doping and performance-enhancing drugs.

Lastly, Chapters 25 and 26 describe the recognition and evaluation of respiratory disease, including the use of exercise challenges and questionnaires in screening programs.

I wish to thank all the authors for their diligence in providing chapters that blend to provide the reader with a full spectrum of information on allergic and respiratory diseases in sports medicine. I thank Ted Allen at Marcel Dekker, Inc., for his help in performing the tasks necessary to complete this text. Finally, I offer my thanks to those investigators and authors who have paved the way, in the 1970s and 1980s, with their pioneering work. I wish to thank Dr. William E. Pierson, chair of the Sports Medicine Committee of the American Academy of Allergy and Immunology in the 1980s, who lent his support to our early prevalence studies.

And so we must move on. We must answer the challenge to improve our understanding of the mechanisms for these disorders, explain the increase in prevalence of these conditions, and always strive to produce better treatments. In the end, the athletes will measure their successes in gold, silver, and bronze, in championships, in individual titles, and even in the ability to compete. We the practitioners will measure our successes when we provide the athletes, from recreational to highly competitive, with the opportunities to participate without respiratory impairment.

John M. Weiler

Contents

Contributors

Sandra D. Anderson, Ph.D., D.Sc. Department of Respiratory Medicine, Royal Prince Alfred Hospital, Sydney, Australia

William H. Baker, M.D. Division of Allergy/Immunology, Department of Internal Medicine, University of Iowa, Iowa City, Iowa

Kenneth C. Beck, Ph.D. Division of Pulmonary and Critical Care Medicine, Department of Internal Medicine, Mayo Clinic and Foundation, Rochester, Minnesota

Robert K. Bush, M.D. Department of Medicine, University of Wisconsin—Madison, and William S. Middleton Memorial Veterans Hospital, Madison, Wisconsin

William W. Busse, M.D. Department of Medicine, University Hospitals—CSC, University of Wisconsin Medical School, Madison, Wisconsin

Ernest N. Charlesworth, M.D. Brenham Clinic, Brenham, Texas

Christodoulos S. Christodoulou, M.D. Division of Allergy/Immunology, Department of Internal Medicine, University of Texas Health Science Center at San Antonio, San Antonio, Texas

Robert E. Coifman, M.D. Allergy & Asthma of South Jersey, Vineland, New Jersey

Evangelia Daviskas, M.Biomed.E., Ph.D. Department of Respiratory Medicine, Royal Prince Alfred Hospital, Sydney, Australia

Joseph D. Diaz, M.D. Division of Allergy/Immunology, Department of Internal Medicine, University of Texas Health Science Center at San Antonio, San Antonio, Texas

Lawrence M. Du Buske, M.D. Department of Allergy and Clinical Immunology, Harvard Medical School and Brigham and Women's Hospital, Boston, Massachusetts

Wade F. Exum, M.D., M.B.A. United States Olympic Committee, Colorado Springs, Colorado

Barbara Fraser, L.P.N., CRC St. Mary's Hospital Regional Department of Pediatrics, Division of Yale University Medical Center, Waterbury, Connecticut

Stephen T. Holgate, M.D. Southampton General Hospital, Southampton, United Kingdom

Richard F. Horan, M.D. Harvard Medical School and Brigham and Women's Hospital, Boston, Massachusetts

William C. Howland III, M.D. Allergy Center of Austin, and HealthQuest Research, Austin, Texas

Bruce D. Johnson, Ph.D. Division of Cardiovascular Diseases, Department of Internal Medicine, Mayo Clinic and Foundation, Rochester, Minnesota

Roger M. Katz, M.D. Department of Pediatrics, UCLA School of Medicine, Los Angeles, California

Gregory L. Landry Department of Pediatrics, University of Wisconsin—Madison, Madison, Wisconsin

David M. Lang, M.D. Division of Allergy/Immunology, Department of Medicine, Allegheny University of the Health Sciences, Philadelphia, Pennsylvania

Jeffrey R. Leipzig, M.D. Division of Allergy and Immunology, Department of Internal Medicine, Saint Louis University School of Medicine, Saint Louis, Missouri

Himender K. Makker, M.D. Southampton General Hospital, Southampton, United Kingdom

Hemalini Mehta, M.D. Department of Medicine, University of Wisconsin Medical School, Madison, Wisconsin

Pope L. Moseley, M.D., M.S. Pulmonary, Allergy, and Critical Care Division, Department of Medicine, School of Medicine, University of New Mexico, Albuquerque, New Mexico

Mark T. O'Hollaren, M.D. Department of Medicine, Oregon Health Sciences University, Portland, Oregon

Nancy K. Ostrom, M.D. Allergy and Asthma Medical Group and Research Center, San Diego, California

David B. Peden, M.D. The School of Medicine, The University of North Carolina at Chapel Hill, Chapel Hill, North Carolina

Margaret M. Peter, M.S., A.T.C. Division of Sports Medicine, United States Olympic Committee, Colorado Springs, Colorado

Joan M. Price, B.A., BSN Department of Drug Control Administration, United States Olympic Committee, Colorado Springs, Colorado

Christopher Randolph, M.D. St. Mary's Hospital Regional Department of Pediatrics, Division of Yale University Medical Center, Waterbury, Connecticut

Robert C. Roach, Ph.D. Copenhagen Muscle Research Center, Copenhagen, Denmark

Albert L. Sheffer, M.D. Harvard Medical School and Brigham and Women's Hospital, Boston, Massachusetts

William S. Silvers, M.D. Allergy, Asthma, and Immunology Clinic of Colorado, Greenwood Medical Center, Englewood, Colorado

Raymond G. Slavin, M.D. Division of Allergy and Immunology, Department of Internal Medicine, Saint Louis University School of Medicine, Saint Louis, Missouri

Sheldon L. Spector, M.D. University of California—Los Angeles, and Allergy Research Foundation, Los Angeles, California

William W. Storms, M.D. Department of Medicine, Asthma and Allergy Associates, University of Colorado Health Sciences Center, Colorado Springs, Colorado

Faye L. Thompson, M.A., A.T.C., L.A.T. Department of Athletic Training Services, University of Iowa, Iowa City, Iowa

Frank J. Twarog, M.D., Ph.D. Children's Hospital and Harvard Medical School, Boston, Massachusetts

Arthur E. Varner, M.D. Department of Medicine, University of Wisconsin—Madison, and William S. Middleton Memorial Veterans Hospital, Madison, Wisconsin

Frank S. Virant, M.D. University of Washington School of Medicine, and Northwest Asthma and Allergy Center, Seattle, Washington

John M. Weiler, M.D. Division of Allergy/Immunology, Department of Internal Medicine, University of Iowa, Iowa City, Iowa

Noe Zamel, M.D., F.R.C.P.C., F.C.C.P. Department of Medicine, University of Toronto, Toronto, Canada

1

Respiratory System Responses to Dynamic Exercise

Bruce D. Johnson and Kenneth C. Beck
Mayo Clinic and Foundation, Rochester, Minnesota

I. INTRODUCTION

The transition from rest to exercise requires a host of acute adaptations in the respiratory system to maintain homeostasis. These adaptations include (a) the regulation of the depth and frequency of breathing, through the activation of the respiratory muscles; (b) the conditioning of the airways, through warming and humidification of the air; (c) the minimization of the work and oxygen cost of breathing by increases in extra- and intrathoracic airway diameter and by regulating end-expiratory lung volume; and (d) the optimization of pulmonary O_2 transfer by increases in alveolar–capillary surface interface and by increases in lymphatic circulation which minimizes lung water accumulation. These adaptations, for the most part, occur as a result of precise humoral and neuromechanical regulation, with an ultimate goal of maintaining oxygenation and pH of the arterial blood at minimal respiratory muscle cost. In health, this regulation is amazingly precise and occurs essentially without perception. However, in disease, these seemingly trivial, but complex, adaptations are challenged. The focus of this brief review will be on the adaptations of the healthy respiratory system to brief dynamic exercise.

II. COUPLING OF INTERNAL TO EXTERNAL RESPIRATION

A. Muscle Fiber Type and the Bioenergetics of Skeletal Muscle

Muscles are generally composed of different fiber types, with diverse metabolic as well as functional properties. Most commonly, fiber types have been differentiated based on histochemical classification after staining for myofibrillar adenosine triphosphatase (mATPase) activity (after alkaline and acid preincubation) and have been divided into type I, IIa, IIb [17] and, more recently, IIx muscle fibers [41]. Although there is considerable overlap in the metabolic and functional properties of muscle fibers, type I fibers tend to stain more richly for oxidative enzymes and less so for glycolytic enzymes, whereas type IIb fibers tend to stain in a reverse pattern [34]. Type IIa and IIx fibers typically stain intermediately for these enzymes [100]. Genetic predisposition largely governs the fiber-type makeup of a muscle; however, training alters the enzymatic profile of muscle fibers [42,47,86].

Muscle fibers have also been classified based on motor unit properties [18]. The motor unit (Fig. 1) includes the motor nerve and the muscle fibers they innervate [70]. Motor units have been separated, based on twitch characteristics and fatigue properties into slow fatigue-resistant units (S), fast fatigue-resistant units (FR), fast fatigue-intermediate units (FI) and fast-fatigable units (FF) [19,23]. A relation has been established between the functional motor unit properties and the histochemical classification of fiber type, such that type I fibers tend to be slow and fatigue-resistant, type IIb tend to be fast and are more fatigable, whereas IIa and IIx fibers tend to have intermediate twitch profiles and fatigue resistance [18,68,100,101].

The recruitment order of the different fiber types has important implications for exercise performance as well as for ventilatory demands. Typically motor units are thought to be recruited based on the motoneuron size (size principle) [52]. The small, S units tend to be recruited first for most tasks, followed by the FR, FI, and finally, the FF units. The recruitment of faster units is likely linked to the increased force demands as well as increased demands for high-velocity movements. Thus, at low levels of activity, only the S and, perhaps, some FR units would be recruited.

Human skeletal muscle fibers generate force by a series of myofibrillar interactions (cycling) between actin and myosin (contractile proteins). Shortening is thought to be the result of a pulling action on the actin by a sweep-like action of the head of the myosin molecule when it is in the linked position [31]. The interaction, or link, is then broken, allowing the

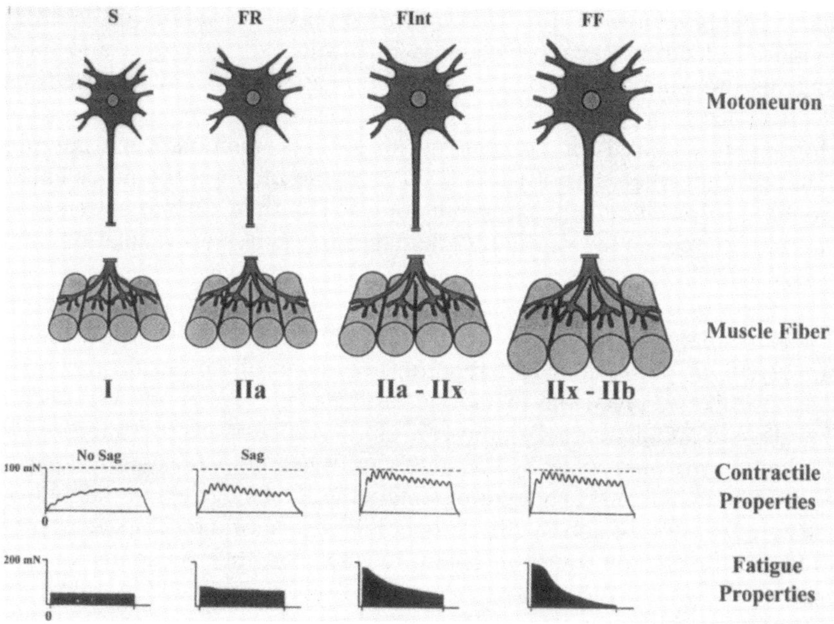

Fig. 1 Motor units comprise a motoneuron and the muscle fibers it innervates (i.e., the muscle unit). Motor units are subclassified based on contractile and fatigue properties into slow (S), fast fatigue-resistant (FR), fast fatigue-intermediate (FI), and fast fatigable (FF) units. Muscle unit fibers display histochemical-staining profiles for myofibrillar ATPase after alkaline and acid preincubations, which permits classification as type I, IIa, IIx, and IIb. The recruitment of the various muscle fiber subtypes plays a role in the observed ventilatory responses during exercise. (From Ref. 101a.)

process to be repeated at the next available link site. This attachment–detachment and reattachment of the actin and myosin causes the muscle to shorten and to produce force generation [76,94]. The recruitment of muscle fibers and the interaction and release of actin and myosin require energy supplied by the hydrolysis (splitting) of the terminal phosphate bond(s) of ATP [65].

The available store of ATP in skeletal muscle is extremely small and can fuel contraction for only a few seconds at high work rates [109]. The concentration of ATP does not fall, however, owing to a breakdown of creatine phosphate into creatine and inorganic phosphate [57]. Creatine, though, acts only as a temporary sink to sustain energy needs, and the major energy source results from oxidative phosphorylation in the mitochondrial electron transport chain, which relies on glycogen and fatty acids as fuel sources. When oxygen (O_2) is available to act as the final electron acceptor, two to three ATPs are formed per oxygenation [97]. More O_2 is required for a given rate of ATP production when fats are oxidized than when carbohydrates serve as the fuel. On the other hand, fats tend to produce less carbon dioxide (CO_2) than carbohydrates and thus tend to reduce the ventilatory demands for acid–base regulation (discussed later).

If oxygen transport does not deliver sufficient O_2 to the electron transport chain, ATP can be formed through the low ATP-yield anaerobic–glycolytic pathway, which requires use of carbohydrates for fuel [57]. It is also likely, given the metabolic profile of the faster muscle fibers, that despite an adequate O_2 delivery, as these fibers are recruited, ATP production will also occur by this pathway. When O_2 is present, the pyruvic acid formed from carbohydrate enters the Krebs cycle and the hydrogens are transferred across the mitochondrial membrane to serve as substrate for the electon transport chain. If, however, there is an inadequate amount of O_2, or if the ability to shuttle hydrogens is exceeded, pyruvate is converted to lactate [65]. At the pH of muscle during exercise, lactic acid is almost completely dissociated into lactate ions and protons. During heavy exercise, it is likely that some of the lactate produced in the more glycolytic fibers is taken up and oxidized by the fibers that contain greater oxidative potential.

The cost of the recruitment of fibers that produce ATP primarily through the glycolytic pathways is a greater stress to acid–base regulation as a result of the increase in cellular proton load with lactate. The advantage is that faster fibers with greater force-generating potential are recruited and the glycolytic process can continue to produce ATP. The initial buffering of the acid load is achieved through intracellular buffers, including proteins and phosphates [67]. The predominant buffering of lactic acid, however, is provided by the bicarbonate system. For every proton that combines with a bicarbonate molecule, one additional molecule of CO_2 is formed. As shown in Fig. 2, this CO_2 production is in addition to the ongoing metabolic CO_2 load produced in the aerobic breakdown of fuels and provides an additional load for pulmonary clearance. Aerobic fibers produce CO_2 in units approximately equal to O_2 consumption; however, the more glycolytic fibers use little O_2 and produce CO_2 at approximately fourfold higher rates [116]. Thus, as these fibers are recruited with progressive exercise, a substantially greater CO_2 load will be presented to the lung for clearance. An inadequate ventilatory response results in enhanced metabolic acidosis and premature cessation of activity.

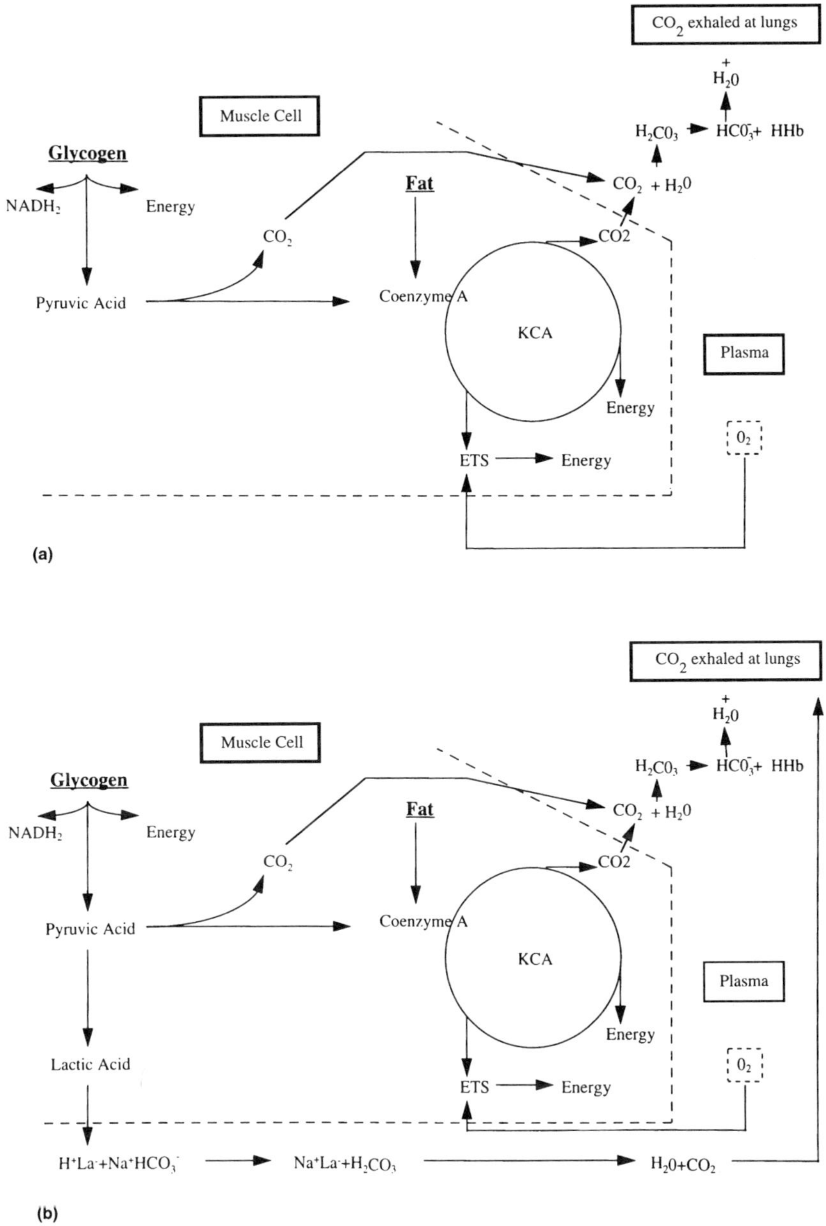

Fig. 2 Proposed mechanism of cellular respiration (a) at rest and (b) during intense exercise, leading to enhanced CO_2 production and increased ventilation. KCA, Krebs citric acid cycle; ETS, electron transport chain.

B. Relation of Ventilation to Metabolic Demand

The recruitment of the muscle fibers and the interaction of actin and myosin thus require an increased demand for blood flow to supply oxygen and to buffer and remove lactate and CO_2. A tight relationship exists between metabolic rate (i.e., oxygen consumption, $\dot{V}O_2$, and carbon dioxide production, $\dot{V}CO_2$) and the ventilatory response. This relationship is demonstrated in Fig. 3, which shows the exercise associated changes in minute ventilation ($\dot{V}E$), $\dot{V}O_2$, and $\dot{V}CO_2$ with increases in work rate. At low levels of exercise intensity, $\dot{V}E$ rises linearly with both $\dot{V}O_2$ and $\dot{V}CO_2$ as the work rate (and the muscle fiber recruitment) increases. However, as the work rate increases further, $\dot{V}CO_2$ and $\dot{V}E$, which remain linearly linked, rise out of proportion to $\dot{V}O_2$. At this point, typically 40–65% $\dot{V}O_2$max, it is likely that intermediate (type IIa) in addition to type I muscle fibers are recruited. Undoubtedly, some lactate is produced, causing the

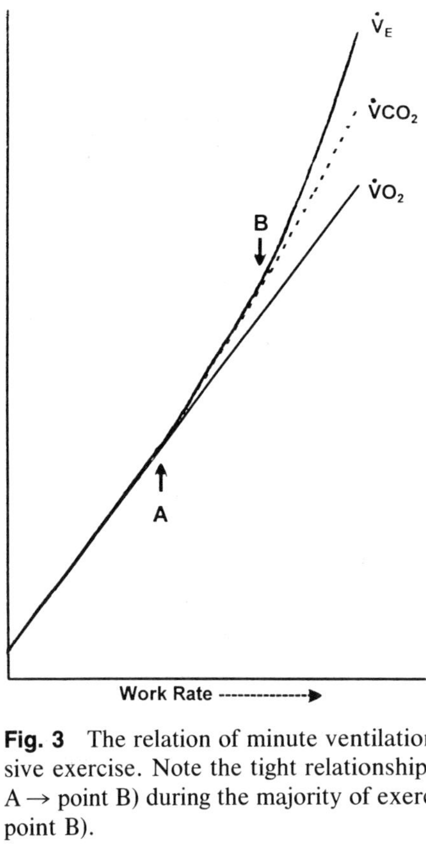

Fig. 3 The relation of minute ventilation ($\dot{V}E$) to $\dot{V}CO_2$ and $\dot{V}O_2$ during progressive exercise. Note the tight relationship observed between $\dot{V}E$ and $\dot{V}CO_2$ (point A → point B) during the majority of exercise until the heavier intensities (beyond point B).

$\dot{V}CO_2$ and $\dot{V}E$ to increase out of proportion to $\dot{V}O_2$ as the respiratory exchange ratio ($\dot{V}CO_2/\dot{V}O_2$) exceeds 1.0. With further increases in work rate, faster fibers are recruited, and more lactate and CO_2 are produced, which further stimulates ventilation. However, at this point, at 70–90% $\dot{V}O_2max$, $\dot{V}E$ begins to increase out of proportion to $\dot{V}CO_2$. It is likely that, at this point, the acid load increases out of proportion to the ventilatory compensation and hydrogen ions stimulate peripheral chemoreceptors (see later) [27,28].

The relation of VE to metabolic demand has been summarized in the alveolar air equation.

$$\dot{V}E = \frac{[K^*\dot{V}CO_2]}{[PaCO_2(1 - VD/VT)]}$$

As noted, $\dot{V}E$ is dependent not only on metabolic demand ($\dot{V}CO_2$) but also on the arterial CO_2 ($PaCO_2$) regulation and the ventilatory dead space to tidal volume ratio (VD/VT, see section on gas exchange). K represents a constant to correct for transformation of fractional concentration to the partial pressure and to express gas volumes at body temperature and pressure saturated with water vapor.

The relationship of ventilation to metabolic demand and the increased ventilation coincident with changes in acid load in the arterial blood forms the basis for noninvasive estimates of the so-termed anaerobic threshold [114,117]. Although the terminology remains controversial, the measurement of ventilatory compensation for metabolic acidosis remains a clinical tool to evaluate fitness, training influences, and clinical disease.

C. Additional Factors Influencing the Ventilatory Response to Exercise

Despite the notable tight relationship of metabolism to ventilation, it is unclear how ventilation is precisely controlled, particularly during exercise. For the most part $PaCO_2$ levels are held almost precisely within 2–4 mmHg through the course of most daily activities. Even during exercise, $PaCO_2$ levels are maintained near resting levels until extremely heavy exercise, when it begins to fall, likely secondary to increased ventilation associated with lactic acidosis and a falling pH [28,116]. Respiratory centers in the brain stem control the periodic nature of inspiration and expiration [91,92] and are likely influenced by afferent inputs sensed predominantly by, but not restricted solely to, the respiratory system [reviews 27,30].

For example, central chemoreceptors are found in the brain and appear to be responsive to hydrogen ions and dissolved CO_2, primarily within the cerebrospinal fluid (CSF), but are also influenced by local blood flow and metabolism [27]. The peripheral chemoreceptors are located in the carotid bodies, as well as the aortic arch, and respond to decreases in arterial pH and Pa_{O_2} and increases in Pa_{CO_2}, serum K^+ and norepinephrine [5,13,21,83,106]. Lung stretch receptors (vagal feedback) may play a part in terminating a breath and in regulating end inspiratory lung volume. However, studies in heart–lung transplant patients, devoid of stretch receptor feedback, demonstrate only small differences in breathing pattern from normal subjects and only at low levels of exercise [96]. Lung irritant receptors are thought to lie between epithelial cells within the airways, and these appear to play a role in the bronchconstriction of asthma in response to released histamine or bradykinin. Juxtacapillary receptors (J-receptors) are found in the alveolar walls, and respond to chemicals in the pulmonary circulation. These receptors cause rapid, shallow breathing when stimulated, and increased interstitial fluid volume of the alveolar walls may activate them. They may play a role in the dyspnea associated with congestive heart failure and have been implicated in the rapid, shallow breathing noted after heavy exercise [38,105,122]. Additional receptors, found in the nose and upper airways, respond to both mechanical and chemical stimulants. Respiratory muscles also contain muscle spindles, Golgi tendon organs, and nerve endings that may respond to length changes, rate of change, load, or metabolites produced with muscle fatigue.

Although ventilatory responses to various chemical stimuli have been studied, no single factor (CO_2, O_2, lactic acid, pH changes, K^+, or catecholamines) has resulted in a ventilatory response of the magnitude observed during exercise [27]. Other stimuli or receptors have, therefore, been suggested, such as the passive movement of limbs sensed by receptors in the joints and muscle, a centrally mediated stimulus, or temporal oscillations in Pa_{CO_2}, sensed by the carotid bodies or an airway chemoreceptor (as yet unidentified in humans) [30,111]. Each of these mechanisms may account for most of the increase in ventilation during exercise, whereas modulation and precise control is provided by central and peripheral chemoreceptors as well as the stretch receptors and respiratory muscles [27]. Other investigators have suggested a synergistic effect of several chemical or humoral stimuli or an alteration in the normal sensitivity of receptors [30]. An example would be the marked increased ventilatory response to hypoxia during low-level or moderate exercise, relative to resting conditions.

Ultimately, ventilatory control during exercise is a balance between factors stimulating ventilation and factors that modify ventilation [27]. Ventilation cannot increase without limits. The load presented to the respiratory muscles and demand for blood flow become increasingly important, as do the mechanical constraints imposed on ventilation by the characteristics of the lungs and chest wall. The importance of the respiratory load and mechanical constraints to ventilation have been suggested by the work of Hesser et al. [53], Clark et al. [22], and Johnson et al. [60] who demonstrated decreased ventilatory responses during exercise when either the work of breathing was increased through hyperbaric environments or when chemical stimuli were added at high intensities of whole-body exercise.

III. BREATHING MECHANICS

The process of increasing minute ventilation through the alteration of airway diameter, integration and recruitment of respiratory muscles, and the subsequent changes in abdominal and pleural pressures in relation to changes in lung volumes and flow rates is known as *breathing mechanics*.

A. Breathing Pattern

Classically, the onset of light exercise is associated with both an increase in depth (tidal volume; V_T), and frequency of breathing (fb). Typically, however, the breathing depth is the dominant way of increasing ventilation at the lower levels of exertion [36,54]. As exercise progresses, both tidal volume and breathing frequency increase until 70–80% of peak exercise, when the response is primarily a frequency response [36,60]. V_T usually plateaus at 50–60% of vital capacity (VC): however, there is considerable variation [122]. Younger adults typically increase V_T by three- to fivefold, whereas in older adults, V_T tends to increase less (two- to fourfold) [14]. Breathing frequency typically increases one- to threefold in most subjects, but in fitter athletes may be increased by six- to sevenfold at high levels of V_E. In some subjects at extremely high ventilatory demands, V_T actually decreases as fb increases [59]. Figure 4 shows the typical changes in breathing pattern with progressive exercise in a group of young highly fit subjects and older active individuals [60,62]. Note, that V_T tends to plateau at approximately 50% of VC; however, this tends to occur at a slightly higher percentage of VC in the older subjects.

The increase in V_T is due to both a decrease in end-expiratory lung volume (EELV), through encroachment on the expiratory reserve volume, and to an increase in end-inspiratory lung volume (EILV), through a decrease in the inspiratory reserve volume [51,62]. With progressive increases in exercise intensity and V_E, EELV continues to fall to 0.5–1.0

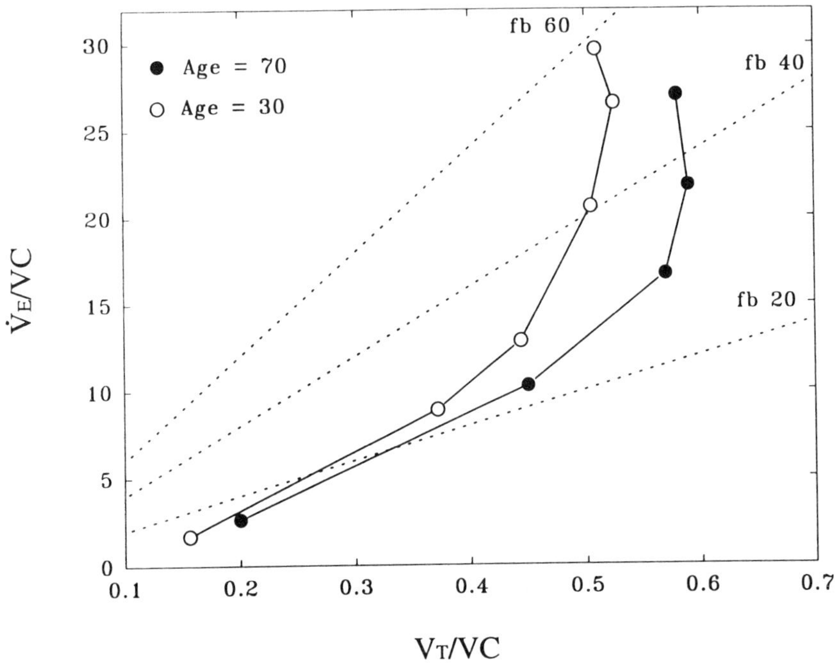

Fig. 4 Ventilation ($\dot{V}_E$) and tidal volume ($\dot{V}_T$) relationship normalized for vital capacity (VC) during progressive exercise in young endurance athletes (○) and moderately trained aged adults (●). Dotted lines represent isofrequency lines. (From Ref. 63.)

L below the resting functional residual capacity (FRC) [51]. It has been hypothesized that the fall in EELV optimizes inspiratory muscle length (for force development) and helps prevent too large an increase in end-inspiratory lung volume (EILV), which would increase the inspiratory elastic load of breathing [26]. In addition, the energy stored in the abdominal wall because of active expiration may provide some passive recoil at the initiation of the ensuing inspiration [93]. In endurance athletes at high ventilatory demands (>150 L/min), EELV may begin to increase, likely secondary to expiratory airflow limitation [60].

The increase in fb with exercise is due to a decrease in inspiratory (t_I) and expiratory time t_E). Typically however, at the moderate to higher ventilatory demands, a greater fractional decrease is noted in t_E so that t_I/t_{TOT} increases from 0.4 at rest to 0.5–0.55 at maximum exercise [75,105].

Owing to the greater decrease in *t*E, the increase in mean expiratory flow rate is greater than the increase in mean inspiratory flow rate.

B. Flow and Pressure–Volume Responses and Changes in Bronchial Tone

Figure 5 shows the typical flow–volume and pressure–volume response to progressive exercise in a healthy young, average fit subject. The flow–volume response is shown within the constraints of the maximal volitional inspiratory and expiratory flow–volume envelope. The pressure–volume response is shown within the constraints of the maximal effective expiratory pressures and the maximal dynamic capacity for inspiratory muscle pressure generation. Pressures are determined by insertion of an air-filled balloon into the lower two-thirds of the esophagus and represent an index of respiratory muscle force production. As shown, expiratory and inspiratory flow continuously increases to maximum exercise. Even at peak exercise, however, little expiratory flow limitation exists (tidal breath does not meet or exceed the expiratory boundary of the MFVL) and inspiratory flow is well within the capacity described by the MFVL [63].

Correspondingly, inspiratory pressure generation gradually increases (becomes more negative) as ventilatory demand increases; however, peak inspiratory pressure reaches only 50% of the dynamic capacity of the inspiratory muscles for pressure production [69] near maximal exercise (in the average fit young adult). Peak inspiratory pressures typically average 20–25% of the static capacity for pleural pressure generation; however, this does not take into account the fall in the capacity for pleural pressure generation caused by an increase in the flow rate (velocity of muscle shortening) and change in lung volume (muscle length) [60]. Similarly, peak expiratory pressures become positive only with heavy exercise and only near EELV. Thus, expiratory pressures for a given lung volume are well below the maximal effective pressures ($Pmax_e$, pressures at which airways begin to narrow or close) even with heavy exercise [60,62,81]. With maximal volitional expiratory efforts, pressures can be generated that are three to four times greater than the $Pmax_e$. However, pressure production in excess of $Pmax_e$ will not produce increases in expiratory airflow (thus termed maximal effective pressures) [81].

Changes in bronchial tone can be inferred from the changes in the expiratory boundary of the MFVL or changes in airway resistance (see later). Figure 6 shows, on average, a small increase in the maximal expiratory airflows in a group of older, fit adults determined immediately after heavy exercise [61]. This has been attributed to an exercise-induced bron-

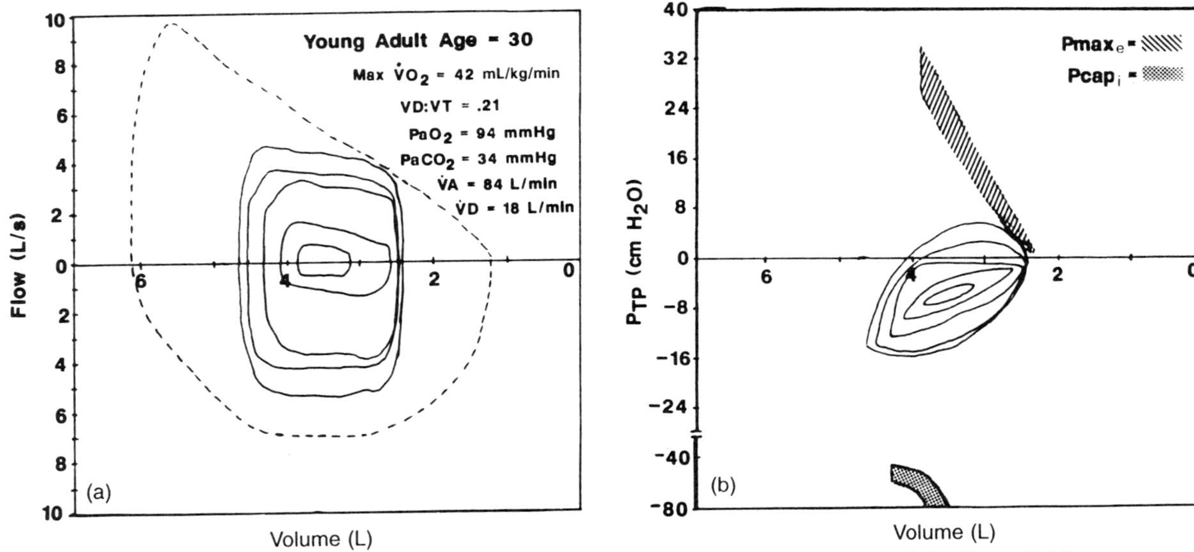

Fig. 5 Typical ventilatory response to progressive exercise in an untrained young adult. The solid lines represent (a) the flow–volume and (b) pressure–volume response at rest and during mild-, moderate-, heavy- and maximum-intensity work loads. Loops were placed on the volume axis according to a measured end-expiratory lung volume (EELV). The flow–volume loops are placed within the maximum volitional postexercise (dashed line) flow–volume loop, and the tidal pressure–volume loops are placed within the shaded area, representing the maximal effective pressures on expiration ($Pmax_e$) and the capacity for inspiratory muscle pressure generation ($Pcap_i$) at the volume and flow rate at which peak pressure occurred during tidal inspiration.

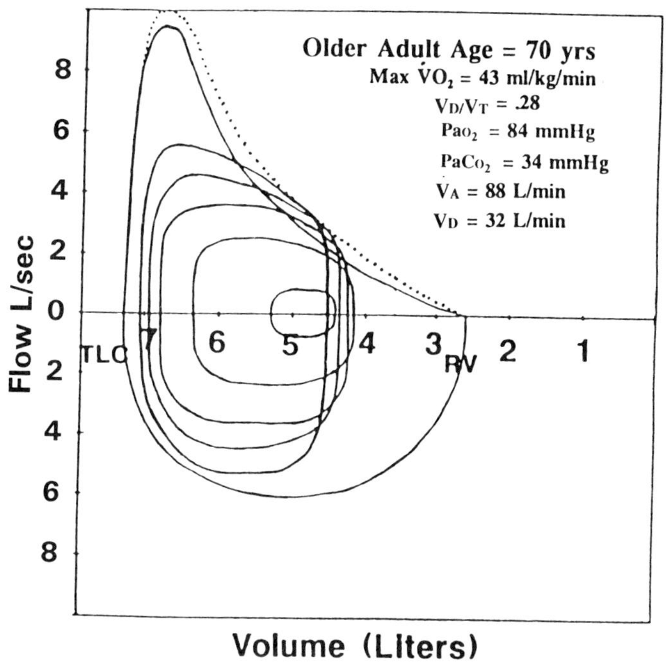

Fig. 6 Ventilatory response to exercise in a group of relatively fit older adults (n = 29, age = 70 yr, V_{O_2}, max = 42 mL kg^{-1} min^{-1}). Tidal breathing exercise flow–volume loops are plotted according to a measured end-expiratory lung volume within the maximal volitional flow–volume envelope (solid line, before exercise; dashed line, after exercise). The increase in maximal volitional flows measured immediately after exercise implies an exercise-induced bronchodilation. (From Ref. 61.)

chodilation secondary to vagal withdrawal [113]. Some controversy continues to exist about the mechanism of exercise-induced bronchodilation; other factors may contribute to the small changes in airway diameter, including sympathetic stimulation or epithelial-derived factors, such as nitric oxide [78]. The later may be induced by lung stretch, or also delivered to the lung from other sources.

C. Changes in Resistance and Compliance, Work, and Oxygen Cost of Breathing

Resistance is defined as a change in pressure for a given flow change, and *compliance* is a volume change for a given pressure change [82,113].

Although difficult to measure with exercise, studies that have controlled for volume and flow rate while measuring resistance, generally find a progressive fall [113]. Conversely, compliance stays relatively constant until heavy exercise, when it tends to fall [122]. The fall in resistance has been used as evidence that airway dilation occurs in healthy subjects with exercise. The fall in compliance near peak exercise, may be due to a high EILV and elastic load, or to an increase in pulmonary vascular fluid volume [122].

The work of breathing has generally been estimated by integrating the area described by the transpulmonary pressure–volume envelope during tidal breathing [82]. Thus, as shown in Fig. 5, as ventilatory demand increases, the area described by the pressure–volume "loop" increases. This measurement of work takes into account flow-resistive work and energy needed to overcome lung tissue resistance. Breaking down work of breathing further into work expended against the chest wall (elastic work) requires measuring the passive elastic properties of the chest wall. The latter is difficult to determine in humans; therefore, the component of work performed against the chest wall has not been thoroughly studied. Elastic work increases during exercise owing to the progressive increase in $\dot{V}_T$; however, reductions in compliance and changes in EELV will also affect the amount of elastic work expended [1,51,53]. The resistive work required to overcome airway resistance to airflow also increases in a nonlinear fashion, going from heavy to maximum exercise as inspiratory flow becomes more turbulent, and as expiratory resistance increases as airways undergo dynamic compression (flow limitation).

Use of the pressure–volume loop analysis does not take into account work components, because of an increased velocity of respiratory muscle shortening, work performed to overcome inertia when switching from inspiration to expiration, or work performed during deformation of the rib cage or abdomen [2]. Because blood flow requirements of working muscles are usually proportional to their energy requirements, the oxygen cost of breathing, therefore, is linked to the rise in the work of breathing, but can diverge from this relationship as factors "unaccounted for" become more significant. The oxygen cost of breathing can be determined by having subjects at rest mimic the essential mechanical components of breathing observed during exercise (i.e., EELV, $\dot{V}_T$, fb, and pressures) and measuring the increment in whole-body $\dot{V}O_2$ [1,2]. Figure 7 shows the increase in respiratory muscle work and O_2 cost with progressive exercise. As shown, the O_2 cost of breathing averages less than 5% of total body $\dot{V}O_2$ at rest and during mild to moderate exercise. During heavy and peak exercise, respiratory muscle oxygen consumption is estimated at 7% of total-body $\dot{V}O_2$ in average fit adults but may be as high as 15–20% in the

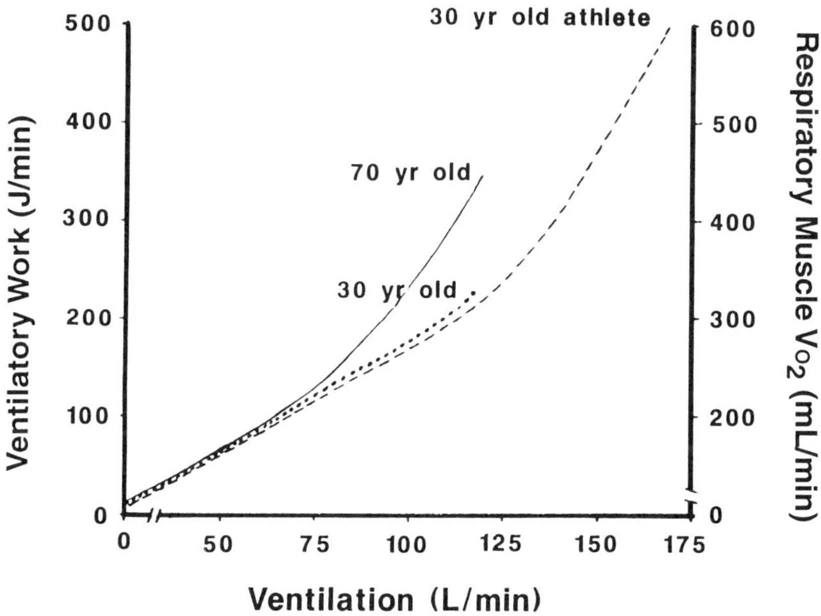

Fig. 7 Ventilatory work and the oxygen cost of breathing during progressive exercise in 30-yr-old, untrained adults (dotted line), 30-yr-old endurance athletes (dashed line), and 70-yr-old moderately fit older adults (solid line).

young and older athletes, respectively, with increased levels of ventilatory demand. Interestingly, in the more highly fit subjects, as ventilatory demand increases and expiratory flow limitation begins to occur, the work and particularly cost of breathing begin to increase disproportionately [2].

D. Nasal Breathing Versus Mouth Breathing

Although variable, most individuals breath through their noses at rest [115]. This occurs despite the fact that nasal airflow resistance is greater than mouth airflow resistance. The switch from primarily nasal breathing to oronasal breathing with exercise appears to occur at a ventilation of 22–44 L/min [70,95,115]. Fregossi and Lansing [34a] demonstrated that the upper limit to nasal ventilation appears to average 30–35 L/min and occurs at a work intensity of approximately 60% of maximum power (using a cycle ergometer). The proportion of nasal to total ventilation varies between 26 and 64% during low level activity [34a,115] and progressively decreases to 25–30% during exercise at 90% of peak power [34a].

Exercise decreases nasal airflow resistance, presumably by dilation of the alai nasi muscles [35,104]. Resistance to airflow can be decreased by 30% with the activation of these muscles [103]. Despite this active dilation, airflow resistance is approximately four times greater through the nose than through the mouth at rest and nine times greater during exercise [115].

E. Indices of Ventilatory Constraint ($\dot{V}_E$ Reserve, Flow Limitation, Δ in EELV and EILV)

Thus far we have examined primarily the response to exercise in the average fit adult ($\dot{V}O_2$max = 100% age predicted). In this population, typically peak ventilation reaches only 50–70% of the 12- to 15-s maximal voluntary ventilation (MVV), little or no flow limitation is typically present along the expiratory border of the tidal flow–volume loop, and EILV approaches only 75% of TLC, and peak inspiratory pressures approach only 50% of that which is available. Thus, substantial reserve is available for increasing minute ventilation during exercise. In contrast, however, endurance athletes may approach these capacities near maximal exercise. Figure 8 shows an example of the flow and pressure–volume response to exercise in two highly trained cross-country runners [60]. As shown, the tidal flow volume loops at peak exercise meet or exceed the expiratory boundary of the MFVL for more than 50% of the tidal breath, which corresponds to tidal expiratory pressures reaching maximal effective pressures over more 30% of the tidal breath. End-expiratory lung volume falls with light to moderate exercise, such as that of the average fit adult (see Fig. 5); however, near peak exercise this begins to increase as the flow limitation increases. As a result of the increase in lung volume at which peak inspiratory pressures occur, the demand for high flow rates (velocity of shortening) and the large pressure demands, peak inspiratory pressures approach a higher percentage of the maximal available pressure (mean peak inspiratory pressure averaged approximated 90% of the maximal available pressures) [60]. Despite the addition of hypercapnic and hypoxic gases to the inspired air near peak exercise, ventilation was generally not increased over that achieved with room air, suggesting that subjects had truly reached mechanical limits to ventilation. However, given the small degree of room available to increase ventilation further in most of these athletes (i.e., the entire tidal breath was not flow-limited and peak inspiratory pressures were typically not 100% of the capacity for pleural pressure generation), a more likely explanation may be that, despite the large chem-

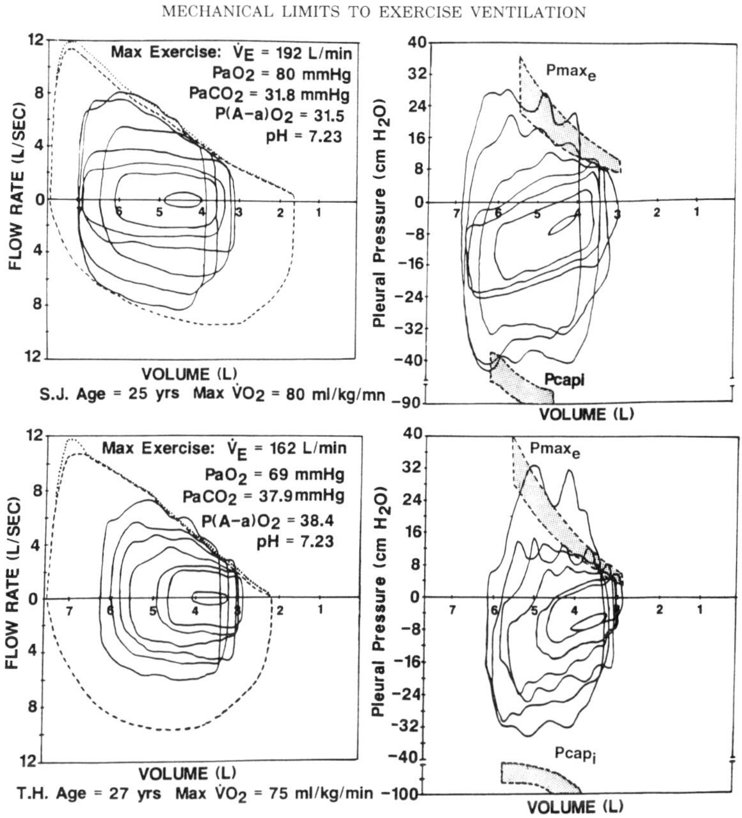

Fig. 8 Ventilatory response to progressive exercise in two young endurance athletes. Tidal flow (left) and pressure (right) volume loops (solid lines) are plotted from rest through maximal exercise. The flow–volume loops are plotted within the before (solid) and after exercise (dashed) maximal volitional flow–volume loops relative to a measured end-expiratory lung volume (EELV). The tidal pressure–volume loops are plotted relative to the maximal effective pressures on expiration and the capacity for pressure generation on inspiration. Because of the much greater $\dot{V}_E$ demands of the endurance athlete, they approach a much greater level of mechanical constraint relative to the untrained adult (see Fig. 5), but similar to that noted in the older relatively fit adult during maximal exercise. (From Ref. 60.)

ical stimulus to increase minute ventilation, the increased work and cost of breathing and demand for blood flow competing with the locomotor muscles, outweigh a ventilatory response. As noted earlier, the oxygen cost of breathing has been estimated to be, on average, 10–15% of total body $\dot{V}O_2$ in these more highly fit subjects, which would require a substantial percentage of the available cardiac output diverted to the respiratory muscles [60].

IV. GAS EXCHANGE

Adequate delivery of oxygen to, and removal of carbon dioxide from, working muscles critically depends on efficiency of gas exchange in the lungs. Oxygen delivery to the tissues is the product of oxygen content of the blood and cardiac output. In situations where oxygen delivery is compromised, exercise may be limited by the ability to deliver oxygen to the tissues. Maintenance of oxygen content of arterial blood ($Pa O_2$) is critical to exercise performance and is dependent on gas exchange efficiency of the lungs. As will be pointed out, the lungs are very efficient gas exchangers at rest, and they become even more efficient at CO_2 removal during exercise. However, the efficiency of oxygenation deteriorates somewhat, which requires compensation through an enhanced ventilatory response.

Gas exchange can be monitored with varying levels of complexity, ranging from observation of the subject's skin color (visible blueness would indicate severe hypoxemia), to use of oximetry or arterial blood gases, to the multiple inert gas elimination technique (MIGET). In the clinical laboratory, use of oximetry and blood gases is most common. MIGET is generally applied only in the research setting, when basic physiological mechanisms are being investigated. In addition, the diffusing capacity of lungs for carbon monoxide can be used either in the clinical setting or for investigating basic mechanisms.

Although a complete discussion of principles of gas exchange cannot be presented in the scope of this review, certain general principles should be emphasized. The fundamental gas-exchanging region of the lung is the pulmonary acinus, which is a few tenths of a millimeter in dimension and is composed of several alveoli. Not all acini have the same amount of ventilation ($\dot{V}_A$) or perfusion (Q), leading to inhomogeneity of gas exchange. The oxygen and carbon dioxide partial pressures in an acinus (P_AO_2, P_ACO_2) reflect a balance between perfusion and ventilation, the $\dot{V}_A/Q$ ratio. An acinus that is well perfused (lower $\dot{V}_A/Q$) will have a lower P_AO_2 and higher P_ACO_2 compared with one that is poorly perfused, but adequately ventilated (high $\dot{V}_A/Q$). We cannot ordinarily measure P_{AO_2} and P_{ACO_2} on an acinar level, especially in humans, so all of our observations are only indirectly related to these fundamental quantities. Expired gas contains information about acinar P_{AO_2} and P_{ACO_2}, and the changes in expired gas P_{O_2} and P_{CO_2} during an expiration partially reflect the sequential emptying of acini. The positive slope of P_{CO_2} versus expired volume and negative slope of P_{O_2} versus expired volume implies that acini with high $\dot{V}_A/Q$ empty early in expiration, leaving the latter part of expiration to those units that are not as well ventilated compared with perfusion. However, the time rate of change of P_{O_2} and P_{CO_2} in expired gas also reflect continued CO_2 output and O_2 uptake. Thus, with higher $\dot{V}_{O_2}$ and $\dot{V}_{CO_2}$ of exercise, the expired gas waveforms become steeper. The end-expired P_{CO_2} (P_{ETCO_2}) usually exceeds arterial Pa_{CO_2} in heavy exercise [64,118]. If P_{ETCO_2} remains below Pa_{CO_2} at moderate to heavy work intensities, there may be larger than normal contribution to expired gas from acini with high $\dot{V}_A/Q$ ratios, such as might occur in pulmonary vascular or parenchymal disorders.

Because the first part of the breath contains gas from the anatomical dead space, which contains inspired gas from the previous breath, the mixture of gas collected over an entire breath (or averaged over many breaths) reflects a mixture of gas from gas-exchanging acini and dead space. Any acinus with $\dot{V}_A/Q$ above the "average" for the lung will contribute gas to the mixed expired sample that is low in CO_2 and high in O_2, and acini with low $\dot{V}_A/Q$ ratios will contribute gas that is higher in CO_2 and lower in O_2 compared with the average acinus. One useful overall index of gas exchange, therefore, is the comparison of partial pressures in mixed expired gas to arterial blood gases. The amount of anatomical dead space and dead space-like effect of regions with higher than average $\dot{V}_A/Q$ will be manifest as a lower mixed expired P_{CO_2} compared with arterial P_{CO_2}. The physiological V_D/V_T ratio, therefore is, obtained from:

$$\frac{V_D}{V_T} = \frac{Pa_{CO_2} - P\bar{E}_{CO_2}}{Pa_{CO_2}}$$

where Pa_{CO_2} is from arterial blood gases, and $P\bar{E}_{CO_2}$ is the partial pressure of mixed expired CO_2. Traditionally, the latter was obtained from a sample of mixed expired gas collected in a large bag or Tissot spirometer. The V_D/V_T ratio should fall to values less than 30% at maximal exercise [63,64,71,118]. As shown in Fig. 9, in healthy, older adults, V_D/V_T is higher at rest, but demonstrates a relative fall with exercise similar to the young adult [63,71]. The fall in V_D/V_T ratio with exercise indicates the lungs become more efficient at eliminating CO_2 during exercise.

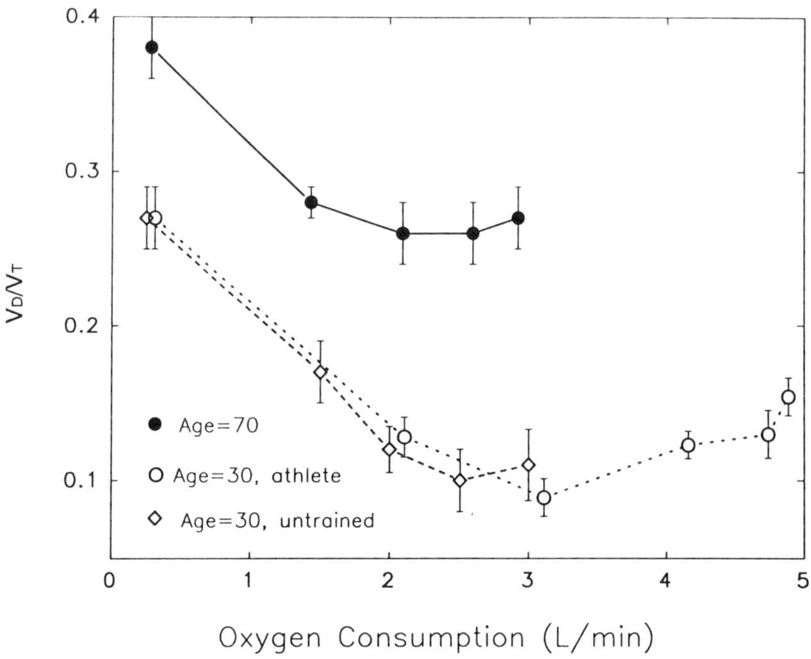

Fig. 9 Dead space ventilation relative to tidal volume (V_D/V_T) during progressive exercise in young untrained adults (◇), young endurance athletes (○), and moderately fit older adults (age = 70 yr) (●). Note that although the aged have a larger V_D/V_T at rest and during exercise, they demonstrate a similar relative decrease. (From Ref. 63.)

With on-line analysis of exercise parameters, the mixed expired gas concentration can be calculated without making an actual collection of mixed expired gas. P_{ECO_2} can be calculated from the total volume of CO_2 expired divided by total volume of expired gas collected over a given time interval, such as 1 min. It is also tempting to derive the V_D/V_T ratio using P_{ETCO_2} in place of Pa_{CO_2}. However, the P_{ETCO_2} is a poor approximation of Pa_{CO_2}, being an overestimate in persons with normal lung function and an underestimate in persons with certain kinds of lung disease. Thus, this parameter should be interpreted very conservatively.

Oxygenation during exercise, as indicated by the Pa_{O_2}, is generally well maintained, although desaturation has been noted in several studies in elite athletes [28,60,87]. Thus, a significant clinical problem in evaluating the athlete with known or suspected lung disease will be deciding if a reduction of arterial oxygenation is within expected normal limits. In normal, nonathletic individuals, Pa_{O_2} near maximal exercise may stay constant or decline by only a few millimeters of mercury [71,88,118]. An example of arterial blood gases obtained during exercise in a highly fit group of young endurance athletes relative to average fit young subjects and fit older adults is shown in Fig. 10. There is conflicting data concerning the effect of age on arterial oxygenation near maximal exercise. In one study, there was no age effect [71], although other studies have suggested a deterioration in oxygenation with age [63,88]. It does appear that some older individuals will demonstrate hypoxemia with exercise at work levels (metabolic demands) at which this is rarely observed in the young adult [63]. However, it should be appreciated that there is a progressive fall in

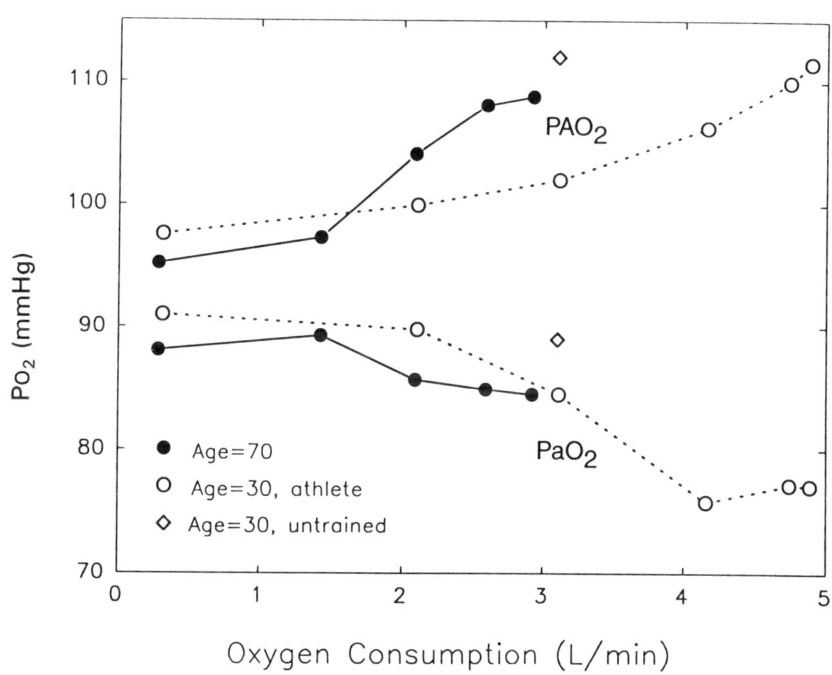

Fig. 10 Alveolar and arterial partial pressures during incremental exercise in an average fit group of subjects (◇, peak exercise only, peak $\dot{V}O_2max$ = 42, mL kg^{-1} min^{-1}) relative to that found in a group of endurance athletes (○, n = 8, peak $\dot{V}O_2max$ = 73 mL kg^{-1} min^{-1}) and a group of relatively fit older adults (●, n = 19, peak $\dot{V}O_2max$ = 42 mL/kg/min). P_{AO_2}, partial pressure of alveolar oxygen; Pa_{O_2}, partial pressure of arterial oxygen. (From Ref. 63.)

$\dot{V}O_2$max with age and those aged athletes who can work at greater metabolic demands than their sedentary counterparts (near those achieved in the average fit young adult), may become hypoxemic for reasons similar to the elite young endurance athlete (see later). Young endurance athletes able to increase demand for $\dot{V}O_2$ may show gas exchange abnormalities that are not present in average fit young adults. Reduction in PaO_2 to less than 70 mmHg or hemoglobin (Hgb) saturation ($HgbO_2\%$) less than 85 at maximal exercise have been reported [28,119], although other studies have shown smaller degrees of gas exchange abnormalities [48]. Which athletes will show desaturation? There is presently insufficient data on the effects of various exercise protocols, subject selection (i.e., age) and level of $\dot{V}O_2$ necessary to induce desaturation to answer this question definitively. It appears that a level of $\dot{V}O_2$ of about 3.5 L/min or $\dot{V}O_2$ expressed per Kg body weight of over 50 will be more likely associated with reduced arterial oxygenation than lower levels of exercise.

Determining why desaturation may occur requires a look at the alveolar air equation for oxygen:

$$P_{AO_2} = P_{IO_2} - Pa_{CO_2}\left[F_{IO_2} - \left(\frac{1 - F_{IO_2}}{R}\right)\right]$$

The average alveolar P_{AO_2} can be reduced by reduced inspired oxygen (P_{IO_2}, e.g., altitude), and by an increase in alveolar and arterial P_{CO_2} (hypoventilation). An important measure of gas exchange efficiency is to compare the P_{AO_2} with Pa_{O_2}, the A − a difference for oxygen (A − a D_{O_2}). Reduced Pa_{O_2}, therefore, is caused by (a) decreased alveolar ventilation relative to CO_2 output, which causes increased Pa_{CO_2} [28], even though A − a D_{O_2} may be normal; (b) diffusion limitation [28,48,49] related to reduction in time the red blood cell is exposed to alveolar gas; (c) an increase in $\dot{V}_A/\dot{Q}$ mismatching as cardiac output increases [48]; and (d) increased contribution of shunted blood. It is possible that these mechanisms may be represented to a variable degree among individuals.

The degree of $\dot{V}_A/\dot{Q}$ mismatching can be completely documented only by the MIGET technique. Although, the increase in $\dot{V}_A/\dot{Q}$ mismatching that has been documented by the MIGET technique is an intriguing finding that would explain some of the reduced Pa_{O_2} in athletes, the observation itself begs for an explanation [110]. Recently, Wilson pointed out that the width of the $\dot{V}_A$ or $\dot{Q}$ peaks obtained by the MIGET technique represent the width of the underlying frequency distributions of $\dot{V}_A/\dot{Q}$ ratios, and are not independent pieces of information [120]. Wilson demonstrated that the width of the $\dot{V}_A/\dot{Q}$ distribution can be viewed as the sum of the widths of the VA and Q distributions, less a component reflecting the degree of correlation between regional VA and Q. Thus, the VA/Q distribution could be widened by either of three mechanisms: widening of the underlying VA distribution, widening of the underlying Q distribution, or a change in the correlation between regional VA and regional Q. In animal studies, increasing cardiac output without changing alveolar ventilation increased the VA/Q dispersion [29], suggesting a widening of the dispersion in regional Q. In humans, the alveolar gas-mixing efficiency decreases as exercise increases [46], consistent with a narrowing of the VA dispersion. Taken together, these indirect results suggest that the widening of the VA/Q distribution seen with exercise is due to a widening of the Q distribution, with little change in VA heterogeneity. VA/Q dispersion can also be caused by inefficient mixing of expired gas in the common dead space (large airways and trachea) as ventilation increases with exercise intensity [108].

V. PULMONARY HEMODYNAMICS

A. Pulmonary Circulation

The role of the pulmonary circulation is to provide for efficient exchange of gases between the mixed venous blood entering the pulmonary capillaries and the alveolar air. This is achieved by an extremely thin interface between the capillaries and the alveoli and by the large network of capillary–alveolar interactions (see Sec. IV). The perfusion of the capillaries has been thought to depend on body position (gravity) and by the driving pressures through the pulmonary capillaries. More recent studies have suggested there may also be inherent regional differences in vascular resistance that dictate a gravity-independent anatomical distribution of blood flow [10]. Ideally, the driving pressure would be determined by the difference between the pulmonary artery pressures (Ppa) and the pulmonary capillary or left atrial pressures. Several studies have measured pulmonary artery pressures at rest and during exercise; however, in exercising humans, it is not possible to measure directly pulmonary capillary or left atrial pressures [12,44,45,58,90]. Thus, this has most often been inferred by pulmonary wedge pressures (Ppw). There is some indication that the major pressure drop in the pulmonary circulation may occur in the pulmonary capillaries. In addition, it is difficult to measure Ppw during exercise owing to large fluctuations in intrathoracic pressures; thus, these measurements need to be viewed with caution. Resting Ppa range between 8 and 28 mm Hg between diastole and systole, with a mean pressure of 14 mm Hg [89]. The Ppw pressures average 3–15 mm Hg, with a mean of 5–8 mm Hg [90]. Thus, the resting driving pressure through the pulmonary circulation is about 7–8 mm Hg.

With moderate exercise ($\dot{V}O_2$ = 1.5–2.0 L/min), the mean Ppa average 21–23 mm Hg, whereas Ppw average 10–12 mm Hg; thus, the driving pressure increases to 11–12 mm Hg. The increase in driving pressure, although small, may increase the number of perfused capillaries and may increase the distention in already perfused capillaries. With heavy exercise ($\dot{V}O_2$ = 3.0–4.0 L/min), Ppa average 31–35 mm Hg, with some subjects higher than 40 mm Hg [90], whereas Ppw rise to 18–21 mm Hg, with some subjects higher than 25 mm Hg. Studies performed on older subjects have noted increased Ppa relative to the young at a given $\dot{V}O_2$; however, the Ppw are also elevated, such that the driving pressures remain essentially unchanged [43,90]. It is thought that in the aged, mild diastolic dysfunction likely contributes to the elevated Ppw.

B. Lung Fluid Balance

Do increases in pulmonary vascular pressures cause the lung to accumulate fluid? Studies using isolated lungs from dogs have suggested that the lungs may begin to accumulate lung water at Ppa higher than 35–40 mm Hg near the maximal values observed in more athletic human subjects [90,121]. In support of this, several earlier studies have demonstrated a fall in the diffusion capacity of the lung for carbon monoxide (D_{LCO}) after heavy endurance exercise, as well as increases in closing volume, decreases in vital capacity (combined with a fall in maximal expiratory airflows), and a relative tachypnea [55,74,77,112,122]. On the other hand, studies in exercising sheep have shown that the large pleural pressure swings likely stimulate the lymphatic flow, which fairly efficiently keeps pace with increased extravascular accumulation of lung fluid in proportion to the rise in cardiac output [23]. Also, when interstitial fluid accumulates, it forms first in the peribronchiolar space and does not inhibit gas exchange [102]. More recent studies examining the fall in D_{LCO} after exercise have suggested the fall may be due to a decrease in thoracic blood volume, rather than an increase in diffusion distance secondary to water accumulation [80]. Thus, although the potential exists for fluid accumulation in the lung during exercise, there is no good evidence to support an increased fluid near the alveolar–capillary interface in humans [37]. It is possible, however, independently of a gas exchange effect, that fluid accumulation in the peribronchial space alone may influence airway diameter in the smaller bronchioles and could lead to early airway closure or a decrease in maximal expiratory airflows.

C. Bronchial Circulation

In addition to the pulmonary circulation, the lung has a second vascular source provided by the bronchial circulation. This vascular supply may originate from branches of the aorta, such as the intercostal, internal mammary, and subclavian arteries, and supplies the bronchi, branching with the airways as far as the terminal bronchioles [85,107]. In many mammals, although uncertain in humans, this circulation plays a role in temperature regulation [3,8]. It also may be involved in lung fluid balance, as implied by its close proximity to the lymphatic circulation [85]. Previous studies have noted marked increases in bronchial blood flow with exercise and with exposure to dry air, such as occurs with hyperventilation [3,73]. In horses, the increase in bronchial blood flow during exercise paralleles the rise in pulmonary arterial temperatures [73]. Interestingly, under extremely adverse conditions, the bronchial circulation has been proposed to play a role in helping prevent pulmonary hypertension and in gas exchange [85,107]. Typically, however, it combines with the thebesian vessels of the heart and contributes to a physiological venoarterial shunt [107].

The bronchial circulation has been estimated to account for approximately 1–1.5% of the total cardiac output at rest and during exercise [7]. Because this circulation probably does not contribute to gas exchange in normal subjects, it results in about one-half the total alveolar–arterial oxygen difference at rest and also for about one-half of the twofold increase observed in the $A\text{–}aD_{O_2}$ during moderate exercise in healthy persons [40]. At the very high metabolic rates achieved by some endurance athletes [28], shunt would be expected to contribute proportionately more to a further widening in the $A\text{–}aD_{O_2}$ because the mixed venous content is probably reduced to less than 2–3 vol% [6]. However, it is unlikely that shunt accounts for all or even a major proportion of the severe exercise-induced hypoxemia observed in some athletes, because mild hyperoxia during heavy exercise causes proportionate increases in alveolar and arterial P_{O_2}, and Pa_{O_2} was normalized even in those subjects who were the most hypoxemic during air breathing [28].

VI. AIRWAY FLUID BALANCE

The lumen side of the airway is a complex tissue, composed of epithelial cells protected by the mucosal surface layer, secretory glands, nerves, smooth muscle, and cells of the immune system, including mast cells and macrophages. In disease, there may be more inflammatory cells populating the airway, including eosinophils and neutrophils [11]. As is true with mast cells [33,84], the ionic milieu of the airway lumenal surface may affect functioning of many of these cell types.

The amount of fluid present and the concentration of ions in the mucosa reflect a dynamic balance between fluid production by glandular structures, fluid transport from alveoli, fluid resorption by airway cells, and fluid evaporation [4,16]. Most of the fluid evaporation probably occurs in the upper airway (oro- and nasopharynx) [39,50]. Although studies have not been done in humans, studies in dogs suggest that increased ventilation does cause an increase in ionic concentration in the airway fluid layer of larger airways [15,72]. The degree to which evaporative water loss extends into smaller airways is a matter of debate, largely because of the difficulty in probing the mucosal layer of smaller airways to determine changes during exercise. Modeling studies have suggested that water loss occurs in smaller airways [39,50]. The ionic milieu may be affected in important ways during exercise as evaporative water loss upsets the normal homeostatic balance. There are both passive and active compensatory mechanisms that activate to restore the ionic milieu. The passive compensations include increases in fluid or ion fluxes across the airway, secondary to changes in concentration gradients for ions, or water as water evaporates from the airways. Active mechanisms include neural and humoral control of both glandular secretion and resorption mechanisms [4]. Mechanical stresses associated with increases in ventilation may cause increases in production of mediators, such as nitric oxide and prostaglandins [32], that have an influence on airway fluid balance [4]. The study of airway fluid balance in humans is really in its infancy. Recent studies suggest that control of airway fluid balance may be different in normal versus asthmatic individuals [24].

VII. SUMMARY

The respiratory system in health thus performs its task of maintaining arterial blood gas homeostasis, at minimal cost during exercise, extremely well. Only with heavy exercise in the highly trained endurance athlete is the respiratory system markedly challenged. Thus, in these individuals, mild changes in airway diameter, lung fluid balance, the oxygen cost of breathing, or breathing pattern may play a role in limiting human performance.

ACKNOWLEDGMENTS

The author would like to thank Audrey Schroeder for preparation of the manuscript and Dr. Dorothy Ainsworth for her helpful comments. This work was supported by the Mayo Foundation and by the General Clinical Research Center Grant MO1-RR00585 from the National Institutes of Health.

REFERENCES

1. Aaron EA, Johnson BD, Seow CK, Dempsey JA. Oxygen cost of exercise hyperpnea: measurement. J Appl Physiol 1992; 72:1810–1817.
2. Aaron EA, Seow KC, Johnson BD, Dempsey JA. Oxygen cost of exercise hyperpnea: implications for performance. J Appl Physiol 1992; 72: 1818–1825.
3. Agostonei P, Arena V, Doria E, Susini G. Inspired gas relative humidity affects systemic to pulmonary bronchial blood flow in humans. Chest 1990; 97:1377–1380.
4. Al-Bazzaz FJ. Regulation of salt and water transport across airway mucosa. Clin Chest Med 1986; 7:259–272.
5. Allen C, Jones N. Rate of change of alveolar carbon dioxide and the control of ventilation during exercise. J Physiol (Lond) 1984; 355:1–9.
6. Astrand PO, Cuddy TE, Saltin B, Stenberg J. Cardiac output during submaximal and maximal work. J Appl Physiol 1964; 19:168–172.
7. Bachofen H, Hobi HJ, Scherrer M. Alveolar arterial N_2 gradients at rest and during exercise in healthy men of different ages. J Appl Physiol 1973; 34:137–142.
8. Baile EM, Dahlby RW, Wiggs BR, Pare PD. Role of tracheal and bronchial circulation in respiratory heat exchange. J Appl Physiol 1985; 58:217–222.
9. Banzett RB, Mead J, Reid MB, Topulos GP. Locomotion in men has no appreciable mechanical effect on breathing. J Appl Physiol 1992; 72: 1922–1926.
10. Beck KC, Rehder K. Difference in regional vascular conductances in isolated dog lungs. J Appl Physiol 1986; 61:530–538.
11. Bentley AM, Menz G, Storz C, Robinson DS, Bradley B, Jeffery PK, Durham SR, Kay AB. Identification of T lymphocytes, macrophages and activated eosinophils in the bronchial mucosa in intrinsic asthma. Am Rev Respir Dis 1992; 146:500–506.
12. Bevegard S. The effects of cardioacceleration by methylscopolamine nitrate on the circulation at rest and during exercise in supine position, with special reference to the stroke volume. Acta Physiol Scand 1963; 57:61–80.
13. Bisgard G, et al. Role of the carotid body in hyperpnea of moderate exercise in goats. J Appl Physiol 1982; 52:1216–1222.
14. Blackie SP, Fairbarn MS, McElvaney NG, Wilcox PG, Morrison NJ, Pardy RL. Normal values and ranges for ventilation and breathing pattern at maximal exercise. Chest 1991; 100:136–142.
15. Boucher RC, Stutts MJ, Bromberg PA, Gatzy JT. Regional differences in airway surface liquid composition. J Appl Physiol 1981; 50:613–620.
16. Boucher RC. Human airway ion transport, Part 1. Am J Respir Crit Care Med 1994; 150:271–281.

17. Brooke MH, Kaiser KK. Muscle fiber types: how many and what kind? Arch Neurol 1970; 23:369–379.
18. Burke RE. Motor units: anatomy, physiology and functional organization. In: Brookhart JM, Mountcastle VB, eds. Handbook of physiology, sec 1, vol III, part 1, the nervous system. Bethesda: American Physiology Society, 1981:345–422.
19. Burke RE, Levine DN, Tsairis P, et al. Physiological types and histochemical profiles of motor units of cat gastrocnemius. J Physiol (Lond) 1973; 234: 723–748.
20. Burke RE, Levine DN, Zajac FE III. Mammalian motor units: physiological–histochemical correlation in three types in cat gastrocnemius. Science 1971; 174:709–712.
21. Busse M, Maassen N, Konrad H. Relation between plasma K^+ and ventilation during incremental exercise after glycogen depletion and repletion in man. J Physiol (Lond) 1991; 443:469–476.
22. Clark JM, Sinclair RE, Lennox JB. Chemical and non-chemical components of ventilation and during hypercapnic exercise in man. J Appl Physiol 1980; 48:1065–1076.
23. Coates GH, O'Bradovich H, Jerreries AL, Gray GW. Effects of exercise on lung lymph flow in sheep and goats during normoxia and hypoxia. J Clin Invest 1984; 74:133–141.
24. Daviskas E, Anderson SD, Gonda I, Chan HK, Cook P, Fulton R. Changes in mucociliary clearance during and after isocapnic hyperventilation in asthmatic and healthy subjects. Eur Resp J 1995; 8:742–751.
25. Dempsey JA. Is the lung built for exercise? Med Sci Sports Exerc 1986; 18:143–155.
26. Dempsey JA, Johnson BD. Demand vs capacity in the healthy pulmonary system. Schweiz Z. Sportmed 1992; 40:55–64.
27. Dempsey JA, Vidruk EH, Mitchell GH. Pulmonary control systems in exercise: update. Fed Proc 1985; 44:2260–70.
28. Dempsey JA, Hanson PG, Henderson KS. Exercise-induced arterial hypoxemia in healthy human subjects at sea level. J Physiol (Lond) 1984; 355: 161.
29. Domino KB, Eisenstein BL, Tran T, Hlastala MP. Increased pulmonary perfusion worsens ventilation–perfusion matching. Anesthesiology 1993; 79:817.
30. Duffin J. Neural drives to breathing during exercise. Can J Appl Physiol 1994; 19:289–304.
31. Ebashi S. Excitation–contraction coupling. Annu Rev Physiol 1976; 38: 293–309.
32. Edmonds JF, Berry EM, Wyllie JH. Release of prostaglandins caused by distension of the lungs. Br J Surg 1969; 56:622–623.
33. Eggleston PA, Kagey-Sobotka A, Schleimer RP, Lichtenstein LM. Interaction between hyperosmolar and IgE-mediated histamine release from basophils and mast cells. Am Rev Respir Dis 1984; 130:86–91.
34. Enad JG, Fournier M, Sieck GC. Oxidative capacity and capillary density of diaphragm motor units. J Appl Physiol 1989; 67:620–627.

34a. Fregossi RF, Lansing RW. Neural drive to nasal dilator muscles. Influence of exercise intensity and oronasal flow partitioning. J Appl Physiol 1995; 79:1330–1337.
35. Forsyth RD, Cole P, Shephard RJ. Exercise and nasal patency. J Appl Physiol 1973; 55:860–865.
36. Gallagher CG, Brown E, Younes M. Breathing pattern during maximal exercise and during submaximal exercise with hypercapnia. J Appl Physiol 1987; 63:238–244.
37. Gallagher CG, Huda W, Rigby M, Greenberg D, Younes M. Lack of radiographic evidence of interstitial pulmonary edema after maximal exercise in normal subjects. Am Rev Respir Dis 1986; 133:581–586.
38. Giesbrecht GG, Younes M. Respiratory response to pulmonary vascular congestion in intact conscious dogs. J Appl Physiol 1993; 74:345–353.
39. Gilbert IA, Fouke JM, McFadden ER. Heat and water flux in the intrathoracic airways and exercise-induced asthma. J Appl Physiol 1987; 63: 1681–1691.
40. Gledhill N, Froese A, Dempsey J. Ventilation to perfusion distribution during exercise in health. In: Dempsey J, Reed C, eds. Muscular exercise and the lung. Madison: University of Wisconsin Press, 1977; 325–344.
41. Gorza L. Identification of a novel type 2 fiber population in mammalian skeletal muscle by combined use of histochemical myosin ATPase and antimyosin monoclonal antibodies. J Histochem Cytochem 1990; 38:257–265.
42. Gosselin LE, Betlach M, Vailas AC, Thomas DP. Training induced alterations in young and senescent rat diaphragm muscle. J Appl Physiol 1992; 72:1506–1511.
43. Granath A, Strandell T. Relationships between cardiac output, stroke volume, and intracardiac pressures at rest and during exercise in supine position and some anthropometric data in healthy old men. Acta Med Scand 1964; 176:447–466.
44. Granath A, Jonsson B, Strandell T. Circulation in healthy old men, studies by right heart catheterization at rest and during exercise in supine and sitting position. Acta Med Scand. 1964; 176:425–446.
45. Gurtner HP, Walser P, Fassler B. Normal values for pulmonary hemodynamics at rest and during exercise in man. Prog Respir Res 1975; 9:295–315.
46. Hale T, Kox WJ. Changes in alveolar mixing efficiency during exercise. Respir Physiol 1991; 86:283.
47. Hammeren J, et al. Exercise training-induced alterations in skeletal muscle oxidative and antioxidative enzyme activity in senescent rats. Int J Sports Med 1992; 13:412–416.
48. Hammond MD, Gale GE, Kapitan KS, Ries A, Wagner PD. Pulmonary gas exchange in humans during exercise at sea level. J Appl Physiol 1986; 60: 1590.
49. Hammond MD, Gale GE, Kapitan KS, Ries A, Wagner PD. Pulmonary gas exchange in humans during normobaric hypoxic exercise. J Appl Physiol 1986; 61:1749.
50. Hanna LM, Scherer PW. A theoretical model of localized heat and water

vapor transport in the human respiratory tract. J Biomech Eng 1986; 108: 19–27.
51. Henke KG, Sharratt M, Pegelow D, Dempsey JA. Regulation of end-expiratory lung volume during exercise. J Appl Physiol 1988; 64:135–146.
52. Henneman E, Mendell LM. Functional organization of motoneuron pool and its inputs. In: Brookhart JM, Mountcastle VB, eds. Handbook of physiology, sec 1 vol III, part 1, the nervous system. Bethesda: American Physiology Society, 1981; 423–507.
53. Hesser CM, Linnarsson D, Fagraeus L. Pulmonary mechanics and work of breathing at maximal ventilation and raised air pressure. J Appl Physiol 1981; 50:747–53.
54. Hey EN, Lloyd BB, Cunningham D, Jukes M, Bolton D. Effects of various respiratory stimuli on the depth and frequency of breathing in man. Respir Physiol 1966; 1:193–205.
55. Hill NS, Jacoby C, Farber HW. Effect on an endurance triathlon on pulmonary function. Med Sci Sports Exerc 1991; 23:1260–1264.
56. Hlastala MP, Domino KB. Role of hypoxia on blood flow in modulating V_A/Q heterogeneity in the lungs. Adv Exp Biol 1994; 345:67–73.
57. Holloszy J. Muscle metabolism during exercise. Arch Phys Rehabil Med 1982; 63:231–234.
58. Holmgren A, Jonsson B, Sjostrand T. Circulatory data in normal subjects at rest and during exercise in recumbant position, with special reference to the stroke volume at different working intensities. Acta Physiol Scand 1960; 49:343–363.
59. Jensen JI, Lyager S, Pedersen OF. The relationship between maximal ventilation, breathing pattern and mechanical limitation of ventilation. J Physiol 1980; 309:521–532.
59a. Johnson BD, Dempsy JA. Demand vs capacity in the aging pulmonary system. In: Holloszy JO, ed. Exercise and sports science reviews. Baltimore: Williams & Wilkins, 1991:171–210.
60. Johnson BD, Saupe KW, Dempsey JA. Mechanical constraints on exercise hyperpnea in endurance athletes. J Appl Physiol 1992; 73:874–886.
61. Johnson BD, Reddan WG, Pegelow DF, Seow KC, Dempsey JA. Flow limitation and regulation of function residual capacity during exercise in a physically active aging population. Am Rev Respir Dis 1991; 143:960–967.
62. Johnson BD, Reddan WG, Seowl KG, Dempsey JA. Mechanical constraints on exercise hyperpnea in a fit aging population. Am Rev Respir Dis 1991; 43:968–977.
63. Johnson BD, Safwan Badr M, Dempsey JA. Impact of the aging pulmonary system on the response to exercise, Clin Chest Med. 1994; 15:229.
64. Jones ND, McHardy GJR, Naimark A, Campbell EJM. Physiological dead space and alveolar–arterial gas pressure differences during exercise. Clin Sci 1966; 31:19.
65. Katz A, Sahlin K. Effect of decreased oxygen availability on NADH and lactate contents in human skeletal muscle during exercise. Acta Physiol Scand 1987; 131:119.

66. Kodama T. Thermodynamic analysis of muscle ATPase mechanisms. Physiol Rev 1985; 65:468–540.
67. Laiken N, Fanestil D. Acid–base balance and regulation of hydrogen ion excretion. In: West J, ed. Physiological basis of medical practice. Baltimore: Williams & Wilkins, 1985.
68. Larsson L, Ansved T, Edstrom L. Effects of age on physiological, immunohistochemical and biochemical properties of fast-twitch single motor units in the rat. J Physiol (Lond) 1991; 443:257–275.
69. Leblanc P, Summers E, Inman MD, Jones NL, Campbell EJM, Killian KJ. Inspiratory muscles during exercise: a problem of supply and demand. J Appl Physiol 1988; 64:2482–2489.
70. Liddell EGT, Sherrington CS. Recruitment and some other factors of reflex inhibition. Proc R Soc Lond (Biol) 1925; 97:488–518.
71. Malmberg P, Hedenström H, Fridriksson HV. Reference values for gas exchange during exercise in healthy nonsmoking and smoking men, Bull Eur Physiopathol Respir 1987; 23:131.
72. Man SFP, Adams GK III, Proctor DF. Effects of temperature, relative humidity and mode of breathing on canine airway secretions. J Appl Physiol 1979; 46:205–210.
73. Manohar M. Blood flow to the respiratory and limb muscles and to abdominal organs during maximal exertion in ponies. J Physiol 1986; 377:25–35.
74. Maron MB, Hamilton LH, Maksud MB. Alterations in pulmonary function consequent to competitive marathon running. Med Sci Sports 1979; 2: 244–249.
75. McParland C, Krishnan B, Lobo J, Gallagher CG. Effect of physical training on breathing pattern during progressive exercise. Respir Physiol 1992; 90: 311–323.
76. Metzger J. Mechanisms of chemomechanical coupling in skeletal muscle during work. In: Lamb D, Gisolfi C, eds. Energy metabolism in exercise and sport. Dubuque IA: Brown & Benchmark, 1992; 1–43.
77. Miles DS, Enoch AD, Grevey SC. Interpretation of changes in DLCO and pulmonary function after running five miles. Respir Physiol 1986; 66: 135–145.
78. Morrison KJ, Gao Y, Vanhoutte PM. Epithelial modulation of airway smooth muscle. Am J Physiol. 1990; 258:L254–L262.
79. Niinimaa V, Cole P, Mintz S, Shephard RJ. The switching point from nasal to oronasal breathing. Respir Physiol 1980; 42:61–71.
80. O'Kroy J, Loy RA, Coast JR. Pulmonary function changes following exercise. Med Sci Sports Exerc 1992; 24:1359–1364.
81. Olafsson S, Hyatt RE. Ventilatory mechanics and expiratory flow limitation during exercise in normal subjects. J Clin Invest 1969; 48:564–573.
82. Otis AB. The work of breathing. In: Fenn WO, Rahn H, eds. The handbook of physiology, sec 3: respiration, vol. I. Philadelphia: Waverly Press, 1964; 463–476.
83. Paterson D. Potassium and ventilation during exercise. J Appl Physiol 1992; 72:811–820.

84. Pearce FL, Flint KC, Leung KBP, Hudspith BN, Seager K, Hammond MD, Brostoff J, Geraint-James D, Johnson NM. Some studies on human pulmonary mast cells obtained by bronchoalveolar lavage and by enzymatic dissociation of whole lung tissue. Int Arch Allergy Appl Immunol 1987; 82: 507–512.
85. Pietra GG, Magno M. Pharmacological factors influencing permeability of the bronchial microcirculation. Fed Proc 1978; 37:2466–2470.
86. Powers S, et al. Diaphragmatic fiber type specific adaptation to endurance training. Resp Physio 1992; 89:195–207.
87. Powers SK, Lawler J, Dempsey JA, Dodd S, Landry G. Effects of incomplete pulmonary gas exchange on V_{O_2} maximal. J Appl Physiol 1989; 66: 2491–2495.
88. Prefaut C, Anselme F, Caillaud C, Masse-Biron J. Exercise-induced hypoxemia in older athletes. J Appl Physiol 1994; 76:120–126.
89. Reeves JT, Groves BM. Approach to the patient with pulmonary hypertension. In: Weir EK, Reeves JT, eds. Pulmonary hypertension. Mt Kisco NY: Futura, 1984; 1–44.
90. Reeves JT, Dempsey JA, Grover RF. Pulmonary circulation during exercise. In: Weirand EK, Reeves JT, eds. Pulmonary vascular physiology and pathophysiology. New York: Marcel Dekker, 1989; 107–133.
91. Richter D, Ballantyne D, Remmers J. How is respiratory rhythm generated? A model. News Physiol Sci 1986; 1:109–111.
92. Richter D. Generation and maintenance of the respiratory rhythm. J Exp Biol 1982; 100:93–107.
93. Road JD, Newman S, Derenee JP, Grassino A. The in vivo length–force relationship of the canine diaphragm. J Appl Physiol 1986; 60:63–70.
94. Ruegg J. Calcium in Muscle Activation. Berlin: Springer-Verlag, 1988.
95. Saibene F, Mognoni P, Lafortuna CL, Mostardi R. Oro-nasal breathing during exercise Pfluegers Arch 1978; 378:65–69.
96. Sciurba FC, Owens GR, Sanders MH, Bartley PG, Hadesty RL, Paradis IL, Costantino JP. Evidence of an altered pattern of breathing during exercise in recipients of heart lung transplants. N Engl J Med 1988; 319:1186–1192.
97. Senior A. ATP synthesis by oxidative phosphorylation. Physiol Rev 1988; 68:177–216.
98. Shephard KL, Rahmoune H. Evaporation-induced changes in airway surface liquid on an isolated guinea pig trachea. J Appl Physiol 1994; 76: 1156–1165.
99. Shephard RJ. The oxygen cost of breathing during vigorous exercise. J Exp Physiol 1966; 51:336–350.
100. Sieck GC. Physiological effects of diaphragm muscle denervation and disuse. Clin Chest Med 1994; 15:641–659.
101. Sieck GC, Fournier M. Diaphragm motor unit recruitment during ventilatory and nonventilatory behaviors. J Appl Physiol 1989; 66:2539–2545.
101a. Sieck GC, Prakash YS. The diaphragm muscle. In: Miller AD, Bianchi AL,

Bishop BP, eds. Neural control of the respiratory muscles. Boca Raton FL: CRC Press, 1996, pp. 7–20.
102. Staub NC, Nagano H, Pearce ML. Pulmonary endema in dogs especially the sequence of fluid accumulation in lungs. J Appl Physiol 1967; 22:227–240.
103. Strohl EP, O'Cain CF, Slutsky AS. Alae nasi activation and nasal resistance in healthy subjects. J Appl Physiol 1982; 52:1432–1437.
104. Syabbalo NC, Bundgaard A, Widdicombe JG. Effects of exercise on nasal airflow resistance in healthy subjects and in patients with asthma and rhinitis. Bull Eur Physiopathol Respir 1985; 21:507–513.
105. Syabbalo NC, Krishnan B, Zintel T, Gallagher CG. Differential ventilatory control during constant work rate and incremental exercise. Respir Physiol 1994; 97:175–187.
106. Syabbalo N, Zintel T, Watts R, Gallagher CG. Carotid chemoreceptors and respiratory adaptations to dead space loading during incremental exercise. J Appl Physiol 1993; 75:1378–1384.
107. Tobin CE. The bronchial arteries and their connections with other vessels in the human lung. Surg Gynecol Obstet 1952; 95:741–750.
108. Tsukimoto K, Arcos JP, Shaffartzik W, Wagner PD, West JB. Effect of common dead space on VA/Q distribution in the dog. J Appl Physiol 1990; 68:2488–2493.
109. Tullson P, Terjung R. Adenine nucleotide metabolism in contracting skeletal muscle. Exerc Sport Sci Rev 1991; 19:507–537.
110. Wagner PD. Ventilation–perfusion matching during exercise. Chest 1992; 101(suppl):192S.
111. Waldrop T. Role of descending neural influences form higher locomotor regions of the CNS. In: Rowell L, ed. Handbook of physiology. New York: Oxford University Press, 1995.
112. Warren GL, Cureton KJ, Sparling PB. Does lung function limit performance in a 24-hour ultramarathon? Respir Physiol 1989; 78:253–264.
113. Warren JG, Jennings SJ, Clark TJH. Effect of adrenergic and vagal blockade on the normal human airway response to exercise. Clin Sci 1984; 66:79–85.
114. Wasserman K, Whipp BJ, Cassaburi R. Respiratory control during exercise. In: Handbook of physiology: respiration. Bethesda: American Physiological Society, 1986; 595–620.
115. Wheatley JR, Amis TC, Engel LA. Oronasal partitioning of ventilation during exercise. J Appl Physiol 1991; 71:546–551.
116. Whipp BJ. The bioenergetic and gas exchange basis of exercise testing. Clin Chest Med 1994; 15(2):173–192.
117. Whipp BJ, Pardy RL. Breathing during exercise. In: Handbook of physiology. The respiratory system, III, sec 3, part 2, Bethesda: American Physiol ogy Society, 1986; 605–630.
118. Whipp BJ, Wasserman K. Alveolar–arterial gas tension differences during graded exercise. J Appl Physiol 1969; 27:361.
119. Williams JH, Powers SK, Kelley Stuart M. Hemoglobin desaturation in

highly trained athletes during heavy exercise. Med Sci Sports Exerc 1986; 18:168.

120. Wilson TA, Beck KC. Contributions of ventilation and perfusion inhomogeneities to the VA/Q distribution. J Appl Physiol 1992; 72:2298.

121. Younes M, Bshouty Z, Ali J. Longitudinal distribution of pulmonary vascular resistance with very high pulmonary blood flow. J Appl Physiol 1987; 62:344–358.

122. Younes M, Kivinen G. Respiratory mechanics and breathing pattern during and following maximal exercise. J Appl Physiol 1984; 57:1773–1782.

2

Evaluating Exercise Capacity and Airway Function in the Athlete

Kenneth C. Beck
Mayo Clinic and Foundation, Rochester, Minnesota

I. INTRODUCTION

In this chapter we will review the practical aspects of setting up and maintaining a laboratory for performing exercise evaluations. This review will be focused on equipment and methods for making various measurements. The reader is referred to other reviews for more thorough discussions of standard exercise protocols and patient preparation [1–5].

II. CONDUCTING THE EXERCISE TEST

Conduct of an exercise evaluation proceeds by first evaluating the patient's ability to safely perform exercise. This involves a limited medical history and, in some persons, a physical examination or preliminary laboratory evaluations such as pulmonary function testing. Exercise testing is generally considered to be safe when performed in a well-equipped laboratory and when the subject is adequately monitored. However, there are not many studies that have addressed the issue of safety [6]. Risk is probably very small in athletes with recent history of moderate to heavy levels of exertion, especially when the exercise is performed with electrocardiogram (ECG) and blood pressure monitoring in an exercise laboratory. Contraindications to exercise testing are listed in various monographs on exercise testing [7–10]. The contraindications are generally based on sound clinical judgment, which should always be the first consideration if conditions exist that are not among the listed contraindications.

Absolute and relative contraindications to exercise testing are listed in Table 1 [7–10]. Systemic hypertension is listed, although there is no agreement about the level (systolic > 200–250 mm Hg and diastolic > 115–120 mm Hg measured at rest). Care should be exercised in testing pregnant women: the American College of Obstetricians and Gynecologists has published guidelines for exercise during pregnancy [11], although they did not address the issue of performing exercise tests to maximal levels during pregnancy. The American College of Sports Medicine has recommended against such testing in pregnant women unless it is clinically indicated [1].

Table 1 Contraindications to Exercise Testing

Absolute contraindications
- Recent myocardial infarction
- Changes in the resting ECG that suggest acute or recent myocardial event
- Unstable angina pectoris
- Uncontrolled cardiac rhythm disturbances, either supraventricular or ventricular, particularly when compromising cardiac output
- Severe aortic stenosis and known or suspected dissecting aortic aneurysm
- Active or suspected acute pericarditis or myocarditis
- Acute congestive heart failure
- Recent systemic or pulmonary embolus
- Acute febrile illness
- Third degree A-V block without pacemaker control
- Pulmonary edema or significant cor pulmonale
- Physical disabilities or other inability to cooperate, such as severe emotional or psychological distress.

Relative contraindications
- Systemic hypertension.
- Resting tachycardia (>120 min^{-1})
- Frequent ventricular or atrial ectopy
- Moderate aortic stenosis
- Moderate to severe pulmonary hypertension
- Moderate valvular heart disease
- Pregnancy
- Known electrolyte abnormalities and severe anemia (Hgb < 10/100 mL)

Note that additional absolute or relative contraindications may exist, and clinical judgment should always be used to determine appropriateness of performing an exercise test.

After satisfactory medical review, the subject should be informed about the procedure. The need for written informed consent is determined by local policies of the institution. Personnel should be trained in basic life support, and it is desirable to have someone also trained in advanced cardiac life support. Whether a physician must be available is a matter of debate, and depends on the clinical history of the subject to be tested: for subjects who are active routinely and have none of the contraindications listed in Table 1, a physician's presence is not routinely required [10]. The subject should not have eaten a heavy meal within about 3 h before testing and should wear comfortable, loose-fitting clothing.

The modality (treadmill versus stationary cycle) and protocol are a matter of individual preference. Exercise protocols designed to determine maximum O_2 consumption ($\dot{V}O_2max$) as one endpoint should be designed to last about 10 min [12]. This target is relatively easy to attain using cycle ergometry, which allows uniform progressive increases in exercise intensity with time. A protocol using cycle ergometry should start with a 3- to 5-min warm-up period at a low intensity (20–50 watts; W). Thereafter, the rapidity of increase in intensity depends on the pretest estimation of the subject's capacity. Pretest estimations can be made by starting with predicted $\dot{V}O_2max$, then adjusting the prediction based on clinical assessment of the subject's capabilities. For instance, a young, fit subject should be able to attain a $\dot{V}O_2max$ of about 45 mL min^{-1} kg^{-1}. A subject weighing 75 kg would, therefore, have an estimated $\dot{V}O_2max$ of 3375 mL min^{-1}. By using a rough rule of thumb that $\dot{V}O_2$ increases about 10 mL $min^{-1}W^{-1}$ of external power output, the estimated maximal power output would be (3375 − 500)/10 = 287 W. A $\dot{V}O_2$ of 500 mL min^{-1} is subtracted from the estimated $\dot{V}O_2max$ to correct for $\dot{V}O_2$ during unloaded cycling. Thus, a 25-W min^{-1} protocol would bring the subject to near maximal within the 10-min guideline. A more fit subject may require 30-, 40- or even 50-W min^{-1} protocols, whereas less fit, smaller, or older subjects may require smaller slopes. The increase in power output can be a steady "ramp," or by incrementing intensity at the end of each 1- or 2-min period.

Treadmill protocols are more complex because there are two variables that affect work intensity, speed and elevation. In the extreme, speed or elevation can be left constant while varying only the other variable (e.g., Balke protocol). The most common treadmill protocol followed is that of Bruce [1,13]. However, there are other alternatives, listed in the guidelines published by the American College of Sports Medicine [1]. A comparison study of treadmill protocols found a slightly larger $\dot{V}O_2max$ using the Taylor versus Bruce and Balke protocols [14]. The Taylor protocol involves 3-min stages of exercise separated by rest periods (5 min) [14] and, therefore, takes much longer to complete than continuous protocols.

During an exercise evaluation, the 12-lead ECG and blood pressure should be monitored as work intensity is increased until the subject cannot continue or other reasons for early termination of the test develop. Reasons for early termination of a test [1] include onset of moderate to severe angina; pronounced ECG changes (>2-mm–horizontal or downsloping ST segment depression or elevation); serious arrhythmias (e.g., second- or third-degree atrioventricular block, sustained ventricular tachycardia, frequent premature ventricular contractions, or atrial fibrillation with a rapid ventricular response); drop in systolic blood pressure with increasing intensity, accompanied by signs or symptoms, or drop below preexercise values; unusual or severe shortness of breath; signs of poor peripheral perfusion (pallor, cyanosis, cold clammy skin); ataxia, vertigo, visual or gait problems, confusion or other signs of central nervous system (CNS) disorder; and acute myocardial infarction. If monitoring fails (e.g., ECG or blood pressure), consideration would be given to stopping, depending on the clinical circumstances. Other changes may prompt stopping a test: physical or verbal manifestations of severe fatigue or shortness of breath; severe wheezing in the chest or upper airways; leg cramps or extreme pain, suggesting claudication; and severe hypertension (systolic pressure > 260 mm Hg; diastolic pressure >115–120 mm Hg).

Quantitative assessments of exercise capacity, whether in athletes or nonathletes, require measurement of maximal external power output, and may involve monitoring of minute ventilation ($\dot{V}_E$) and metabolic rate (oxygen consumption, $\dot{V}O_2$ and carbon dioxide production, $\dot{V}CO_2$). Additional measurements might include flow versus lung volume loops obtained before, during, and following the exercise, and assessment of gas exchange, either by analyzing the gas exchange parameters obtained noninvasively, or by obtaining arterial blood gases during the exercise. The instrumentation for making each of these measurements, with exception of arterial blood gases (presented in Chap. 1) is discussed in the following.

A. Measuring Power Output (Ergometry)

Exercise uses internal energy stores of the body to perform useful external work. The rate of performance of the external work is defined as *power*. In a strictly thermodynamic sense, work is equal to the force times the distance over which it acts. The unit of work is the *joule* (J; equal to one Newton-meter) and power is measured in Joules per second ($J\ s^{-1}$) or watts (W). Power output is also commonly expressed in kilopond meters per minute, where 100 W = 618 kp m min^{-1}. If any of the three fundamental measurements (force, distance, and time) is in error, then the calculated power output will also be in error.

The quantitative assessment of work output is made using either a cycle ergometer or a treadmill. With cycle ergometers, the power output is measured directly by setting or measuring the resistance that must be overcome to turn the pedals of the cycle (torque) and by determining the rate at which the athlete is turning the crank (revolutions per minute; rpm). Power output is the product of these two numbers (power = torque × rpm). With the treadmill, determining the precise power output is more difficult. External power while walking or running on a flat motorized treadmill is essentially zero. The metabolic requirement for walking is derived entirely from work required to move the limbs, and from the up and down motion against gravity. When the treadmill is inclined, power output increases owing to the work against gravity needed to prevent downward motion. Thus, power output is related to body weight in addition to treadmill speed and elevation [1,4].

Because speed and elevation during treadmill testing and power output during cycle ergometry are used to gauge exercise intensity, it is important that the cycle or treadmill be calibrated and operating correctly. When setting up an exercise laboratory, it is worthwhile to validate the exercise equipment, and varying levels of validation are possible, depending on need (Table 2). Treadmill validation is relatively easy, requiring checking of the accuracy of the percentage elevation and speed of the belt, with a subject running on the treadmill, because the weight of the subject can alter treadmill speed. Validation of belt speed is easily performed by counting the number of times a mark or piece of tape affixed to the tread cycles around per minute.

Cycle ergometers (arm or leg) are more difficult to validate. Frictional resistance against which the subject performs work is applied by frictional belts or pads tightened against a rotating wheel, or by electrically braking a flywheel. Either mechanism may be adjusted to a fixed resistance or the setting controlled by an electronic circuit that continuously measures power output and adjusts the resistance mechanism to keep power within a specified range. With or without feedback circuitry, ergometers designed for fitness evaluation generally provide a continuous display of power output. In bikes with a frictional belt mechanism, a calibration table must be provided that allows the user to relate tension and pedal speed to power output in standard units of watts or kp m min^{-1}. With electronic control of power output, the ergometer may compensate for variations in pedal speed by varying braking force, and power output may be relatively constant independent of pedaling speed within a certain range (e.g., 40–150 min^{-1}).

Table 2 Validation of Equipment to Gauge Exercise Intensity

	Treadmill	Cycle ergometers
Level 1 (basic)	1. Verify belt speed by timed count of belt revolutions, with subject walking or jogging. 2. Verify elevation (direct measurement). **Periodic validation**: yearly.	1. From manufacturer: date, method used, acceptable tolerance, and output of delivered instrument. 2. Validation of tachometer: timed counting of pedal revolutions. **Periodic validation**: yearly.
Level 2 (intermediate)	1. Subject walks or runs on treadmill at "standard" settings with measurement of $\dot{V}O_2$. **Periodic validation**: monthly.	1. Subject pedals at "standard" intensity with measurement of $\dot{V}O_2$. 2. Static calibration of internal force transducer. **Periodic validation**: Step 1 repeated monthly; step 2 repeated yearly.
Level 3 (advanced)	(Same as level 2)	1. External calibrator device to confirm power output under dynamic conditions. **Periodic validation**: yearly.

Validation of a cycle ergometer requires validation of the tachometer by timed counting of pedal revolutions, and checking the accuracy of the internal force measuring transducer. Some manufacturers provide a "static" calibration device that allows the user to perform checks of the internal force transducer (see level 2, Table 2). Static calibration does not check the internal resistance of the cycle, nor does it check the accuracy of the controller mechanism. Dynamic calibration is more difficult to perform, and it requires a external means to turn the crank of the cycle while measuring the torque. Calibrators have been designed, and some manufacturers may loan or rent these devices for validation studies [15,16].

A useful final check of equipment is to have someone from the laboratory exercise on the treadmill or ergometer at a given setting while $\dot{V}O_2$ is being measured. A value for $\dot{V}O_2$ that is not within expected limits is an indication of an error somewhere in the system. For instance, while riding a cycle ergometer set at 100 W, a 72-kg person should consume about 1470 mL min^{-1} of $\dot{V}O_2$ [1]. Allowances should be made for variability in these numbers owing to intersubject variability in exercise efficiency and to measurement noise [17]. Day-to-day standard deviation of $\dot{V}O_2$ in our laboratory is about 50 mL min^{-1}. Thus, an acceptable range in the foregoing example might be 1370–1570 mL min^{-1}. If the value obtained is outside the acceptable range, the error could be in the measurement of $\dot{V}O_2$ (discussed in the following section) as well as the ergometer. This procedure is useful for both initial validation and periodic documentation of equipment accuracy.

B. Measuring Metabolic and Ventilatory Responses

The $\dot{V}O_2$, $\dot{V}CO_2$, and $\dot{V}E$, all can be measured by collecting expired gas at the mouth. Historically, these measurements were all made by timed collection of expired gas into large collection bags [18] or a spirometer. Data for gas volume output per unit time ($\dot{V}E$) can be combined with mixed expired and inspired gas concentrations to obtain $\dot{V}O_2$ and $\dot{V}CO_2$. The bag collection procedure is somewhat laborious, requires large bulky equipment, and does not usually yield data until after exercise is completed. Automated methods have been developed allowing rapid calculation of $\dot{V}O_2$, $\dot{V}CO_2$, and $\dot{V}E$ from continuous measurements of expired gas flow and gas concentrations. The two most common methods for providing rapid on-line analysis are the mixing chamber technique [5,19] and breath-by-breath technique [20].

For both techniques, expired gas flow must be measured continuously and integrated to provide a measure of expired minute ventilation. The most common technique for flow measurement is use of a pneumotachograph. Pneumotachographs may have undesirable nonlinearities in the relation between output signal and flow. Furthermore, the calibration curve may be affected by how the pneumotachograph is mounted in the system owing to entrance and exit effects of flowing gases. Thus, pneumotachographs must be carefully validated to ensure accuracy over the flow range expected during exercise (which may approach 10 L s^{-1} in athletes), and in day-to-day use, care must be taken to ensure proper attachment to the exercise equipment. A common means for daily calibration is to use a 3-L gas syringe. In computed systems, the software integrates the flow signal to obtain volume, which is compared with the known gas volume of the syringe. Adequate validation should include pumping the 3-L syringe at various rates to confirm that output of the pneumotachograph is independent of flow [21]. Software that does not allow comparison of integrated syringe volumes across a range of flows is unacceptable. The internal resistance and dead space volume of the instrument must also be taken into consideration. Although good data on the effect of breathing resistance on exercise response are not available, a resistance of more than 1–2 cm H_2O L^{-1} s^{-1} will be sensed by subjects at high levels of exercise. Added dead space of equipment will manifest itself as an increase in ventilatory requirement, particularly at rest and lower levels of exercise.

Measurement of $\dot{V}O_2$ and $\dot{V}CO_2$ requires gas analysis. If the classic bag collection technique is being used, the time taken to analyze the gas is not a critical issue. Instruments that require many minutes per sample analysis include gas absorption methods (Haldane and Scholander techniques) and gas chromatography. On-line data analysis requires more rapid analyzers. Usually, shortening of the response time is associated with reduced stability, and possible decreases in accuracy and precision. Essential requirements for a gas analyzer include speed of response, linearity, stability of calibration, and independence of output (i.e., presence of CO_2 does not affect O_2 measurement). Initial validation of equipment should include validation of these properties. This can be accomplished with a set of three to four precision-grade gas tanks, which can be used to verify linearity, independence, and stability. One potential problem with this procedure is an error in the stated gas concentrations of the calibration gases. In spite of the "guaranteed" precision from the supplier, errors can occur that are difficult to detect if high-precision gas analysis is not available. Testing at least one of these gases both dry and humidified will test how the analyzer is affected by water vapor. If validation cannot be performed in the laboratory, the manufacturer should supply documentation that validation was performed before the equipment was put into use (level 1, Table 3). However, research or large clinical testing laboratories should perform their own initial validation (levels 2 or 3).

With all techniques for measuring $\dot{V}O_2$ and $\dot{V}CO_2$, correction must be made for water vapor in expired air [22]. Rapid gas analyzers used in most commercial systems (with the exception of the few that rely on mass spectrometry) require the gas sample to be dried before analysis. It is common for manufacturers to use drying gas sample lines, in which water vapor is absorbed in transport from the mouth to the gas analyzers. Drying sample lines are prone to failure, and this failure to correct adequately for water vapor in the expired gas can be a surprisingly large (20–25%) source of error in either breath-by-breath or mixing chamber systems [22].

In breath-by-breath and mixing chamber systems, the delay time between gas analysis and expired flow measurement must be adequately handled to obtain accurate results. Gas concentration signals will always

Table 3 Validation of $\dot{V}O_2$, $\dot{V}CO_2$, and $\dot{V}E$

Level 1 (basic)	1. From manufacturer: date, method used, acceptable tolerance, and output of delivered instrument. 2. Compare $\dot{V}O_2$, $\dot{V}CO_2$, and $\dot{V}E$ with normal standards for subject exercising at set intensity. **Periodic Validations**: 1. Daily calibration (pneumotachograph and gas analyzers) 2. Step 2 repeated monthly.
Level 2 (intermediate)	1. Compare $\dot{V}O_2$, $\dot{V}CO_2$, and $\dot{V}E$ with values obtained from simultaneous direct bag collections **Periodic Validations**: Quarterly to yearly.
Level 3 (advanced)	1. Linearity check of gas analyzers. 2. Check of $\dot{V}O_2$ at normal and high breathing rates. **Periodic Validations**: Quarterly to yearly.

lag behind flow signals owing to the transport delay between the mouth and the gas analyzer and because of the time it takes the analyzer to respond to the change in gas concentration. Automated systems usually have a calibration routine that checks the total delay time (transport and analyzer response). Because of the deleterious effect of not knowing the exact delay time [20,23–25], delay time should be checked regularly (daily to at least weekly).

With all systems (bag collection, breath-by-breath, and mixing chamber), initial and periodic validations should include obtaining $\dot{V}O_2$ and $\dot{V}CO_2$ in a subject that can be compared with predicted $\dot{V}O_2$ for the subject's body weight and exercise intensity [1], with the historical normal range established for the subject, or with direct measurement by bag collections. Note that comparison with predicted values is similar to validation recommended for the ergometer, discussed earlier. If comparison is being made with historical averages or predicted values, based on the subject's weight and ergometer settings, one must have confidence in the power output of the ergometer. One advantage of comparing $\dot{V}O_2$ values with values obtained by direct bag collection is that the comparison is independent of power output, and the $\dot{V}O_2$ values obtained by the bag collection permit an indirect validation of the ergometer. The $\dot{V}O_2$ and $\dot{V}CO_2$ must be validated over the full range of conditions likely to occur in the laboratory (i.e., over the range of ventilations and respiratory rates that are expected). Problems can occur at higher ventilations or respiratory rates that are not present at rest because of nonlinearities in the pneumotachograph, or because of small errors in delay time of the analyzer. Because patients with lung disease can achieve respiratory rates of over 60 min^{-1} [2,25], systems should be capable of producing accurate values for $\dot{V}O_2$, $\dot{V}E$, and $\dot{V}CO_2$ in that range. To validate equipment at higher minute ventilations or respiratory rates, an external calibrating device can be used [26], although one can also collect data while a laboratory volunteer increases respiratory rate voluntarily [25]. If care is taken to avoid hyperventilation while performing this procedure and the subject is in steady state, the $\dot{V}O_2$ values obtained should be within a few hundred milliliters per minute at normal and increased respiratory rates when the system is functioning properly.

Table 2 and Table 3 list recommended initial and periodic validation procedures, categorized by level of validation required. Periodic validations are very useful for documentation of accuracy of laboratory equipment and for detecting errors caused by failure of individual components of the system. The periodic validation procedure is similar to that required for quality assurance of blood gas laboratories. When validation data are obtained, the values for $\dot{V}O_2$ and $\dot{V}CO_2$ are compared with historical average. If the current values are outside of the mean ±95% confidence interval for the subject, a second measurement is obtained to confirm the error. If both measurements are out of acceptable limits, steps are taken to determine a cause of the error and repeat validation is performed. The most frequent cause for error in $\dot{V}O_2$ in our experience is failure of the gas analyzers or failure of the mechanism for drying the gas sample. Otherwise, errors can occur in gas flow measurement (which would be revealed if expired gas is collected in a Douglas bag at the same time as the validation run), or in ergometer calibration (rarely). Use of gas exchange simulator devices [26] is not recommended for routine quality checks, because these calibrators do not add water vapor in "expired" gas, and there is no temperature change from inspiration to expiration. Thus, they do not test the integrity of the gas sample-drying circuit and ability to compensate for temperature difference of expired gas. These devices can be useful for validating equipment at higher respiratory rates or for finding the source of error.

C. Assessing Ventilatory Limitations to Exercise

As exercise intensity increases, minute ventilation must increase to meet metabolic demands (Fig. 1). A theoretical upper limit to exercise capacity (a limit that most individuals can *not* attain) is established by the upper limit of the ventilation ($\dot{V}E$,cap) that the lungs can sustain. However, the

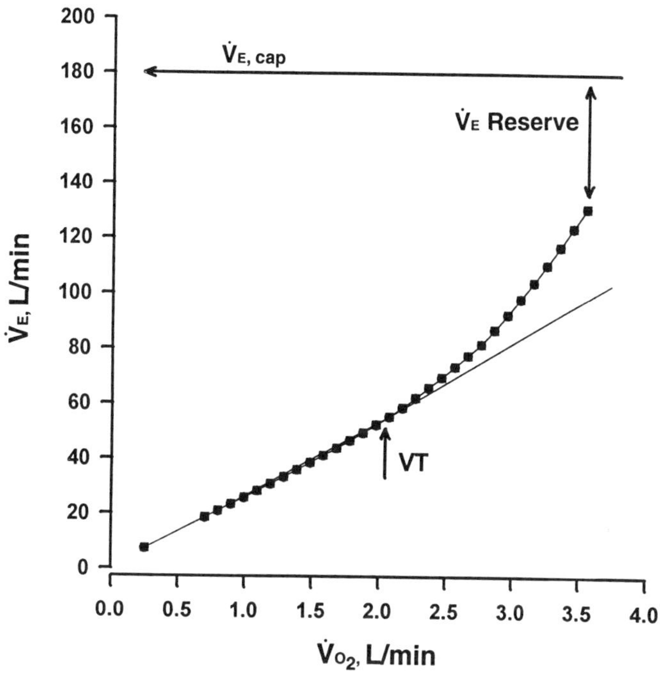

Fig. 1 Ventilatory response to exercise: $\dot{V}_E$ is plotted against $\dot{V}_{O_2}$. Maximal ventilatory capacity ($\dot{V}_{E,cap}$) is defined by the lungs' ability to sustain $\dot{V}_E$. The point of nonlinear increase in $\dot{V}_E$ defines the ventilatory threshold (VT; discussed in text).

maximal $\dot{V}_{E,cap}$ of the lungs is difficult to define in all individuals. A simple method to define it is to use the maximal voluntary ventilation (MVV) [2,5]. The MVV is obtained by having a patient breath in and out of a spirometer as hard as possible for 12–15 s [21]. The MVV probably overestimates "true" $\dot{V}_{E,cap}$ for two reasons: (a) the maneuver is a short, high-intensity effort that cannot be sustained [27]; and (b) the breathing pattern adopted by most subjects is different from exercise ventilation, in that breathing occurs at higher lung volume and at higher respiratory rate [28,29]. Another method commonly used to estimate ventilatory capacity is to use some multiple (typically 35–40) times the 1-S forced expiratory volume (FEV_1) obtained from spirometry. This multiple was obtained by comparing the FEV_1 with the MVV in large populations, as shown in Fig. 2. Note that there is a range of values for the ratio of MVV/FEV_1, indicating some imprecision in use of $FEV_1 \times 40$ to define either MVV

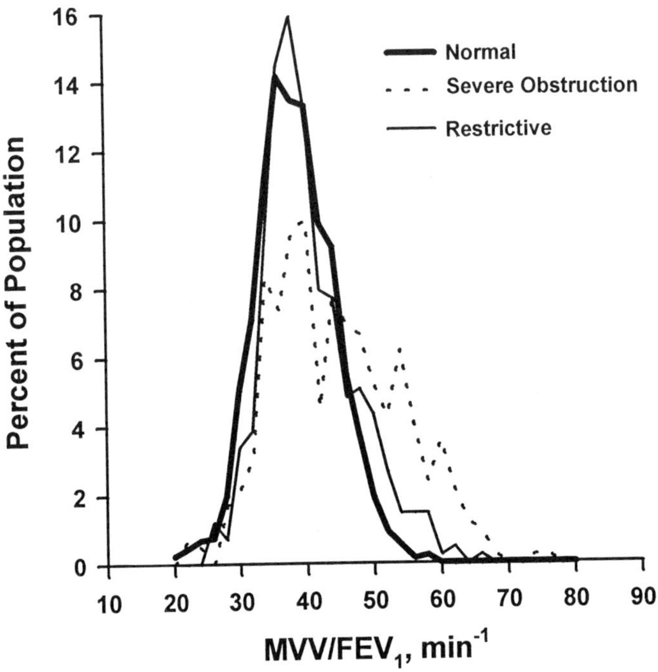

Fig. 2 Relation between MVV and FEV_1, both measured by spirometry: Three line patterns show data from patients with normal lung function, chronic obstructive airways disease, and restrictive lung disease, respectively. Note the most common value of MVV/FEV_1 (peak of curves) occurs between 35 and 40, although a wide range of possible values exists for all groups. Very low values (<30) or very high values (>48) may indicate abnormal lung or chest wall mechanics.

or $\dot{V}_{E,cap}$ in individual patients. If the MVV/FEV_1 ratio is less than 30 or more than 48, other abnormalities, such as upper airway obstruction or respiratory muscle weakness, are suggested, although some subjects will simply be unable to perform the MVV maneuver adequately.

The true maximal $\dot{V}_E$ a given subject is capable of performing during exercise is dependent on several factors, one of which is the breathing pattern adopted by the subject. To understand this, refer to Fig. 3, in which tidal flow (V_T) versus volume (f-V) loops are shown under the maximal expiratory flow versus volume (MEFV) curve for a normal subject. Because the MEFV curve represents the maximal flow the lungs can produce, one should be able to use the MEFV curve to calculate the $\dot{V}_{E,cap}$ [30,31]. Maximal expiratory flow decreases with lung volume

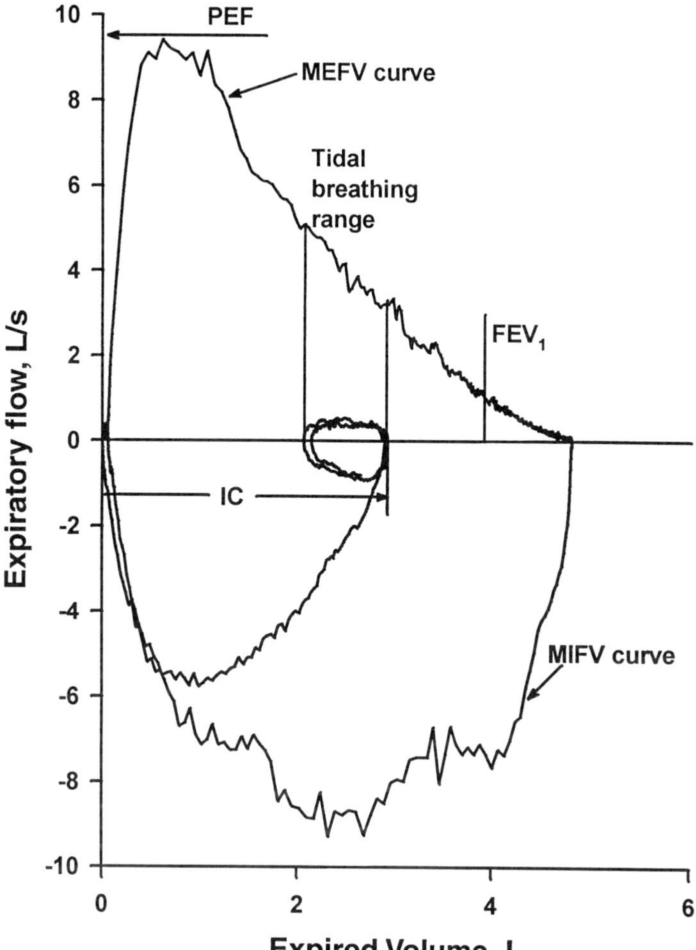

Fig. 3 Maximal expiratory and inspiratory flow versus volume loops (MEFV and MIFV, respectively). Inside the maximal envelope defined by the MEFV and MIFV curves is the flow versus volume loop generated during resting tidal breathing. In the lung volume range of tidal breathing, the maximal ventilation the lungs are capable of would be restricted by the MEFV curve. PEF, peak expiratory flow; IC, inspiratory capacity.

below full inflation, as shown by the downsloping shape of the MEFV curve below peak flow (PEF). Consequently, to estimate $\dot{V}_{E,cap}$, one must know the range over which the subject is breathing (tidal breathing range). The procedure used to determine maximal calculated ventilatory capacity ($\dot{V}_{E,calc}$) is illustrated in Fig. 4b [30–33]. Because of the downsloping shape of the MEFV curve, the $\dot{V}_{E,calc}$ is less if a subject breaths with the same tidal volume at lower lung volume, where MEFV flows are lower. With both tidal volume and end-expiratory lung volumes varying with exercise intensity [34,35], $\dot{V}_{E,calc}$ becomes a dynamic quantity that varies with breathing pattern during exercise [30,32,33]. Furthermore, in individuals with hyperreactive airways, the $\dot{V}_{E,calc}$ varies more

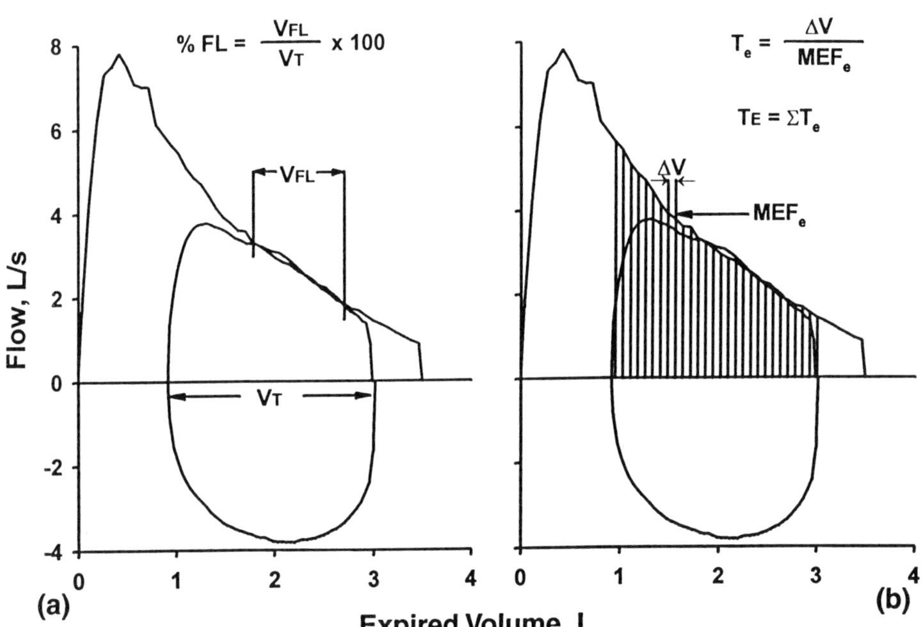

Fig. 4 Calculation of flow limitation (a) and calculated ventilatory capacity ($\dot{V}_{E,calc}$) (b). The %FL is quantified by measuring the fraction of the tidal volume (V_T) over which expiratory flows meet or exceed the MEFV curve. $\dot{V}_{E,calc}$ is quantified by first dividing the V_T into small incremental volume ranges, ΔV, within which a minimal incremental time contribution, t_e, to the breath is calculated. Minimal expiratory time, t_E is the sum of the t_e, and $\dot{V}_{E,calc}$ is the V_T divided by the minimal expiratory time, multiplied by $(1 - t_I/t_{TOT})$, where t_I is time spent in inspiration and t_{TOT} is total respiratory cycle time.

than in normal individuals because of variations in the MEFV curve during exercise, particularly exercise of variable intensity [33]. Although $\dot{V}_{E,calc}$ can be used to quantify $\dot{V}_{E,cap}$ and $\dot{V}_E$ reserve at various times during exercise, a somewhat simpler means of quantifying the degree to which $\dot{V}_E$ is approaching the $\dot{V}_{E,cap}$ is to look at the degree of flow limitation (%FL; see Fig. 4a) during exercise. Paralleling the changes in $\dot{V}_{E,calc}$ during exercise, the %FL is higher and more variable in persons with a history of exercise-induced asthma than in normal individuals [33]. Example tidal f-V and MEFV curves for one normal and one asthmatic subject at rest and exercising near 50% of their maximal capacity are shown in Fig. 5. Note the exercise-related bronchodilation (dashed MEFV curve, shifted up) in the asthmatic, and the tidal expiratory flows exceeding the MEFV flows in this subject. The latter phenomenon is discussed further in the following.

Although the techniques outlined in the foregoing can be used to document degree of flow limitation with exercise more accurately and with higher time resolution than traditional methods, there are some technical pitfalls to keep in mind. To make quantitative estimates of $\dot{V}_{E,calc}$ and %FL requires a means for continuously recording flow at the mouth, which can be integrated to register volume changes. The flow signal can be obtained from a single pneumotachograph connected directly to the mouthpiece, or by means of separate pneumotachographs connected to the inspiratory and expiratory ports of a nonrebreathing valve. In either event, the flowmeter(s) must be carefully calibrated and linearized to avoid drift of the volume signal to higher or lower lung volumes during the recording. The source of drift can be from the fact the $\dot{V}O_2 \neq \dot{V}CO_2$, from effects of changing gas viscosity, temperature, or water vapor content between inspired and expired air, or from nonlinearities of the pneumotachographs. Once drift is minimized, the tidal flow versus volume loops can be aligned with the MEFV curve only if the inspiratory capacity (IC) is known (see Fig. 3). The IC should be measured immediately after recording tidal flow–volume curves. It is not appropriate to assume that IC does not change during exercise because numerous studies have shown that end-expiratory lung volume (EELV) and, therefore, IC changes with exercise intensity [33,35,36]. Improper alignment of the tidal f-V loop with the MEFV curve will lead to errors in $\dot{V}_{E,calc}$ and in %FL. The most likely error in alignment is due to underestimation of the IC because of incomplete inspiratory effort on the part of the subject. However, if there is considerable drift on the integrated volume signal, it is possible to overestimate IC. With an underestimate of IC, the tidal f-V loop will be aligned at a volume that is too high; $\dot{V}_{E,calc}$ will be overestimated, and %FL will be underestimated.

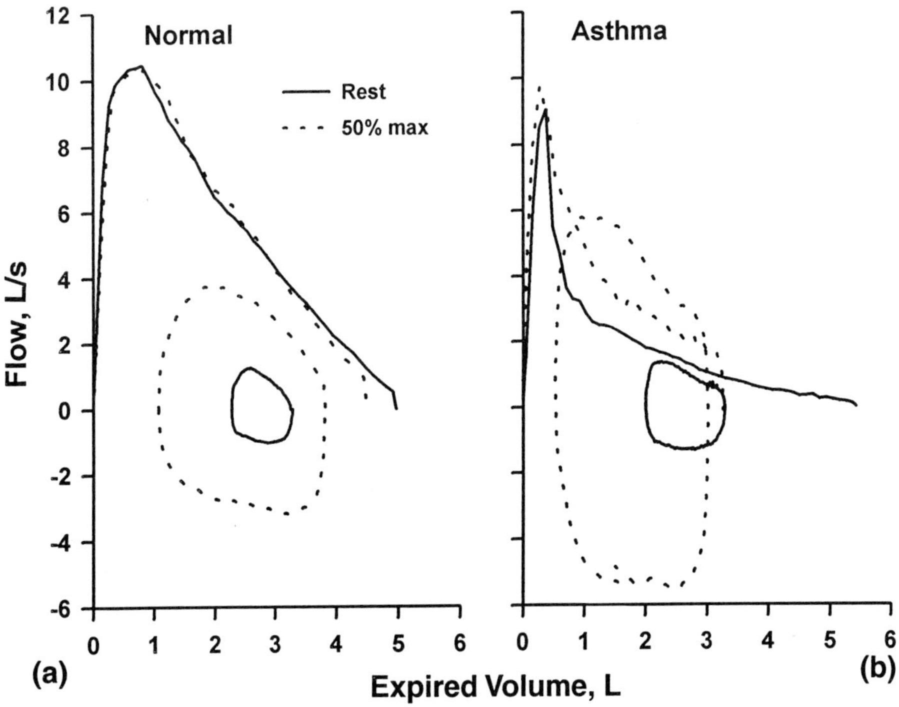

Fig. 5 Maximal expiratory flow versus volume curves (MEFV) and tidal breathing curves for a normal (a) and asthmatic (b) subject. Solid curves indicate MEFV and tidal-breathing curves obtained before exercise and dashed curves indicated MEFV and tidal-breathing curves obtained at about 50% of the subjects' maximal exercise capacity. Note the drop in end-expiratory lung volume and absence of flow limitation during exercise in the normal subject, but increase in end-expiratory lung volume and tidal flows exceeding MEFV flows in the patient with asthma. In addition, the exercise MEFV curve shows evidence for exercise-related bronchodilation in the patient with asthma. In this patient, the %FL is >80% and $\dot{V}_{E,calc}$ underestimates actual ventilation.

Even after proper alignment, the tidal f-V loop may occasionally appear to exceed the MEFV loop during exercise (see Fig 5) [37]. Tidal flows exceeding the MEFV flows can be from various causes: (a) the "gas compression" artifact associated with MEFV curves will underestimate MEFV flows at all lung volumes [38,39]; (b) exercise-induced bronchodilation will cause tidal f-V flows to exceed the preexercise MEFV curve [40–42]; and (c) unequal time constants of emptying within the lung will allow tidal f-V flows to exceed the MEFV flows [37,43,44]. In most situations, documenting that tidal flows meet or exceed the MEFV flows, particularly if the MEFV flows are also obtained during exercise, allows one to conclude that the patient is probably experiencing flow limitation.

Although these techniques were initially described many years ago, they have not been in widespread use in clinical laboratories. Recent introduction of instrumentation allowing recording of tidal f-V loops during exercise will make these measurements more commonplace. Normal ranges for values are not available for large populations of individuals. The %FL is essentially zero in normal [29,33,45] and mildly asthmatic persons at rest and up to moderate levels of exercise [33]. Patients with mild airflow limitation on preexercise spirometry may show some degree of FL at rest, with increasing FL during exercise [45]. Older athletes may also show varying degrees of FL during moderate to high-level exercise [46]. We have studied several obese patients who breathe with lower than normal (EELV) at rest and who show significant %FL even at rest. These individuals complain of symptoms suggestive of asthma, even though their spirometry and methacholine challenge tests are often normal [47,48].

D. Assessing Asthmatic Response to Exercise

In this section, we will outline how an athlete would be worked up specifically to document the degree of exercise-induced asthma. Although the physiology of exercise-induced asthma is reviewed elsewhere in this volume (see Chaps. 5 and 6), we must emphasize some key points for the purpose of this discussion. First, incremental exercise protocols are used in most exercise laboratories; the typical asthmatic when performing an incremental protocol will experience bronchoconstriction only *after* exercise is terminated. Several studies have documented that bronchodilation occurs during exercise [40–42]. This bronchodilation may turn to mild bronchoconstriction if constant-load exercise is performed for longer than about 10–15 min [42,49], although the finding of bronchoconstriction during prolonged exercise is not universal [50]. Second, the degree of bronchoconstriction that occurs after exercise is directly related to the intensity and duration of exercise, and is related to either heat or water exchange in the airways [51–53].

To test adequately for exercise-induced asthma in the laboratory requires monitoring of airway function *after* exercise (although monitoring airway function during exercise may provide additional useful information), and requires exercise of adequate intensity and duration. To maximize the response, the subject should breath either frigid or dry air. Unless the exercise study is being performed to test adequacy of medications, the subject should withhold medications before the test. The time necessary for "washout" of existing medications ranges from a few hours for short-acting β-agonists, such as isoproterenol, to at least 12 h for the long-acting β-agonists [55], and up to few days for inhaled steroids. A standard exercise protocol calls for before exercise spirometry, followed by exercise at about 70–80% of the subjects' maximum predicted heart rate for 5–10 min while breathing frigid or dry gas. Following this exercise, spirometry is performed every 3–5 min for up to 30 min. The maximal response usually occurs between 5 and 10 min following exercise [42,51–53], although recent evidence indicates a few individuals may not reach maximal fall in FEV_1 for up to 20 min after exercise [54]. The source of inspired gas can be either from a cold air generator (available from a number of commercial sources), or a tank of compressed air. Compressed air is essentially void of water vapor. Even if the vapor pressure of water within the tank was near the 20 mm Hg expected for typical room temperatures; this pressure is trivial compared with the total pressure of the gas in the tank, making the fractional water content essentially zero. If the standard protocol cannot be followed (lower intensity or duration of exercise; room air breathing instead of dry or frigid gas), then the test results could be falsely negative. For instance, we will occasionally perform spirometry before and after a standard incremental exercise protocol (about 10-min duration, with intensity increasing 15–30 W/min^{-1} to subject's volitional fatigue) while breathing room air (50% humidity). Although less sensitive, when positive results are obtained, there is good evidence for exercise-induced asthma. If the exercise is performed outdoors, air temperature, air humidity, and concentration of pollen in the air (for atopic subjects) on the day of the test will affect test results [56]. In addition, levels of air pollution may have an effect [57–59]. Although there is a reasonable correlation between exercise response and methacholine responsiveness, some patients will respond to exercise, but not to methacholine, and others will respond to methacholine, but not to exercise [60].

Firm standards are not available for interpretation of the fall in MEFV flows following exercise. It appears that the FEV_1, rather than the peak flow or other isovolume flows, such as expiratory flow at 50% or 75% of the vital capacity, is the most reliable parameter to follow for interpreting the changes [61]. A fall in FEV_1 after exercise compared with before exercise of between 10 [62] and 15% [60] is generally considered a positive test. A larger percentage fall in PEF is needed to be considered positive. In a large population (N = 5700) study of school children who underwent a challenge by hyperventilating cold dry air for 4 min (isocapnic hyperventilation with cold dry air induces bronchoconstriction in a way similar to exercise), the 95% confidence interval for percentage fall in

FEV_1 in children without history or symptoms of asthma was about 9% [61]. Similarly, a study of 527 children and adolescents showed that those without asthma dropped their FEV_1 at most 7% after exercise breathing room air, whereas those with asthma dropped their FEV_1 at least 8% [63]. Thus, a fall of 10–15% is probably reasonable to be considered as an abnormally positive response to exercise, indicative of asthma.

The *lability index*, defined as the percentage increase during exercise plus percentage fall after exercise in FEV_1 or PEF was defined by Godfrey [52] and Anderson [51]. Because MEFV flows generally improve to a variable degree during exercise in asthmatics, the lability index will in general be larger than the more standard calculation of percentage change in expiratory flows after exercise. We have studied a few individuals whose bronchodilatory response during exercise dominated over the bronchoconstriction that occurred after exercise (e.g., see Fig. 5), and in whom the degree of exercise asthma would have been considerably underestimated without measuring MEFV flows during exercise. The bronchodilator response is probably inversely correlated with flows before exercise; individuals with a mild or moderate flow limitation or increased airway resistance before exercise are more likely to show the bronchodilation during exercise [51]. Although measuring MEFV flows during exercise adds complexity to the exercise assessment, both in terms of patient effort and technical difficulty of measuring MEFV curves during exercise, it can be useful in some situations to document more completely the exercise response.

E. Detection of Anaerobic Threshold

As exercise intensity increases, the fuel used by the muscles changes from fats to carbohydrates and, finally, as oxygen supply to the muscles becomes inadequate, ATP is generated from carbohydrate stores by anaerobic metabolism, producing lactic acid. The detailed physiology of metabolic response to exercise is covered in Chapter 1. In this section, the techniques used to determine the exercise intensity above which anaerobic metabolism becomes significant will be reviewed. It should be stated at the outset, however, that the "anaerobic threshold" is probably not a true threshold; the level of lactic acid in the tissues and the blood is a reflection of the balance between production and metabolism of lactate, and both production and uptake are affected by the type of muscle fibers that are active, by regional distribution of blood perfusion, and by humoral factors. When lactic acid levels in the blood increase, the change in pH may induce a change in ventilation as the body attempts to buffer the acid by respiratory compensation. However, it is unclear if the change in pH itself is the stimulus to ventilation, or some other factor, perhaps correlated with acidosis, is the final stimulus.

Although the mechanisms leading to buildup of lactic acid in the blood and the mechanism for the stimulation of ventilation that is closely associated with the this buildup are a matter of continued debate, it is clear that the $\dot{V}O_2$ at which lactate begins to accumulate significantly is an important parameter that describes an individual's capacity for exercise: there is a stronger correlation between the $\dot{V}O_2$ at which lactate begins to increase and running times in middle- to long-distance races than there is between VO_2max and running times [64].

Two events related to the buildup of lactic acid in the blood can be detected by analyzing the pattern of change in $\dot{V}E$, $\dot{V}O_2$, and $\dot{V}CO_2$ during exercise. The first is the increase in $\dot{V}CO_2$ relative to $\dot{V}O_2$ owing to the buffering of blood acid by the CO_2–HCO_3^--buffering system. The second is an increase in minute ventilation relative to $\dot{V}CO_2$, the respiratory compensation for metabolic acidosis. In the discussion that follows, I will outline the techniques used to determine the $\dot{V}O_2$ at which buildup of lactic acid in the blood becomes significant (lactate threshold; LT) and to determine the $\dot{V}O_2$ at which ventilatory consequences of lactic acid buildup become evident (ventilatory threshold; VT). It must be kept in mind that the LT and VT, although roughly equivalent, may not be the same in all individuals.

To determine the LT, multiple blood samples must be taken during exercise and analyzed for levels of lactic acid. Because tissues can take up lactic acid, levels in venous blood may differ from those in arterial blood [65]. Because of the complex lactate kinetics near and above the LT, the duration of each exercise intensity during a progressive incremental exercise study is important in determining the level of lactic acid achieved and the LT [65]. Partly because of the debate over whether the buildup of lactate is a "threshold" rather than continual increase phenomenon [66], there is no universal agreement for determining the $\dot{V}O_2$ or work intensity above which lactate accumulation is "significant." Some laboratories use the $\dot{V}O_2$ or work intensity above which lactate concentration exceeds a fixed value, such as 4 mM, or 1 mM above the value obtained before exercise [67] as the LT. However, others fit the lactate versus $\dot{V}O_2$ curve to mathematical models and use the fit to determine the point at which blood lactate concentration begins to build up [68,69]. A log–log transformation helps identify a breakpoint in many cases [70]. Determinations of LT using either the log–log transformation method or using a lactate level of 1 mM above preexercise values are probably the best methods to use for identifying the LT for clinical purposes.

Because the LT determination requires multiple blood samples to be drawn during exercise, the VT is often used as an estimate of the LT.

Picking the VT can be based on three methods, ranging from simple to complex: (a) the $\dot{V}O_2$ or work intensity above which the respiratory exchange ratio (RER = $\dot{V}CO_2/\dot{V}O_2$) exceeds 1.0; (b) the $\dot{V}O_2$ at which the ventilatory equivalents for oxygen ($\dot{V}E/\dot{V}O_2$) begins to increase; and (c) the breakpoint in the plot of $\dot{V}CO_2$ versus $\dot{V}O_2$, identifying the $\dot{V}O_2$ at which $\dot{V}CO_2$ begins to increase out of proportion to the $\dot{V}O_2$. These three methods are explained in the following.

To understand the basis for the VT, three equations must be presented. The first describes the buffering capacity of the blood:

$$[H^+] + [HCO_3^-] \Leftrightarrow [H_2CO_3] \overset{ca}{\Leftrightarrow} [CO_2] + [H_2O] \quad (1)$$

The source of the H^+ on the left side of the equation is lactic acid. The breakdown of carbonic acid to gaseous CO_2 and water (the second reaction in the sequence) is catalyzed by the enzyme carbonic anhydrase (ca). This reaction leads to an increase in $\dot{V}CO_2$ above the $\dot{V}CO_2$ generated by metabolism. Eqs. (2) and (3) describe the efficiency of gas exchange in the lungs:

$$\dot{V}_A = \frac{\dot{V}CO_2}{Pa,CO_2} \times 863 \quad (2)$$

$$\dot{V}_E = \frac{\dot{V}_A}{(1 - V_D/V_T)} \quad (3)$$

Equations (2) and (3) can be combined to form an equation that describes the changes in $\dot{V}_E$ with changes in $PaCO_2$ and V_D/V_T:

$$\dot{V}_E = \frac{(\dot{V}CO_2/PaCO_2)\cdot 863}{[1 - (V_D/V_T)]} = \frac{\dot{V}CO_2\cdot 863}{PaCO_2\cdot[1 - (V_D/V_T)]} \quad (4)$$

And finally, two important equations can be generated from Eq. (4) by dividing by $\dot{V}CO_2$ to obtain the ventilatory equivalents for CO_2 ($\dot{V}E/\dot{V}CO_2$) and multiplying by RER = $\dot{V}CO_2/\dot{V}O_2$ to obtain the ventilatory equivalents for O_2 ($\dot{V}E/\dot{V}O_2$):

$$\frac{\dot{V}_F}{\dot{V}CO_2} = \frac{863}{PaCO_2\cdot[1 - (V_D/V_T)]} \quad (5)$$

$$\frac{\dot{V}_E}{\dot{V}O_2} = \frac{RER\cdot 863}{PaCO_2\cdot[1 - (V_D/V_T)]}$$

The pattern of changes in lactate, arterial pH, $\dot{V}E/\dot{V}CO_2$, $\dot{V}E/\dot{V}O_2$ during an incremental exercise study are shown in Fig. 6. Note that in early stages of exercise the $\dot{V}E$ increases nearly linearly and lactate and pH are constant. In these early stages, both $\dot{V}E/\dot{V}O_2$ and $\dot{V}E/\dot{V}CO_2$ decline as gas exchange becomes more efficient (V_D/V_T falls). At about 100–120 W in this example, the blood lactate concentration increases, although end tidal CO_2 (P_{ET,CO_2}) stays constant, indicating no extra increase in ventilation in response to the acid. In this period of isocapnic buffering, $\dot{V}CO_2$ increases more than $\dot{V}O_2$ owing to the extra production of CO_2 by the blood-buffering system (see Eq. 1). During this period, the $\dot{V}E/\dot{V}CO_2$ is relatively constant because both Pa_{CO_2} and V_D/V_T are constant (first Eq. 5), though $\dot{V}E/\dot{V}O_2$ increases because of the increase in RER. When lactate increases above about 4 mEq/L, P_{ET,CO_2} begins to decline as the body starts to add respiratory compensation for the acidosis by increasing $\dot{V}E$. At this point, both the ventilatory equivalents for $\dot{V}O_2$ and $\dot{V}CO_2$ increase.

The three main methods for determining ventilatory threshold (VT) noninvasively are based on Eqs. (1) and (5). The first method is simply to pick the point where RER exceeds 1.0, the maximal value that can be obtained in steady state during aerobic metabolism of fat, carbohydrate, or protein. This technique is often useful to pick the approximate VT during an exercise study, before the complete pattern of response is evident. The second method uses the changes in $\dot{V}E/\dot{V}O_2$ and $\dot{V}E/\dot{V}CO_2$: The VT is taken as the point where $\dot{V}E/\dot{V}O_2$ starts to increase, although $\dot{V}E/\dot{V}CO_2$ is still constant or decreasing (Fig. 7). The last condition is necessary because both $\dot{V}E/\dot{V}O_2$ and $\dot{V}E/\dot{V}CO_2$ can increase with hyperventilation [reduced Pa_{CO_2}, see Eqs. (5)]. Picking this point is sometimes difficult in practice owing to breath-by-breath variation in the data. Smoothing by averaging groups of five to ten breaths or in 20- to 30-s windows is useful to reduce such scatter. Mathematical techniques can be used to fit the data to curves that allow objective picking of the VT, although it is important that such fitting procedures be verified by visual inspection of the data before the VT is accepted.

The last method involves plotting of $\dot{V}CO_2$ against $\dot{V}O_2$ to find the point at which $\dot{V}CO_2$ increases out of proportion to $\dot{V}O_2$ (see Fig. 7b). In its simplest form, this method is easy to implement and apply; one simply plots $\dot{V}CO_2$ against $\dot{V}O_2$ and fits (either manually or automatically by minimizing sums of squared errors about the regression lines) the data to two straight-line segments. However, the original description of this "V-slope" method is more involved: data collected before and for the first minute of the incremental increase in work intensity are discarded, as are data from the highest exercise levels, and a correction is made for brief

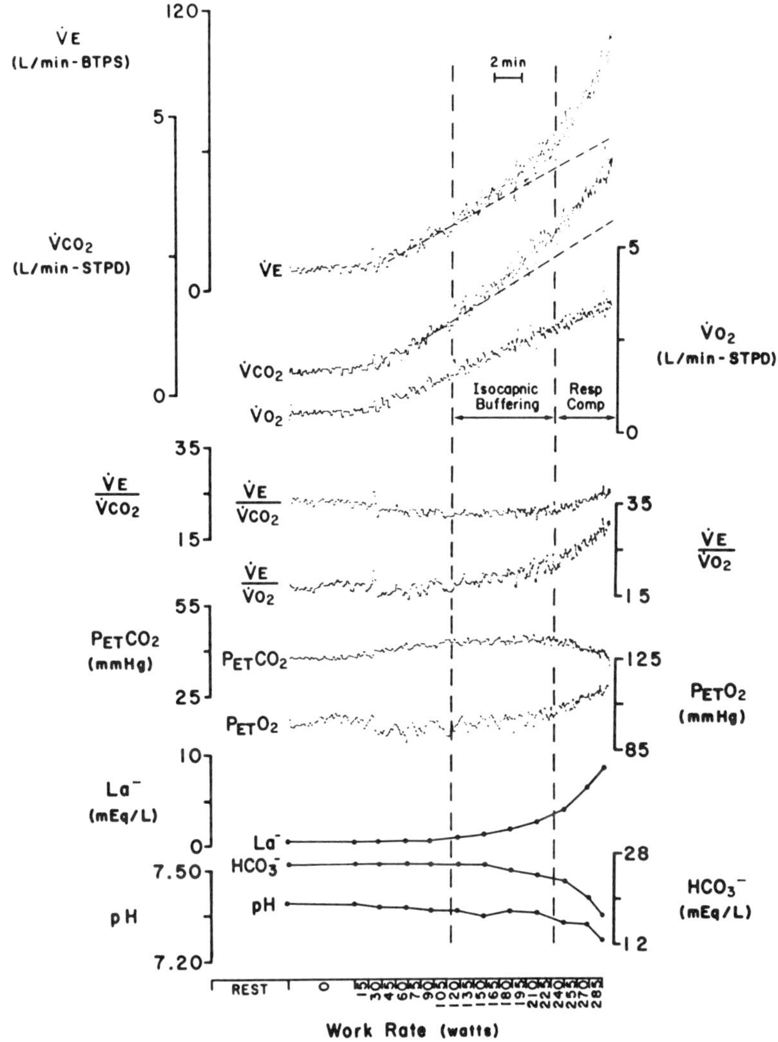

Fig. 6 Pattern of response to exercise, showing ventilation ($\dot{V}E$), $\dot{V}O_2$, $\dot{V}CO_2$, $\dot{V}E/\dot{V}O_2$, $\dot{V}E/\dot{V}CO_2$, end tidal PO_2($PETO_2$) and PCO_2($PETCO_2$), lactate (La^-) and pH. See text for explanations. (From Ref. 2).

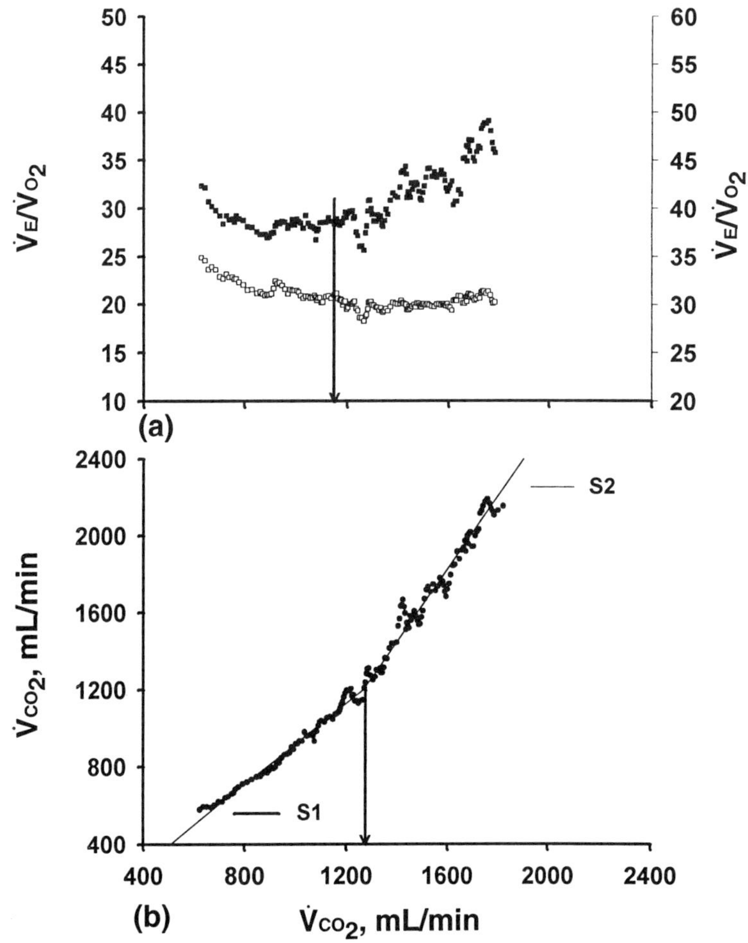

Fig. 7 Breath-by-breath variations in $\dot{V}_E/\dot{V}_{O_2}$, $\dot{V}_E/\dot{V}_{CO_2}$, and $\dot{V}_{CO_2}$ plotted against $\dot{V}_{O_2}$ during a maximal exercise study. Arrows show the VT defined by ventilatory equivalents criteria (a) and V-slope method (b).

periods of hyper- or hypoventilation [71]. It is unclear what effect such corrections have on the resultant VT, although users should be provided documentation by manufacturers of the methods used if the V-slope technique is made available.

All of the methods for determining the VT critically depend on a typical response to exercise (see Fig. 5). Patients who show atypical ventilatory responses, such as hyperventilation before the VT or hypoventilation, may have an indeterminate VT. An example is shown in Fig. 8. This patient had moderate obstructive pulmonary disease and was unable to increase his ventilation in response to metabolic acidosis. In fact, there was an *increase* in his Pa_{CO_2} at the higher levels of exercise. Because of the CO_2 retention, the $\dot{V}_{CO_2}$ measured at the mouth was less than metabolic $\dot{V}_{CO_2}$, and the plot of $\dot{V}_{CO_2}$ versus $\dot{V}_{O_2}$ failed to show the increasing slope that is expected. This type of pattern cannot be sustained for long: if $\dot{V}_{CO_2}$ at the mouth underestimates $\dot{V}_{CO_2}$ from the working muscles, then CO_2 stores must be accumulating, leading to further acidosis. $\dot{V}_{O_2}$ at the mouth is probably also underestimated, although to a smaller degree than the underestimate of $\dot{V}_{CO_2}$ owing to differences in O_2 and CO_2 capacity of blood and tissues. Though VT is indeterminate in these cases, the unusual pattern is important to document.

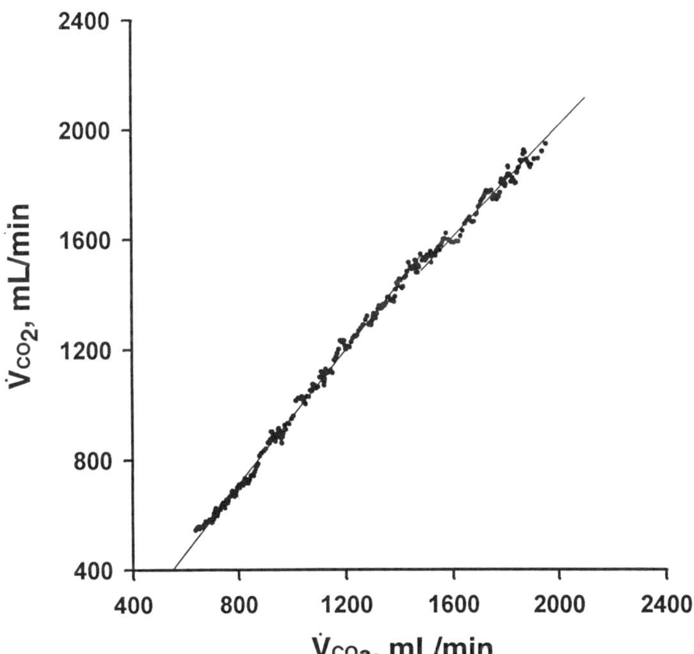

Fig. 8 Example of V-slope method applied to patient with chronic obstructive pulmonary disease who was ventilatory-limited to the point of retaining CO_2 at maximal exercise. Note the slope of $\dot{V}_{O_2}$ versus $\dot{V}_{CO_2}$ shows slight *reduction* instead of the expected increase at higher levels of $\dot{V}_{O_2}$.

III. SUMMARY

Obtaining the exercise response of athletes with known or suspected lung disease can present numerous technical challenges. With advent of commercially available computed data acquisition, documenting the exercise response is becoming easier and more commonplace. However, to obtain accurate and reproducible data requires adequate initial validation and regular quality control measures. Computed technology makes data analysis techniques that used to be available only in research laboratories available to clinical laboratories and fitness centers. These techniques include identification of onset the ventilatory threshold (usually associated with switch from predominantly aerobic to anaerobic metabolism), and quantification of flow limitation and abnormal-breathing patterns. These techniques should only be used with knowledge of the underlying physiological mechanisms and the possible technological difficulties that may arise.

LIST OF ABBREVIATIONS

$\dot{V}O_2max$	Maximal oxygen consumption
$\dot{V}O_2$	Oxygen consumption
ECG	Electrocardiogram
$\dot{V}E$	Minute ventilation (expired)
$\dot{V}CO_2$	Carbon dioxide production
CO_2	Carbon dioxide
O_2	Oxygen
$\dot{V}E$,cap	Ventilatory capacity
FEV_1	Forced expiratory volume in 1 s
f-V	Submaximal flow versus volume curves
MEFV	Maximal expiratory flow versus volume curves
PEF	Peak expiratory flow
$\dot{V}E$,calc	Calculated $\dot{V}E$,cap, using MEFV loops
%FL	Percentage flow limitation, obtained from comparing f-V to MEFV curves
IC	Inspiratory capacity
LT	Lactate threshold
VT	Ventilatory threshold
RER	Respiratory exchange ratio, $\dot{V}CO_2/\dot{V}O_2$
H^+	Hydrogen ion
HCO_3^-	Bicarbonate ion
H_2CO_3	Carbonic acid
H_2O	Water
ca	Carbonic anhydrase

pH	Log of hydrogen ion concentration
V_D/V_T	Dead space to tidal volume ratio
Pa_{CO_2}	Arterial partial pressure of CO_2
P_{ET,CO_2}	End tidal partial pressure of CO_2

REFERENCES

1. American College of Sports Medicine. Guidelines for exercise testing and prescription, 5th ed. Philadelphia: Williams & Wilkins, 1995.
2. Wasserman K, Hansen JE, Sue DY, Whipp BJ. Principles of exercise testing and interpretation. Philadelphia: Lea & Febiger, 1987.
3. Powers SK, Howley ET. Exercise physiology. Theory and application to fitness and performance. Dubuque, IA, WC Brown Publishers, 1990.
4. Astrand PO. Textbook of work physiology. New York: Mcgraw-Hill, 1977.
5. Jones NL, Campbell EJM. Clinical exercise testing. Philadelphia: WB Saunders, 1982.
6. Bell MM. Five-year experience with exercise stress testing in a family practice program. Fam Med 1994; 26:290.
7. Froelicher VF, Marcondes GD. Manual of exercise testing. St Louis: Mosby Year Book, 1989.
8. Jones NL. Clinical exercise testing. Philadelphia: WB Saunders, 1988.
9. Zavala DC. Manual on exercise testing: a training handbook. 3rd ed. Iowa City: University of Iowa, 1993.
10. Pina IL, Balady GJ, Hanson P, Labovitz AJ, Madonna DW, Myers J. Guidelines for clinical exercise testing laboratories. A statement for healthcare professionals from the Committee on Exercise and Cardiac Rehabilitation, American Heart Association. Circulation 1995; 91:912.
11. American College of Obstetricians and Gynecologists Technical Bulletin. Exercise during pregnancy and the postpartum period. Number 189, February 1994.
12. Buchfuhrer MJ, Hansen JE, Robinson TE, Sue DY, Wasserman K, Whipp BJ. Optimizing the exercise protocol for cardiopulmonary assessment. J Appl Physiol 1983; 55:1558.
13. Bruce RA, Kusumi F, Hosmer D. Maximal oxygen intake and nomographic assessment of functional aerobic impairment in cardiovascular disease. Am Heart J 1973; 85:546.
14. Froelicher VF Jr, Brammell H, Davis G, Noguera I, Stewart A, Lancaster MC. A comparison of the reproducibility and physiologic response to three maximal treadmill exercise protocols. Chest 1974; 65:512.
15. Russell JC, Dale JD. Dynamic torquemeter calibration of bicycle ergometers. J Appl Physiol 1986; 61:1217.
16. Van Praagh E, Bedu M, Roddier P, Coudert J. A simple calibration method for mechanically braked cycle ergometers. Int J Sports Med 1992; 13:27.
17. Howley ET, Bassett DR Jr, Welch HG. Criteria for maximal oxygen uptake: review and commentary. Med Sci Sports Exerc 1995; 27:1292.

18. Mitchell JH, Sproule BJ, Chapman CB. The physiological meaning of the maximal oxygen intake test. J Clin Invest 1958; 37:538.
19. Hughson RL, Kowalchuk JM, Prime WM, Green HJ. Open-circuit gas exchange analysis in the non-steady-state. Can J Appl Sports Sci 1980; 5:15.
20. Beaver WL, Wasserman K, Whipp BJ. On-line computer analysis and breath-by-breath graphical display of exercise function tests. J Appl Physiol 1973; 34:128.
21. American Thoracic Society. Standardization of spirometry, 1994 update. Am J Respir Crit Care Med 1995; 152:1107.
22. Beaver WL. Water vapor corrections in oxygen consumption calculations. J Appl Physiol 1973; 35:928.
23. Hughson RL, Northey DR, Xing HC, Dietrich BH, Cochrane JE. Alignment of ventilation and gas fraction for breath-by-breath respiratory gas exchange calculations in exercise. Comp Biomed Res 1991; 24:118.
24. Beaver WL, Lamarra N, Wasserman K. Breath-by-breath measurement of true alveolar gas exchange. J Appl Physiol 1981; 51:1662.
25. Proctor DN, Beck KC. Delay time adjustments to minimize errors in breath-by-breath measurement of $\dot{V}O_2$ during exercise. J Appl Physiol 1996; 81: 2495–2499.
26. Huszczuk A, Whipp BJ, Wasserman K. A respiratory gas exchange simulator for routine calibration in metabolic studies. Eur Respir J 1990; 3:465.
27. Freedmen S. Sustained maximum voluntary ventilation. Respir Physiol 1970; 8:230.
28. Hyatt RE. The interrelationships of pressure, flow and volume during various respiratory maneuvers in normal and emphysematous subjects. Am Rev Respir Dis 1961; 83:676.
29. Olafsson S, Hyatt RE. Ventilatory mechanics and expiratory flow limitation during exercise in normal subjects. J Clin Invest 1969; 48:564.
30. Jensen JI, Lyager S, Pedersen OF. The relationship between maximal ventilation, breathing pattern and mechanical limitation of ventilation. J Physiol (Lond) 1980; 309:521.
31. Bartlett RG, Jr, Phillips NE, Wolski G. Maximum voluntary ventilation prediction from the velocity–volume loop. Dis Chest 1963; 43:382.
32. Beck KC, Staats BA, Babb TG, Hyatt RE. Dynamics of breathing during exercise. In: Whipp BJ, Wasserman K, eds. Exercise: pulmonary physiology and pathophysiology, New York: Marcel Dekker, 1991; 67.
33. Johnson BD, Scanlon PD, Beck KC. Regulation of ventilatory capacity during exercise in asthmatics. J Appl Physiol 1995; 79:892.
34. Sharratt MT, Henke KG, Aaron EA, Pegelow DF, Dempsey JA. Exercise-induced changes in functional residual capacity. Respir Physiol 1987; 70:313.
35. Lind F, Hesser CM. Breathing pattern and lung volumes during exercise. Acta Physiol Scand 1984; 120:123.
36. Henke KG, Sharratt M, Pegelow D, Dempsey JA. Regulation of end-expiratory lung volume during exercise. J Appl Physiol 1988; 64:135.
37. Potter WA, Olafsson S, Hyatt RE. Ventilatory mechanics and expiratory flow limitation during exercise in patients with obstructive lung disease. J Clin Invest 1971; 50:910.

38. Coates AL, Desmond KJ, Demizio D, Allen P, Beaudry PH. Sources of error in flow–volume curves. Effect of expired volume measured at the mouth vs that measured in a body plethysmograph. Chest 1988; 94:976.
39. Hyatt RE. Effort independence and forced expiratory flow. Chest 1980; 77: 246.
40. Stirling DR, Cotton DJ, Graham BL, Hodson WC, Cockcroft DW, Dosman JA. Characteristics of airway tone during exercise in patients with asthma. J Appl Physiol 1983; 54:934.
41. Inman MD, Watson RM, Killian KJ, O'Byrne PM. Methacholine airway responsiveness decreases during exercise in asthmatic subjects. Am Rev Respir Dis 1990; 141:1414.
42. Beck KC, Offord KP, Scanlon PD. Bronchoconstriction occurring during exercise in asthmatic subjects. Am J Respir Crit Care Med 1994; 149:352.
43. Melissinos CG, Webster P, Tien YK, Mead J. Time dependence of maximum flow as an index of nonuniform emptying. J Appl Physiol 1979; 47:1043.
44. Wilson TA, Fredberg JJ, Rodarte JR, Hyatt RE. Interdependence of regional expiratory flow. J Appl Physiol 1985; 59:1924.
45. Babb TG, Viggiano R, Hurley B, Staats BA, Rodarte JR. Effect of mild-to-moderate airflow limitation on exercise capacity. J Appl Physiol 1991; 70: 223.
46. Johnson BD, Reddan WG, Seow KC, Dempsey JA. Mechanical constraints on exercise hyperpnea in a fit aging population. Am Rev Respir Dis 1991; 143:968.
47. Harmon KR, Davies SF, Duane P, Dunitz J, Leatherman JW. A distinct cause of wheezing: functional pseudoasthma solely from exaggerated expiratory activity. Am J Respir Crit Care Med 1995; 151:A674.
48. Chiba M, Beck KC, Scanlon PD, Staats BA, Mottram CD. Cardiopulmonary exercise testing in pseudoasthma associated with obesity. Am J Respir Crit Care Med 1996; 153:A513.
49. Suman OE, Babcock MA, Pegelow DF, Jarjour NN, Reddan WC. Airway obstruction during exercise in asthma. Am J Respir Crit Care Med 1995; 152: 24.
50. Mansfield L, McDonnell J, Morgan W, Souhrada JF. Airway response in asthmatic children during and after exercise. Respiration 1979; 38:135.
51. Anderson SD, Silverman M, Konig P, Godfrey S. Exercise-induced asthma. Br J Dis Chest 1975; 69:1.
52. Godfrey S. Exercise induced asthma—clinical, physiological, and therapeutic implications. J Allergy Clin Immunol 1975; 56:1.
53. Godfrey S, Silverman M, Anderson SD. Problems interpreting exercise-induced asthma. J Allergy Clin Immunol 1973; 52:199.
54. Brudno DS, Wagner JM, Rupp NT. Length of postexercise assessment in the determination of exercise-induced bronchospasm. Ann Allergy 1994; 73: 227.
55. Kemp JP, Dockhorn RJ, Busse WW, Bleecker ER, VanAs A. Prolonged effect of inhaled salmeterol against exercise-induced bronchospasm. Am J Respir Crit Care Med 1994; 150:1612.
56. Karjalainen J, Lindqvist A, Laitinen LA. Seasonal variability of exercise-

induced asthma especially outdoors. Effect of birch pollen allergy. Clin Exp Allergy 1989; 19:273.
57. Fernandes ALG, Molfino NA, McClean PA, Silverman F, Tarlo S, Raizenne M, Slutsky AS, Zamel N. The effect of pre-exposure to 0.12 ppm of ozone on exercise-induced asthma. Chest 1994; 106:1077.
58. Spektor DM, Lippmann M, Thurston DG, Lioy PJ, Steckol J, O'Connor G, Garshick E, Speizer FE, Hayes C. Effects of ambient ozone on respiratory function in healthy adults exercising outdoors. Am Rev Respir Dis 1988; 138: 821.
59. Linn WS, Shamoo DA, Avol EL, Whynot JD, Anderson KR, Venet TG, Hackney JD. Dose–response study of asthmatic volunteers exposed to nitrogen dioxide during intermittent exercise. Arch Environ Health 1986; 41:292.
60. Haby MM, Anderson SD, Peat JK, Mellis CM, Toelle BG, Woolcock AJ. An exercise challenge protocol for epidemiological studies of asthma in children: comparison with histamine challenge. Eur Respir J 1994; 7:43.
61. Nicolai T, Mutius EV, Reitmeir P, Wist M. Reactivity to cold-air hyperventilation in normal and in asthmatic children in a survey of 5,697 schoolchildren in Southern Bavaria. Am Rev Respir Dis 1993; 147:565.
62. Backer V, Ulrik CS. Bronchial responsiveness to exercise in a random sample of 494 children and adolescents from Copenhagen. Clin Exp Allergy 1992; 22:741.
63. Backer V, Dirksen A, Bach-Mortensen N, Hansen KK, Laursen EM, Wendelboe D. The distribution of responsiveness to histamine and exercise in 527 children and adolescents. J Allergy Clin Immunol 1991; 88:68.
64. Kumagai S, Tanaka K, Matsuura Y, Matsuzaka A, Hirakoba K, Asano K. Relationships of the anaerobic threshold with the 5 km, 10 km, and 10 mile races. Eur J Physiol 1982; 49:13.
65. Yoshida T. Effect of exercise duration during incremental exercise on the determination of anaerobic threshold and the onset of blood lactate accumulation. Eur J Appl Physiol 1984; 53:196.
66. Morton RH. Detection of a lactate threshold during incremental exercise? J Appl Physiol 1989; 67:885.
67. Kowalchuk JM, Heigenhauser GJF, Jones NL. Effect of pH on metabolic and cardiorespiratory responses during progressive exercise. J Appl Physiol 1984; 57:1558.
68. Ribeiro JP, Hughes V, Fielding RA, Holden W, Evans W, Knuttgen HG. Metabolic and ventilatory responses to steady state exercise relative to lactate thresholds. Eur J Appl Physiol 1986; 55:215.
69. Green HJ, Hughson RL, Orr GW, Ranney DA. Anaerobic threshold, blood lactate, and muscle metabolites in progressive exercise. J Appl Physiol 1983; 54:1032.
70. Beaver WL, Wasserman K, Whipp BJ. Improved detection of lactate threshold during exercise using a log–log transformation. J Appl Physiol 1985; 59: 1936.
71. Beaver WL, Wasserman K, Whipp BJ. A new method for detecting the anaerobic threshold by gas exchange. J Appl Physiol 1986; 60:2020.

3

The History of Exercise-Induced Asthma and Definition of the Syndrome

Frank S. Virant
University of Washington School of Medicine, and
Northwest Asthma and Allergy Center, Seattle, Washington

I. INTRODUCTION

The phenomenon of exercise-induced asthma was first recognized nearly 2000 years ago. It has been only over the last three decades, though, that we have been able to accurately characterize exercise asthma as a consequence of careful clinical observation, pharmacological studies, and direct airway measurement of heat and water content after prolonged activity.

Exercise-induced asthma is defined as the clinical occurrence of cough, wheeze, shortness of breath, chest pain, or an "itching or scratching" sensation within the chest that occurs 5 min after the cessation of exercise. Typically, exercise for 5–8 min at a workload of at least 80% of maximal predicted oxygen consumption, is required to generate objective symptoms and concurrent airflow obstruction. A subset of patients may experience a "late-phase" bronchospasm occurring 4–12 h after the initial activity as described in Chapter 7. The magnitude of the late-phase reaction is generally much less than the early-phase response, although there may be a direct relation between the severity of these events. Exercise-induced asthma is commonly encountered in clinical medicine, occurring in over 90% of patients with nonspecific bronchial hyperresponsiveness.

II. HISTORICAL PERSPECTIVE

A. Exercise as an Asthma Trigger

Exercise as a cause for asthma was first noted by Aretaeus, the Cappadocian, in the second century AD [1]. Writing in his treatise on the treatment of acute and chronic diseases, Aretaeus stated "If from running, gymnastic exercises, or any other work, the breathing becomes difficult, it is called asthma. . . ." Writing in the year 150 AD, he described the clinical presentation of asthma: "The symptoms of its approach are heaviness of the chest; sluggishness to one's accustomed work, and to every other exertion; difficulty of breathing in running or on a steep road; they are hoarse and troubled with cough. . . ." Finally, Arataeus also made some interesting clinical observations relating to the pathophysiology of asthma: "The cause is a coldness. . .of the spirit. There is a postponement of death to those in whom the lungs are warmed and heated in the exercise of their trade, from being wrapped in wool such as the workers in gypsum, or braziers, or blacksmiths, or the heaters of baths."

Aretaeus, it appears, had little influence on the medical profession of his time. He was rarely quoted, presumably because the bulk of his writings reflected the teachings of his predecessor Hippocrates [2]. Incredibly, over 1500 years would pass before the next significant writing on the subject of exercise-induced asthma.

B. Effect of Exercise Type

Sir John Floyer, writing in London near the end of the 17th century, reported that different types of exercise caused different amounts of exercise-induced asthma [3]. For many years, it was generally assumed that this was because the severity of exercise was also different. This point was not clarified until 1975, when a careful review of published data about exercise testing suggested that exercise-induced asthma was more severe and more frequently demonstrable after running than other forms of exercise [4]. This ultimately led to elegant studies comparing different types of exercise of similar physiological intensity [5]. This research demonstrated that free-range running was the most potent stimulus for exercise-induced asthma, resulting in an average 47% decrease in peak expiratory flow rate after exercise. Running on a treadmill was slightly less potent, causing a 33% decrease, and cycling even less so, resulting in an average 25% decrease in airflows after activity. Several other forms of exercise, including swimming, kayaking, and walking, even though strenuous enough to require the same oxygen consumption as free-range running, created relatively little exercise-induced asthma, resulting in a 13–15% decrease in airflows. This important research not only clarified the observations of Floyer in the late 1600s, but also had important implications relative to the pathophysiology of exercise-induced asthma, the best types of exercise to use for tolerance testing (free-range running or treadmill), and in predicting what types of exercise might be best tolerated by the unmedicated asthmatic (swimming, walking, and kayaking).

C. Airway Dynamics with Exercise

Over 200 years after Sir John Floyer's observations, several authors described exercise-induced asthma, including Herbst in 1928, Kaltrieder in 1937, Eskildsen in 1945, and Pearson in 1952 [6]. In reviewing these modern descriptions of exercise-induced asthma, a major area of controversy emerged: some authors reported that exercise decreased airway obstruction, whereas others reported that airway obstruction increased with activity in asthmatics. This issue was finally clarified, in 1962 by Jones and colleagues, when they reported that the effect of exercise on the asthmatic airway was dependent on the duration of activity [7]. Relatively brief exercise of 1- or 2-min duration typically resulted in bronchodilation. In contrast, prolonged exercise of 4- to 12-min duration created bronchoconstriction. This research formed an important part of our current understanding of the exercise-induced asthma syndrome and laid the framework for subsequent pharmacological studies.

D. Exercise-Induced Asthma Severity and Hyperventilation

In the early 1970s, Chan-Yeung and co-workers were the first to recognize an association between the level of ventilation and the severity of exercise-induced asthma [8]. At the same time, this group demonstrated that hyperventilation with 5.6% CO_2 at high flow rates could also induce marked bronchospasm. These initial studies ultimately prompted further investigation of other factors likely to be linked to hyperventilation and, hence, to exercise-induced asthma, including heat and water loss. Deal et al. reported that reductions in the temperature and water content of inspired air enhanced airway response to isocapneic hyperventilation [9]. Simultaneously, it was also demonstrated that isocapneic hyperventilation with dry air at ambient temperatures could provoke potent bronchoconstriction and that the reduction in flow rates was similar to that induced by exercise under the same inspired air conditions [10].

E. History of Pharmacological Studies in Exercise-Induced Asthma

1. β-Adrenergic Agonists

In 1896, Solomon Solis-Cohen introduced the use of "adrenal substance" in the treatment of allergic rhinitis and asthma [11]. Although Solis-Cohen did not realize what the active agent was, or how much or how little of the active agent was absorbed, the fairly predictable clinical response of patients to this substance led to increase in research and ultimate identification of epinephrine. Concurrent research by Langley in 1905 demonstrated that substances such as epinephrine (adrenaline) did not act on nerve endings, but rather, through specific receptors [12]. Subsequent research by Alquist in 1948, in which he observed the effects of six sympathomimetic amines on different organs, led to the theory of α- and β-receptors [13]. This was further clarified by Lands in 1967, who proposed that there were two different types of β-adrenergic receptors: β_1 and β_2 [14]. With the discovery that bronchial smooth-muscle relaxation was a β_2-adrenoreceptor attribute, researchers began experimenting with substitutions of the epinephrine molecule to decipher which portion was important for α-, β_1-, and β_2-receptor stimulation.

McNeil and colleagues in 1965 administered epinephrine before exercise and demonstrated some degree of inhibition in an uncontrolled study [15]. Subsequently, Heimlick and colleagues showed a response to a combination of ephedrine and theophylline, but again, this was uncontrolled [16]. Subsequent work pointed out the importance of using a placebo in such studies [17]. Bierman et al. [18] observed that ephedrine itself had no greater protective value than placebo, although when administered with theophylline, it did enhance the theophylline effect.

Early studies with isoproterenol, one of the first epinephrine derivatives, showed that, although this agent could block exercise-induced asthma, it had two drawbacks similar to epinephrine itself: (a) it had a relatively short half-life, such that exercise an hour or more after administration had the same decrease in the forced expiratory volume in 1 s (FEV_1) as after placebo; and (b) it had significant β_1-receptor stimulation (and potential for side effects) [19,20].

The development of longer-acting, more β_2-specific agonists offered the promise of a clinically useful agent. Metaproterenol was demonstrated to be effective either when inhaled 10 min before exercise [21], or when administered orally 2–3 h before activity [22]. Terbutaline administered orally was initially similar to metaproterenol, but could still be protective up to 6 h later when metaproterenol no longer had an effect [23]. Godfrey and colleagues [24] showed that albuterol (salbutamol) could be effective when administered by aerosol 10 min before exercise, or orally 2 h before exercise.

The development of even longer-acting β_2-agonists, such as bitolterol [25], formoterol [26], and salmeterol [27] has led to the possibility of agents that can block exercise-induced asthma for 6, 8, or even 12 h.

2. Cromolyn

For years it had been appreciated that plant extracts containing khellin could relax smooth muscle. A systematic search for synthetically similar drugs capable of diminishing asthma attacks led to the introduction of cromolyn sodium as a potential therapeutic antiasthmatic agent in 1968.

Although cromolyn appeared to be quite beneficial, based on initial studies on allergic asthma, studies of efficacy in exercise-induced asthma have been quite variable. Simonson et al. [28] noted that only one of six patients responded to cromolyn when administered before exercise. Sly and co-workers using treadmill exercise [29], and Eggleston et al. employing cycloergometer exercise [30], were able to demonstrate only minimal protective effect using cromolyn before exercise. In contrast, Silverman and co-workers [31] showed that cromolyn produced a highly significant degree of protection, and in 14 of 31 patients exercise-induced asthma was completely inhibited. In attempting to explain the dichotomy of results, Silverman and Godfrey criticized the Sly and Eggleston studies in that the exercise stimulus may not have been sufficient to induce maximal bronchoconstriction, and that the cromolyn may have been administered too long before activity. Further studies by Shapiro et al. [32] suggested that the beneficial effects of cromolyn were preferentially apparent in the larger airways, and only apparent when subjects were maximally stressed, such as with a free-running system.

3. Methylxanthines

Theophylline is effective in reversing small and large airway exercise-induced asthma when administered as a 3.5 mg/kg dose 1–2 h before exercise. Weinberger and colleagues [33] showed that a theophylline dose adequate to produce a serum concentration of 10–20 μg/mL has appreciable activation in exercise-induced asthma. Simons et al. demonstrated that, at theophylline doses that create serum concentrations above 20 μg, no further beneficial effect on exercise-induced asthma occurs.

Dyphyllin, a less potent theophylline analogue that is more soluble and has a shorter half-life, does demonstrate some beneficial activity in exercise-induced asthma [34]. This agent was evaluated because it can be useful in patients who are intolerant to theophylline, but frequently require doses above the recommended 15 mg/kg to achieve efficacy.

4. Anticholinergics

In 1963, Jones et al. [35] reported two subjects who appeared to respond to intravenous atropine, 20–30 μg/kg. Sly and co-workers [36] were unable to identify a response to 100 μg/kg in ten children. Kiviloog [37] found atropine effective when administered by aerosol in five of nine subjects with exercise-induced asthma. Kershnar and colleagues [38] reported that aerosolized atropine and isoproterenol significantly modified exercise-induced asthma, but when administered together, showed a synergistic positive response.

The lack of concordance of these studies suggested that either the cholinergic effect of exercise was variable in some patients, or that the potential benefit of such drugs was limited by the inability to administer large enough doses without observing untoward side effects, such as dryness of the mouth. The development of ipratropium bromide, an antimuscarinic agent that is administered by aerosol, but is poorly absorbed, has allowed subsequent studies to clarify this point. When ipratropium is administered in a dose of 40 μg, it is an effective bronchodilator and antagonist of asthma, although it is not as potent as the β-agonists [39]. Although the slowness of onset of ipratropium action makes it less attractive for reversing bronchoconstriction, interestingly this agent can be immediately effective in preventing exercise-induced asthma [40].

5. Corticosteroids

A great deal of controversy surrounds the area of corticosteroids and exercise-induced asthma. McNeil et al. [15] observed that exercise-induced asthma was unchanged after administering 100 mg hydrocortisone parenterally to five adult asthmatics 15 min before exercise. Konig [41] found that the degree of exercise-induced asthma was lessened after administering oral prednisone to nine asthmatics for 1 week, although only three of the nine had a change greater than that which could have been due to random variation alone.

The administration of aerosolized betamethasone (single dose) showed no significant difference over placebo and, even with repeated administration, failed to modify exercise-induced asthma in five of six children studied [41]. In contrast, Hodgson et al. [42] found some protection from exercise-induced asthma on long-term administration of aerosolized betamethasone. When approaching the issue from a different perspective, Frears and co-workers [43] showed increased exercise-induced asthma and lability when placebo was substituted for betamethasone aerosol therapy on a long-term basis.

In summary, it would appear that corticosteroids have little effect on exercise-induced asthma when administered as single therapy before activity. In concert with our current view of the inflammatory component of asthma, it would appear, however, that long-term corticosteroid therapy can modify the severity and lability of exercise-induced asthma by reducing bronchial hyperresponsiveness in general.

6. Antihistamines

The observation in the early 1970s that cromolyn could effectively inhibit exercise-induced asthma if administered in adequate doses soon enough before to exercise, suggested an important role for mast cells and their mediators in the pathogenesis of exercise-induced asthma [31]. This suggested that the blockade of histamine might have a significant therapeutic benefit in alleviating this type of asthma [44]. Holgate and colleagues [45] showed that a single oral dose of 180 mg of terfenadine could inhibit exercise-induced immediate responses by approximately 35%. This group achieved almost identical results with astemizole [46] and azelastine [47]. The authors point out [48] that when the dose of terfenadine is increased from 180 to 600 mg, protection against challenge is not increased. This would suggest that histamine may contribute 35% of the immediate airway response to exercise challenge with other mediators contributing the remainder. In these studies, optimal doses of terfenadine (180 mg) and azelastine (8.8 mg) produced a three- to fivefold protection of the airways during the immediate response—roughly equivalent to the protection produced by therapeutic doses of cromolyn.

In contrast, a study by Gong et al. [49] failed to show any protective effect of the administration of oral cetirizine before allergen or exercise challenge. Possible explanations for the surprising lack of effect of cetirizine in these studies include (a) the optimal cetirizine dose was not used (maximum only 20 mg); (b) four out of ten patients participated in both allergen and exercise-induced arms of the study and allergen reactions may have induced a heightened bronchial hyperresponsiveness (potentially mitigating the effect of cetirizine on subsequent exercise challenge); and (c) exercise challenge was performed in cold air to generate a final temperature at the subject's mouth of approximately −18°C (and cold air may induce more of a cholinergic response, potentially decreasing the relative importance of histamine release).

7. Nedocromil

The search for an agent that would have similar, but more potent, properties than cromolyn led to the development of nedocromil sodium. A comprehensive review of available studies suggests that nedocromil is probably more effective than cromolyn against a variety of neurogenic and chemical stimuli, such as sodium metabisulfite [50] and AMP [51–53]. In contrast, the effect of nedocromil at doses up to 8 mg appears to be equal to that observed after 10 mg of cromolyn for protection against allergen or physical stimuli challenges such as "fog" [54] and cold, dry air [55]. A study of the effect of nedocromil versus cromolyn in the inhibition of exercise-induced asthma in children showed that nedocromil was slightly more efficacious, although not at a statistically significant level [56]. Further studies using higher doses of nedocromil (8–12 mg) remained to be performed to see if this might confer an enhanced protective effect against exercise challenge.

F. Exercise-Induced Asthma Pathophysiology

Weinstein and co-workers in 1976 [57] reported that exercise-induced asthma could be prevented by the inhalation of nebulized normal saline during exercise. The following year, Chen and Horton [58] demonstrated the beneficial effect of inspiring hot, humid air during exercise—the degree of bronchospasm was determined by the amount of heat lost in bringing the inspired air to alveolar ideal conditions (37°C, 44 mg of water per liter). In this study, it was noted that water loss was proportional to heat loss; therefore, either drying or cooling of the airways could be the primary stimulus to exercise-induced asthma. This theory was confirmed when Strauss et al. later in 1977 reported [59] that exercise-induced asthma was enhanced when cold, dry air was inspired during activity.

In the late 1970s and early 1980s, Deal et al. examined the airway response to a wide range of ambient temperatures and humidity [9]. Ultimately they demonstrated that cooling of the airways could occur in response to hyperpnea, such as might occur during exercise.

Simultaneously, in the early 1980s, research by Anderson and colleagues in Australia [60–63] suggested that the rate and amount of water loss, rather than heat loss, determines the magnitude of the airway response to exercise. Evidence for this theory came from reanalysis of previous studies suggesting that changing the inspired temperature was less critical than previously thought, and exercise-induced asthma could occur when the inspired temperature was 37°C [9] (suggesting than a stimulus other than airway cooling was contributing to asthma).

A series of elegant experiments by McFadden et al. in 1985 [64] suggested that the severity of exercise-induced asthma was dependent not only on airway cooling and drying, but also on the rapidity and magnitude of airway rewarming and rehydration after challenge. This provides our contemporary view of the pathophysiology—bronchospasm after exercise is due to a gradient effect (i.e., the rate of change of inspired air water and heat content).

III. DEFINITIONS

A. Classic Exercise-Induced Asthma

Classic or "early-phase" exercise-induced asthma describes the airway obstruction that occurs after an exercise stimulus. Generally, exercise from 5 to 8 min at a workload representing at least 80% of the maximal predicted oxygen consumption is required to generate bronchospasm [65]. The typical patient demonstrates transient bronchodilation [66] during the period of exercise, whereas the appearance and symptoms of obstruction occur 5 min after the cessation of activity (Fig. 1). In the absence of bronchodilator therapy or alteration of ambient air conditions, most patients spontaneously recover to preexercise airflows within a period of

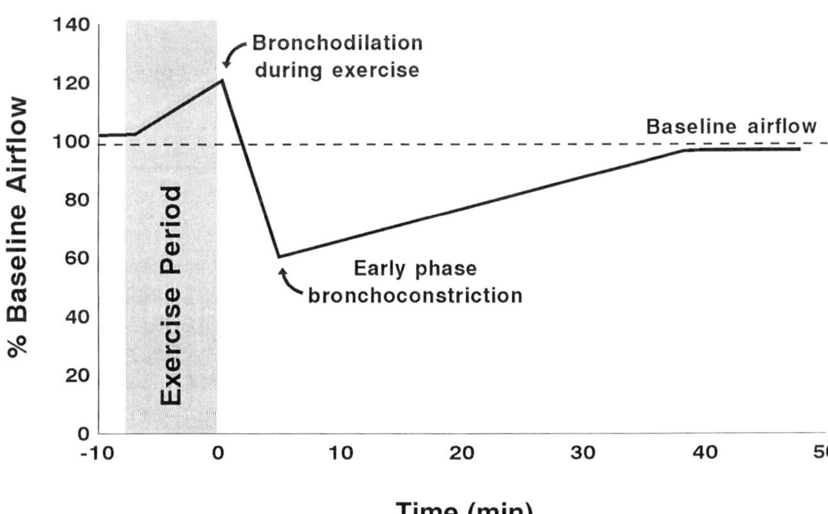

Fig. 1 Classic (early-phase) exercise-induced asthma.

20–60 min [65]. Common symptoms described by patients with exercise-induced asthma include cough, wheeze, shortness of breath, chest pain, and an "itching or scratching" sensation within the chest [67]. The severity of exercise-induced asthma is directly proportional to the rate of heat and water loss during the activity, which is influenced by the workload and ambient air conditions. This accounts for the observation that vigorous running outdoors on a cool, dry day is a severe stimulus for exercise-induced asthma. In contrast, walking indoors at room temperature at 50% relative humidity is unlikely to create airway changes during exercise [5].

The precise mechanism by which respiratory heat and water loss during exercise creates bronchospasm is unclear. Nonetheless, pharmacological studies involving exercise pretreatment with β-agonists, cromolyn, nedocromil, antihistamines, and anticholinergics suggest that airway obstruction following exercise involves mast cell activation, with subsequent histamine release and at least some degree of cholinergic stimulation.

B. Late-Phase Reactions

In 1980, Bierman and colleagues [68] originally described late reactions to exercise asthma occurring 4–12 h after the initial exercise stimulus (Fig. 2). The occurrence of such a phenomenon was subsequently also reported

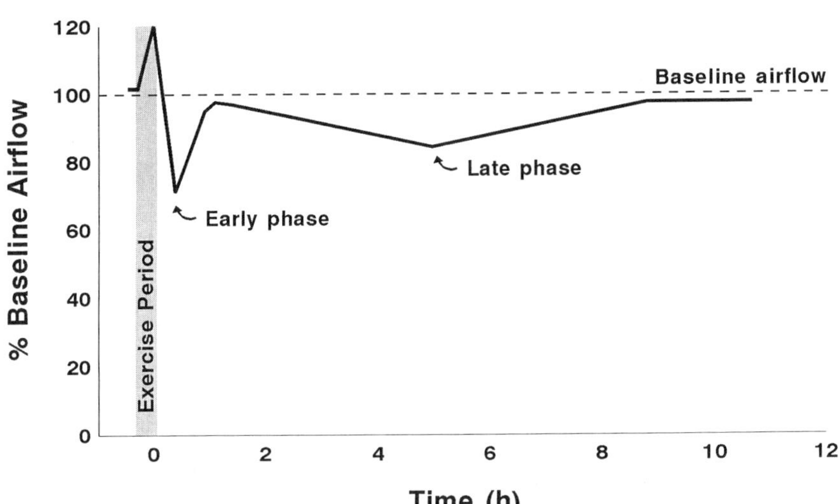

Fig. 2 Exercise-induced asthma with late-phase reaction.

by Feldman et al. in 1982 [69], and Boulet and his group in 1987 [70]. Collectively, these studies, as well as work done by Horn et al. [71], suggest that the frequency of late-phase reactions varies from 30 to 55%. The prevalence of these late-phase reactions appears to be similar to that observed after antigen challenge (33–73%) [72]. Late-phase reactions after exercise are not determined by the severity of disease or baseline bronchial hyperresponsiveness [73]. There is a significant correlation between the magnitude of the early and late reactions, which emphasizes the direct relation of these events [74] This is described in more detail in Chapter 7.

IV. SUMMARY

Although exercise has been appreciated as a stimulus for asthma for nearly 2000 years, the bulk of our understanding of this process has occurred over the last three decades. In the early 1960s we learned that during exercise, bronchodilation occurs, whereas constriction occurs within 5 min after cessation of activity. Observations in the early 1970s made it apparent that exercise-induced asthma was very similar to isocapneic hyperventilation. Pharmacological studies in the late 1960s and the subsequent decade demonstrated many similarities between antigen-induced asthma and exercise-induced asthma: constriction of bronchial smooth muscle (β-agonists), mast cell activation (cromolyn, nedocromil, antihistamines), and cholinergic stimulation (anticholinergics). Collectively, the research done in the 1970s provided the impetus for subsequent research by McFadden et al. [64] and Anderson and colleagues [61–63], demonstrating the dual importance of heat and water loss from the respiratory tree in the induction of exercise-induced asthma.

Concurrently, over the last 30 years, the syndrome of exercise-induced asthma has been well characterized. Nearly 90% of patients with bronchial hyperresponsiveness will experience exercise-induced asthma. The occurrence of this type of asthma is influenced by the intensity and duration of exercise, and generally requires a workload of at least 80% of maximal oxygen consumption over a minimum period of 5–8 min. The magnitude of airway obstruction is also dependent on the water and heat content of the inspired air. All patients with exercise-induced asthma experience an early phase of obstruction, typically 5 min after the cessation of exercise, with slow resolution to preexercise airflows over a period of 20–60 min. Fewer patients may additionally experience a late phase of bronchospasm occurring 4–12 h after exercise. The intensity of the late-phase response, if it occurs, is generally less than the early response, but there may be a direct correlation between the magnitude of these two events. There is now no one parameter by which one can predict who will experience a late reaction after exercise, because this does not appear to depend on age, sex, degree of atopy, severity of asthma, or baseline airway hyperresponsiveness.

REFERENCES

1. Adams F, ed and trans. The extant works of Aretaeus the Cappadocian. London: The Syndenham Society, 1856.
2. Sampter M, ed. Excerpts from classics in allergy. Columbus OH: Ross Laboratories, 1969.
3. Floyer J. A treatise of the asthma. London: R Wilkin & W Innis, 1698.
4. Anderson SD, Silverman M, Konig P, Godfrey S. Exercise-induced asthma. Br J Dis Chest 1975; 69:1–39.
5. Fitch KD, Godfrey S. Asthma and athletic performance. JAMA 1976; 236: 152–157.
6. Ghory JE. Exercise and asthma: overview and clinical impact. Pediatrics 1975; 56(suppl):844–846.
7. Jones RS, Wharton JJ, Bustong OH. The effect of ventilatory function in the child with asthma. Br J Dis Chest 1962; 56:78.
8. Chan-Yeung MMW, Vyas MN, Grzybowski S. Exercise-induced asthma. Am Rev Respir Dis 1971; 104:915.
9. Deal EC Jr, McFadden ER Jr, Ingram RH Jr, Jaeger JJ. Hyperpnea and heat flux: initial reaction sequence in exercise-induced asthma. J Appl Physiol 1979; 46:476.
10. Kilham H, Tooley M, Silverman M. Running, walking, and hyperventilation causing asthma in children. Thorax 1979; 34:582.
11. Solis-Cohen S. The use of adrenal substance in the treatment of asthma. JAMA 1900; 34:1164–66.
12. Langley JN. On the reaction of cells and of nerve endings to certain poisons, chiefly as regards the reaction of striated muscle to nicotine and to curari. J Physiol 1905; 33:374.
13. Ahlquist RP. A study of the adrenotropic receptors. Am J Physiol 1948; 153: 586.
14. Lands AM, Arnold A, McAuliff JP, et al. Differentiation of receptor systems activated by sympathomimetic amines. Nature 1967; 214:597.
15. McNeill RS, Nairn JR, Millar JS, Ingram CG. Exercise-induced asthma. Q J Med 1965; 35:55–67.
16. Heimlich EM, Strick L, Busser RJ. An exercise response test in childhood asthma [abstract]. J Allergy 1966; 37:103.
17. Godfrey S, Silverman M, Anderson S. Problems of interpreting exercise-induced asthma. J Allergy Clin Immunol 1973; 52:199–209.
18. Bierman CW, Pierson WE, Shapiro GG. Exercise-induced asthma: pharma-

cological assessment of single drugs and drug combinations. JAMA 1975; 234:295–298.
19. Tattersfield AE, McNicol MW. Salbutamol and isoproterenol: a double blind trial to compare bronchodilator and cardiovascular activity. N Engl J Med 1969; 281:1323.
20. Snider GL, Laguarda R. Albuterol and isoproterenol aerosols. JAMA 1972; 221:682.
21. Sly RM, Heimlich EM, Ginsburg J, et al. Exercise-induced bronchospasm evaluation of metaproterenol. Ann Allergy 1968; 26:253.
22. Sly RM, Mayer J. Exercise-induced bronchospasm: evaluation of metaproterenol syrup. Ann Allergy 1969; 27:158.
23. Morse JL, Jones NL, Anderson GD. The effect of terbutaline in exercise-induced asthma. Am Rev Respir Dis 1976; 113:89–92.
24. Godfrey S, Konig P. Suppression of exercise-induced asthma by salbutamol, theophylline, atropine, cromolyn and placebo in a group of asthmatic children. Pediatrics 1975; 56:930–934.
25. Walker SB, Bierman CW, Pierson WE, Shapiro GG, Furukawa CT, Mingo TS. Bitolterol mesylate in exercise-induced asthma. J Allergy Clin Immunol 1986; 77:32–36.
26. Arvidsson P, Larsson S, Lofdahl CG, et al. Formoterol, a new long-acting bronchodilator for inhalation. Eur Respir J 1989; 2:325–330.
27. Ramage L, Lipworth BJ, Ingram CG, Cree IA, Dhillon DP. Reduced protection against exercise induced bronchoconstriction after chronic dosing with salmeterol. Respir Med 1994; 88:363–368.
28. Simonsson BG, Skoogh BE, Ekstrom JB. Exercise-induced airways constriction. Thorax 1972; 27:169–180.
29. Sly RM. Effect of cromolyn sodium on exercise-induced airway obstruction in asthmatic children. Ann Allergy 1971; 29:362.
30. Eggelston PA, Bierman CW, Pierson WE, et al. A double-blind trial of the effect of cromolyn sodium on exercise-induced bronchospasm. J Allergy Clin Immunol 1972; 50:57.
31. Silverman M, Konig P, Godfrey S. Use of serial exercise tests to assess the efficacy and duration of action of drugs for asthma. Thorax 1973; 28:574–578.
32. Shapiro GG, Pierson WE, Bierman CW. The effect of cromolyn sodium on exercise-induced bronchospasm using a free running system. Pediatrics 1975; 56(suppl):923–926.
33. Kiechel F, Pollack J, Cooper D, Swinberger M. The comparative efficacy of theophylline (T) and cromolyn (C) in suppressing exercise-induced bronchospasm (EIB) [abstract]. J Allergy Clin Immunol 1976; 57:250.
34. Simons FER, Bierman CW, Sprenkle AC, Simons KJ. Efficacy of dyphylline (dihydroxyprophyltheophylline) in exercise-induced bronchospasm. Pediatrics 1975; 56:916–918.
35. Jones RS, Wharton JJ, Buston MH. The place of physical exercise and bronchodilator drugs in the assessment of the asthmatic child. Arch Dis Child 1963; 38:539–545.
36. Sly RM, Heimlick EM, Busser RJ, Strick L. Exercise-induced broncho-

spasm: effect of adrenergic or cholinergic blockade. J Allergy Clin Immunol 1967; 40:93–99.
37. Kiviloog J. The effect of pretreatment with atropine in exercise-induced bronchoconstriction. Pediatrics 1975; 56(suppl):940–941.
38. Kershnar H, Katz R, Tashkin D, Rachelefsky G, Siegel S. Comparison of cromolyn sodium (CS), aerosolized atropine (A), isoproterenol (I), and A + I in the prevention of exercise-induced asthma [abstract]. J Allergy Clin Immunol 1976; 57:261.
39. Pakes GE, Brogden RN, Heel RC, Speight TM, Avery GS. Ipratropium bromide: a review of its pharmacological properties and therapeutic efficacy in asthma and chronic bronchitis. Drugs 1980; 20:237.
40. Anderson SD. Issues in exercise-induced asthma. J Allergy Clin Immunol 1985; 76:763–772.
41. Konig P, Jaffe P, Godfrey S. Effect of corticosteroids on exercise-induced asthma. J Allergy Clin Immunol 1974; 54:14–19.
42. Hodgson SV, McPherson A, Friedman M. Effect of betamethasone valerate aerosol on exercise-induced asthma in children Postgrad Med J 1974; 50(suppl 4):69–73.
43. Frears J, Hodgson S, Friedman M. Effect of placebo substitution during long-term betamethasone valerate aerosol treatment in asthmatic children. Arch Dis Child 1975; 50:387–392.
44. Patel JR. Terfenadine in exercise-induced asthma. Br Med J 1984; 288: 1496–1497.
45. Finnerty JP, Holgate ST. Role of histamine and prostaglandins in EIA. J Allergy Clin Immunol 1988; 81:240.
46. Howarth PH, Holgate ST. Astemizole, an H_1 antagonist in allergic asthma. J Allergy Clin Immunol 1985; 75:166.
47. Rafferty P, Harrison PJ, Aurich R, Holgate ST. The in vivo potency and selectivity of azelastine as an H_1-histamine receptor antagonist in human airways and skin. J Allergy Clin Immunol 1988; 82:1113–1118.
48. Holgate St, Finnerty JP. Antihistamines in asthma. J Allergy Clin Immunol 1989; 83:537–547.
49. Gong H Jr, Taskhin DP, Dauphinee B, Djahed B, Wu TC. Effects of oral cetirizine, a selective H_1 antagonist, on allergen- and exercise-induced bronchoconstriction in subjects with asthma. J Allergy Clin Immunol 1990; 85: 632–641.
50. Dixon CMS, Ind PW. Inhaled sodium metabisulphite induced bronchoconstriction: inhibition by nedocromil sodium cromoglycate. Br J Clin Pharmacol 1990; 30:371–376.
51. Crimi N, Palermo F, Oliveri R et al. Comparative study of the effects of nedocromil sodium (4 mg) and sodium cromoglycate (10 mg) on adenosine-induced bronchoconstriction in asthmatic subjects. Clin Allergy 1988; 18: 367–374.
52. Phillips GD, Scott VL, Richards R, Holgate ST. Effect of nedocromil sodium and sodium cromoglycate against bronchoconstriction induced by inhaled adenosine 5′-monophosphate. Eur Respir J 1989; 2:210–217.

53. Richards R, Phillips GD, Holgate ST. Nedocromil sodium is more potent than sodium cromoglycate against AMP-induced bronchoconstriction in atopic asthmatic subjects. Clin Exp Allergy 1989; 19:285–291.
54. del Bufalo C, Fasano L, Patalano F, Gunella G. Inhibition of fog-induced bronchoconstriction by nedocromil sodium and sodium cromoglycate in intrinsic asthma: a double-blind, placebo-controlled study. Respiration 1989; 55:181–185.
55. Juniper EF, Kline PA, Morris MM, Hargreave FE. Airway constriction by isocapnic hyperventilation of cold, dry air: comparison of magnitude and duration of protection by nedocromil sodium and sodium cromoglycate. Clin Allergy 1987; 17:523–528.
56. Novembre E, Frongia FG, Veneruso G, Vierucci A. Inhibition of exercise-induced asthma (EIA) by nedocromil sodium and sodium cromoglycate in children. Pediatr Allergy Immunol 1994; 5:107–110.
57. Weinstein RE, Anderson JA, Kvale P, Sweet LC. Effects of humidification on exercise-induced asthma (EIA). J Allergy Clin Immunol 1976; 57:250.
58. Chen WY, Horton DJ. Heat and water loss from the airways and exercise-induced asthma. Respiration 1977; 34:305.
59. Strauss RH, McFadden ER, Ingram RH, Jaegar JJ, Stearns DR. Enhancement of exercise-induced asthma by cold air. N Engl J Med 1977; 297: 743.
60. Anderson SD, Schoeffel RE, Follet R, Perry CP, Daviskas E, Kendall M. Sensitivity to heat and water loss at rest and during exercise in asthmatic patients. Eur J Respir Dis 1982; 63:459.
61. Anderson SD, Schoeffel RE. Respiratory heat and water loss during exercise in patients with asthma: effect of repeated exercise challenge. Eur J Respir Dis 1982; 63:472.
62. Anderson SD, Scheoffel RE, Black JL, Daviskas E. Exercise-induced asthma without airway cooling? [abstract]. Am Rev Respir Dis 1983; 127: 228.
63. Anderson SD, Hahn AG, Black JL, Morton A, Fitch K. Reinterpretation of the effect of temperature and water content of the inspired air in exercise-induced asthma (EIA). Am Rev Respir Dis 1984; 130:575–579.
64. McFadden ER JR, Lenner KAM, Strohl KP. Postexertional airway rewarming and thermally induced asthma: new insights into pathophysiology and possible pathogenesis. J Clin Invest 1986; 78:18–25.
65. Godfrey S. Clinical variables of exercise-induced bronchospasm. In: Dempsey JA, Reed CE, eds. Muscular exercise and the lung. Madison: The University of Wisconson Press, 1977:247–288.
66. Silverman M. MD thesis, University of Cambridge, England, 1973.
67. Weins L, Sabath R, Ewing L, Gowdamarajan R, Portnoy J, Scagliotti D. Chest pain in otherwise healthy children and adolescents is frequently caused by exercise-induced asthma. Pediatrics 1992; 90:350–353.
68. Bierman CW, Spiro SG, Petheram I. Late response to exercise-induced asthma [abstract]. J Allergy Clin Immunol 1980; 65:206.
69. Feldman CH, Fox J, Kraut E, Feldman BR, Davis WJ. Exercise-induced

asthma (EIA): treatment for early and late responses [abstract]. Am Rev Respir Dis 1982; 125:195.

70. Boulet LP, Legris C, Turcotte M, Hebert J. Prevalence and characteristics of late asthmatic responses to exercise. J Allergy Clin Immunol 1987; 80: 655–662.
71. Horn CR, Jones RM, Lee D, Brennan R. Late response in exercise-induced asthma. Clin Allergy 1984; 14:307–309.
72. MacIntire D, Boyd G. Factors influencing the occurrence of a late reaction to allergen challenge in atopic asthmatics. Clin Allergy 1984; 14:311–317.
73. Iikura Y, Inui, Nagakura T, Lee TH. Factors predisposing to exercise-induced late asthmatic responses. J Allergy Clin Immunol 1985; 75:285–289.
74. Bierman CW, Spiro SG, Petheram I. Characterization of the late response in exercise-induced asthma. J Allergy Clin Immunol 1984; 74:701–706.

4

Prevalence of Exercise-Induced Asthma in the Athlete

Hemalini Mehta and William W. Busse
University of Wisconsin Medical School, Madison, Wisconsin

I. INTRODUCTION

Exercise-induced asthma (EIA) is a syndrome characterized by transient airway obstruction, usually occurring 5–15 min following physical exertion. Symptoms consist of wheezing, coughing, shortness of breath, chest discomfort, or a combination thereof lasting up to 15–30 min following exercise cessation. However, if exercise is prolonged, asthma can develop during physical exertion. Furthermore, if a patient has severe asthma, even minimal exertion can provoke airflow obstruction. An estimated 12–15% of the general population suffer from exercise-induced asthma [1]. Although this is noted to be a problem for children and young adults because of their increased activity level, the recent heightened awareness of the additional benefits of fitness and exercise in older adults makes exercise-induced asthma of relevance to all aged groups. Additionally, exercise-induced asthma is the most common exercise pulmonary syndrome observed in recreational as well as competitive athletes.

II. PREVALENCE OF EIA IN INDIVIDUALS WITH ASTHMA

Several factors can trigger acute attacks of asthma; exercise is one of the more common. Exercise-induced asthma has been reported to affect 50–80% of patients with asthma [2]. This condition is more prevalent in children than in adults, probably related to children being more active.

Table 1 Prevalence of Exercise-Induced Asthma

Author [Ref]	Population		Asthma	Allergies	Prevalence (%)
Kattan [3]	Children	Overall	Yes	—	71.4
		+ EIA hx			77.2
		− EIA hx			50.0
Cropp [4]	Children	Boys	Yes	—	46–90
		Girls			36–77
Bransford [5]	Children	Symptomatic asthma	Yes	—	43.0
		Asymptomatic asthma			0.0
Kawabori [2]	Children	—	—	Yes	35–40
Bransford [5]	Children	—	—	Yes	14.6
Custovic [7]	Children	FEV_1 and FEF_{25-75}	—	Yes	0.0
Rupp [11]	Adolescent athletes	Risk of EIA by history	—	—	17.0
		No risk of EIA by history			12.0
Shield [12]	Adolescent athletes	Risk of EIA by history	—	—	66.0
Weiler [13]	College football players	Response to methacholine	—	—	42.8
		Response to exercise challenge			3.3
Weiler [14]	College football players	Response to methacholine	18/78 athletes	—	50.0
Rice [15]	College athletes	Exercise challenge	—	—	2.8
Huftel [16]	College athletes	Response to methacholine	8/50 athletes		16.4
Pierson [17]	1976 Olympic athletes			—	14.0
Voy [18]	1984 Olympic athletes		26/67 athletes	—	11.0

In a study by Kattan et al. in 1978 [3], 25 normal and 105 children with asthma were exercised on a treadmill. The incidence of EIA in the asthmatic population was 71.4%, whereas none of the 25 normal children responded to exercise (Table 1). Surprisingly, of those with a positive history of EIA, only 77.2% showed a response; in contrast, 50% of those with a negative history responded. This demonstrates that the patient's history may be an unreliable predictor of a response. Additionally, Cropp et al. [4] have shown that strenuous exercise elicited a significant deterioration in clinical and physiological measurements of airflow in 36–77% of asthmatic girls and 46–90% of boys with asthma. In a recent study of 12- and 13-year-old schoolchildren, Bransford et al. [5] demonstrated a 43% incidence of EIA in those persons with symptomatic asthma in the 6 months before the study; none of six children with asymptomatic asthma developed EIA. It is now generally believed that EIA affects all patients with asthma, if challenged with exercise of sufficient intensity [6].

III. PREVALENCE OF EIA IN ATOPIC, NONASTHMATIC POPULATION

Although several studies have documented a relation between asthma and EIA, the prevalence of exercise-induced symptoms in the atopic population is still controversial. Kawabori and colleagues [2] demonstrated exercise-induced bronchoconstriction in 35–40% of those with allergic rhinitis or hay fever symptoms if exercise challenged. A more recent study showed a 14.6% incidence of airflow obstruction with exercise in children with allergic rhinitis and no history of clinical asthma, when tested during a nonpollen season [5]. Custovic et al. [7] evaluated 26 atopic nonasthmatic children and showed, when using 1-S forced expiratory volume (FEV_1) and 25–75% forced expiratory flow (FEF_{25-75}) criteria, that none of the subjects demonstrated bronchoconstriction in response to exercise. These observations suggest that the selection criteria, for a population, study is critical to address the prevalence of EIA in the nonasthmatic population.

Exercise-induced asthma has also been elicited in "normal" persons. Approximately 9% of persons with EIA have no history of asthma or allergy [8]. The maximum fall in postexercise PEFR in normal children, may vary from 12.5 to 15%. A decrease of >15% in PEFR is often taken as diagnostic of exercise-induced bronchospasm [3,9]. Thus, a major source of variation in the incidence of EIA may result from the use of arbitrarily criteria to determine abnormality.

IV. PREVALENCE OF EIA IN ATHLETES

In 1972, exercise-induced asthma cost an American swimmer participating in the XXI Olympiad, a gold medal when it was discovered that he used an oral ephedrine-containing bronchodilator before his race. Over the last decade, there has been a heightened awareness of EIA in recreational as well as competitive athletes. In this select population, the prevalence of EIA is in the range of 3–10% and is common even among highly trained and competitive athletes [10].

Previous studies and screening programs have usually focused on highly trained competitive athletes, such as college or Olympic team participants. Few studies have involved the adolescent population, for whom identification of EIA may beneficially influence later participation in sports. In high school athletes, Rupp et al. [11] have shown an incidence of 17% in students considered at risk for EIA by history or baseline spirometry. Of those students with no risk factors, 12% demonstrated EIA after exercise. Shield and colleagues [12], as part of a preparticipation screening evaluation, evaluated 516 high school players using a questionnaire designed to elicit risk factors for EIA. They then exercise-challenged 65 of 181 individuals who had responded positive to at least one item, and found that 66% demonstrated a significant degree of airflow obstruction with exercise.

On examining the college athlete, Weiler and colleagues [13] became interested in evaluating college football players after members of university football team were noted to have significant problems with wheezing and chest tightness during pregame preparation in California for the 1982 Rose Bowl. Ninety-one players were evaluated with a methacholine bronchial challenge, resulting in a positive response in 39 and an equivocal response in an additional 7 players [13]. Two-thirds of the participants were then challenged with exercise (running wind sprints), with a resultant greater than 20% reduction in FEV_1 in 3 individuals. Further studies by Weiler have shown a history of asthma in 12% of the university football players, with a 7% incidence in comparable age-matched students [14]. The prevalence of nonspecific hyperresponsiveness to inhaled methacholine occurred in 50% of the players. To determine the incidence of EIA in all intercollegiate athletes, Rice et al. [15] studied 983 participants at the University of Washington. Athletes with a history of exercise-induced respiratory symptoms were then challenged. Only 2.8% of the 983 athletes had positive challenges before arrival at college. However, athletes without a positive history were not exercise challenged, and this rate of positive challenges would have been expected to have been higher. Interestingly, those athletes with symptoms of EIA did not appear to select sports with less aerobic activity or less asthma provocation potential. Most recently, Huftel et al. studied 304 intercollegiate athletes over a 3-year period at the University of Wisconsin—Madison [16]. They demonstrated bronchial responsiveness to methacholine in 50 of these athletes. Eight of these individuals had a history of asthma and routinely used a bronchodilator before exercising. Sixteen additional athletes had symptoms consistent with EIA, but were taking no medications, illustrating the important fact that some athletes may not be aware of bronchoconstriction associated with exercise.

Since the 1972 Olympiad incident, there has been an increase in efforts to ascertain the occurrence of EIA in the Olympic athlete population. Studies of the last five Australian Olympic teams have demonstrated a prevalence rate of asthma or EIA as high as 14% [17]. Subsequent studies from the 1984 and 1988 summer Olympic Games disclosed that between 8 and 11% of United States athletes suffered from EIA. During the 1984 Olympic Games, 597 athletes were screened, and 67(11%) had symptoms consistent with EIA [18]. Only 26 of these individuals reported a history of previously documented asthma, again emphasizing the importance of screening for EIA in nonasthmatic, conditioned athletes. Forty-one medals, including 15 golds and 21 silvers, were awarded to individuals with EIA, which was comparable with athletes without EIA, demonstrating that with appropriate therapy, this condition can be controlled and should not compromise an individual's performance, even in world class competition.

Exercise-induced asthma is a common clinical problem affecting almost all individuals with asthma and possibly as many as 40 of those who suffer from nonasthmatic allergic diseases. Exercise-induced bronchoconstriction appears to affect 3–14% of athletes and is common even among those who are highly skilled and successful. Early recognition and treatment of exercise-induced asthma is of vital importance, especially in young athletes, because effective management may ensure that these individuals will continue to participate in and enjoy physical activity.

REFERENCES

1. McCarthy P. Wheezing and breezing through exercise-induced asthma. Phys Sportsmed 1989; 17(7):125–130.
2. Kawabori I, et al. Incidence of exercise-induced asthma in children. J Allergy Clin Immunol 1976; 58:447–455.
3. Kattan M, et al. The response to exercise in normal and asthmatic children. J Pediatr 1978; 92:718–721.

4. Cropp GJA, et al. Grading, time course, and incidence of exercise-induced airway obstruction and hyperinflation in asthmatic children. Pediatrics 1975; 56:868–879.
5. Bransford RP, et al. Exercise-induced asthma in adolescent gym class population. Int Arch Allergy Appl Immunol 1991; 94:272–274.
6. McFadden ER, et al. Exercise-induced asthma. Assessment of current etiologic concepts. Chest 1987; 91:151S–157S.
7. Custovic A, et al. Exercise testing revisted. The response to exercise in normal and atopic children. Chest 1994; 105:1127–1132.
8. Afrasiabi R, et al. Exercise-induced asthma. It needn't sideline your patients. Phys Sportsmed 1991; 19(5):49–62.
9. Burr ML, et al. Peak expiratory flow rates before and after exercise in schoolchildren. Arch Dis Child 1974; 49:923–926.
10. Godfrey S. Symposium on special problems and management of allergic athletes. International Symposium on Special Problems and Management of Allergic Athletes. J Allergy Clin Immunol 1984; 73:630S–632S.
11. Rupp NT, et al. The value of screening for risk of exercise-induced asthma in high school athletes. Ann Allergy 1993; 70:339–342.
12. Shield S, et al. Incidence of exercise-induced bronchospasm (EIB) in high school football players. J Allergy Clin Immunol 1991; 87:166.
13. Weiler JM, et al. Prevalence of bronchial hyperresponsiveness within a university football team. J Allergy Clin Immunol 1983; 71:108.
14. Weiler JM, et al. Prevalence of bronchial hyperresponsiveness in highly trained athletes. Chest 1986; 90:23–28.
15. Rice SG, et al. Identification of exercise-induced asthma among intercollegiate athletes. Ann Allergy 1985; 55:790–793.
16. Huftel MA, et al. Finding and managing asthma in competitive athletes. J Respir Dis 1991; 12:1110–1122.
17. Pierson WE, et al. Exercise-induced bronchospasm in children and adolescents. Pediatr Clin North Am 1979; 35:1031–1040.
18. Voy RO. The U.S. Olympic committee experience with exercise-induced bronchospasm, 1984. Med Sci Sports Exerc 1986; 18:328–330.

5

Pathophysiology of Exercise-Induced Asthma: The Role of Respiratory Water Loss

Sandra D. Anderson and Evangelia Daviskas
Royal Prince Alfred Hospital, Sydney, Australia

I. INTRODUCTION

A. Definition

Exercise-induced asthma (EIA), exercise-induced bronchoconstriction (EIB), and exercise-induced bronchospasm are the names used to describe the transient increase in airways resistance that occurs following vigorous exercise [1]. The increase in resistance has traditionally been measured indirectly by recording a reduction in peak expiratory flow (PEF) or forced expiratory volume in 1 second (FEV_1).

A reduction of 10% or more in PEF or FEV_1 from the preexercise value is considered abnormal when the exercise is performed under standardized conditions in a laboratory [1]. A reduction of 15% or more in PEF or FEV_1 is considered abnormal when the exercise is performed under field conditions [2].

B. Exercise-Induced Asthma and Exercise-Induced Bronchoconstriction in Patients with Asthma

Exercise-induced asthma has been most commonly studied in persons with clinically recognized asthma. EIA occurs in persons with mild, moderate, or severe asthma. It appears as one of the first symptoms or signs of asthma, but is also the last symptom to disappear after treatment with aerosol steroids [3].

It is well documented that EIA is associated with lung hyperinflation, gas trapping [4,5], and arterial hypoxemia [6,7] in patients with asthma. The increase in resistance, hyperinflation, gas trapping, and arterial hypoxemia are usually rapidly reversed by administering a β_2-adrenoceptor agonist. However, these physiological consequences of exercise make it uncomfortable for many asthmatics to take part in sports and other strenuous activity. Consequently, attention has been on prevention, rather than reversal, of EIA. This approach is aimed at encouraging persons with asthma to take part regularly in sports and other vigorous activities.

C. Prevention of Exercise-Induced Asthma in Asthmatic Subjects

Exercise-induced asthma is inhibited or prevented by taking one to two times the clinically recommended dose of a β_2-adrenoceptor agonist [1,8–10] cromolyn sodium (10–20 mg) [1,9,11,12], or nedocromil sodium (4–8 mg) [13,14] immediately before exercise. Prolonged treatment with aerosol corticosteroids usually reduces the severity of EIA. However, 50% of patients who are otherwise well-controlled with aerosol steroids will still have EIA [3]. Treatment with aerosol steroids usually reduces the dose of β_2-adrenoceptor agonist required to prevent EIA [15]. The results of studies using hyperosmolar saline challenge, a surrogate challenge for EIA, suggest that cromolyn sodium and nedocromil sodium would give an additional benefit to steroids, thereby reducing the severity of EIA [16,17].

D. Stimulus and Mechanism of Exercise-Induced Asthma and Exercise-Induced Bronchoconstriction

The stimulus whereby exercise induces an attack of asthma is the loss of water from the respiratory tract while bringing large volumes of air to alveolar conditions in a short time period [18,19]. The severity of EIA is directly related to the rate of water loss (Fig. 1) and this rate can be altered by changing both the amount of water in the inspired air (Fig. 2) and the rate of ventilation. In the 1970s several investigators showed that the airway response to exercise was prevented by inhaling air fully conditioned to body temperature and water vapor in persons with mild to moderate EIA [18,20–22] and with severe EIA [23] (Fig. 3).

During exercise, when ventilation is high and breathing is through the mouth, the lower airways must be recruited to humidify and heat the

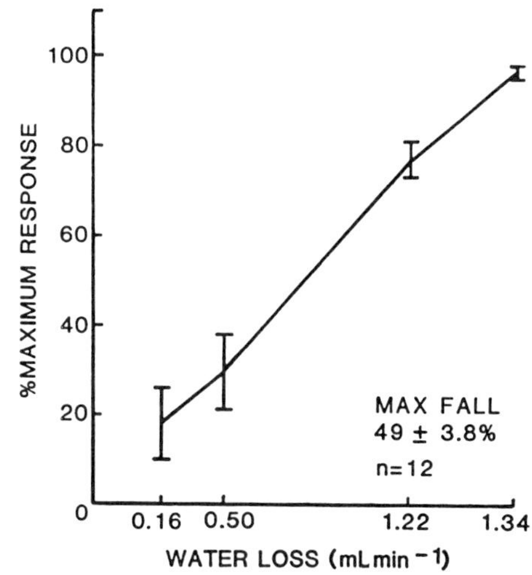

Fig. 1 Rate of water loss in relation to the fall in forced expiratory volume in 1 s (FEV_1), expressed as a percentage of the maximum fall observed in FEV_1. The maximum percentage fall in FEV_1 for the group was 49 ± 3.8. This was observed during exercise at the highest rate of water loss. Only 2% of the maximum response was observed when the inspired water concentration was close to body conditions. (Data from Ref. 19.)

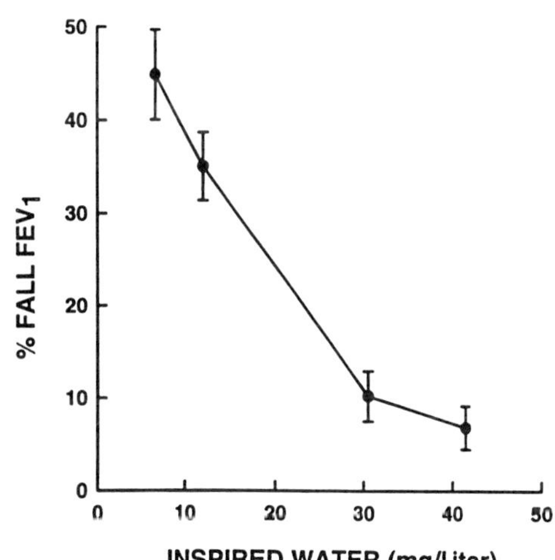

Fig. 2 Mean ± 1 SEM values for the percentage fall in FEV_1 observed in relation to the inspired water concentration in the same group of children performing the same exercise challenge as that described in Fig. 1. (Data from Ref. 19.)

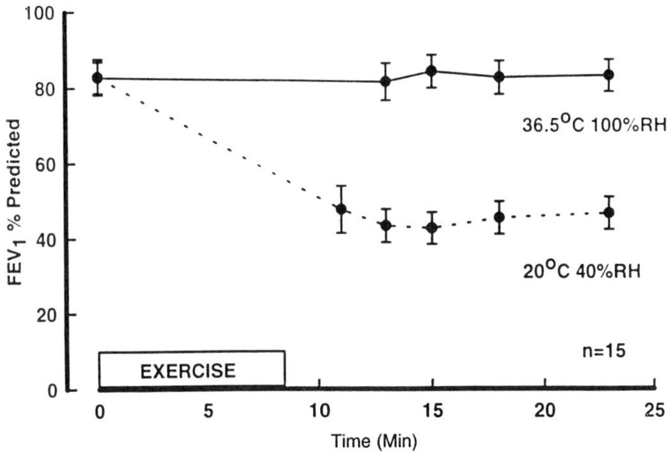

Fig. 3 Mean ± 1 SEM values for FEV_1 expressed as a percentage of the predicted normal value, before and after 5.5–8 min of treadmill running in 15 patients with severe exercise-induced asthma (age range 9–42 yr). Exercise was performed on two occasions 17–20 min apart. The first exercise test was always performed breathing warm humid air, and the second test, room air. The subjects inhaled through a Hans Rudolph 2700 valve. When expressed as a percentage of the prechallenge value, the percentage fall in FEV_1 after the warm humid air was 6.5 ± 5.2 SD and 53.9 ± 11.5 SD after the room air. (Data from Ref. 23.)

inspired air. This results in significant loss of water by evaporation from the lower airways. Unless the lost water is replaced instantaneously, dehydration of the airway surface will occur. Heat loss, which results from the conditioning of inspired air, is mostly due to vaporization of water. The mechanism whereby the water lost by evaporation causes the airways of asthmatics to narrow is thought to relate to the osmotic [9,24–26] and thermal effects [18,19,27].

Airway narrowing in response to the osmotic effects of evaporative water loss is thought to involve the release of mediators from mast cells [30–34] and neuropeptides from sensory nerves [35]. There is evidence that histamine is released into arterial blood when it is sampled at the same time that the airways narrow in response to exercise [30,36]. However, it has been difficult to obtain direct evidence for histamine release into the airways [37,38]. This failure may relate to the difficulty, when using lavage, to make measurements at the same time that the airway response to exercise occurs. Histamine may be diluted, rapidly degraded, or simply not released into the airways, and this may account for these negative findings. The finding that specific antihistamines [39] and leukotriene antagonists inhibit EIA [40–43] supports the role for these mediators in the pathogenesis of EIA. These mediators are thought to cause the airways to narrow by causing the airway smooth muscle to contract. The effects of the subsequent airway narrowing on lung function (e.g., FEV_1 and PEF) would be amplified in the presence of edema caused by the same mediators.

Airway narrowing in response to thermal effects of evaporative water loss (i.e., airway cooling and rapid rewarming) is thought to be due to engorgement of the bronchial vasculature and mucosal edema, but is independent of bronchial smooth-muscle contraction and mediator release [28,29,44]. However, abnormal airway cooling and rapid rewarming are not prerequisites for the airways to narrow in response to dry air hyperpnea, especially when hot dry air is inspired [26,45,46]. Rather, they appear to be epiphenomena of exercising while breathing air of subfreezing temperature. Many investigators and reviewers agree that it is more likely to be the osmotic, rather than thermal, effects of evaporative water loss that determine the occurrence of EIA [47–50]. Furthermore, the effectiveness of β_2-adrenoceptor agonist, both in preventing and reversing EIA, makes it difficult to accept that the airway narrowing seen in this condition is solely due to vascular engorgement and edema, and is independent of bronchial smooth-muscle contraction. Therefore, we will consider hyperpnea with cold air for its potential to increase the surface area over which evaporative water loss occurs in the airways, rather than for its potential to cause airway cooling as a result of evaporation of water. We will consider vascular events for their potential to change water transport to the airways, rather than for their currently disputed effects on airways resistance [51–54].

E. Exercise-Induced Asthma and Exercise-Induced Bronchoconstriction in "Healthy" Subjects

The results of epidemiological studies have shown that the prevalence of EIA or EIB is high and that EIA occurs in persons not recognized as having asthma by other criteria, such as symptoms and questionnaires [55,56]. In particular, abnormal reductions in PEF and FEV_1 have been reported after strenuous exercise in elite athletes [57–59], school children [60–62], skaters [63], and defense force recruits [64,65].

These are important findings, and they raise several questions. Does the demand for water exceed supply in the airways in some healthy subjects when they perform strenuous exercise? Does chronic dehydration of the airways, by hyperpnea, lead to inflammation and lung function changes consistent with asthma? Do the physiological changes of hyperinflation and hypoxemia occur in healthy persons who have EIA? Do medications, such as cromolyn sodium and nedocromil sodium, given immediately before exercise prevent airway response in healthy persons? Do β_2-adrenoceptor agonists alter the response to exercise if used long-term? Does chronic treatment with aerosol steroids prevent the response? Does stopping exercise, and thus airway dehydration for a prolonged period, improve lung function or reduce the airway response to exercise? Finally, are these persons asthmatic or at risk of developing clinically recognized asthma? If they are asthmatic, how should they be treated medically, and how should they be treated in terms of entry into occupations such as the defense forces?

This chapter provides an explanation for changes in lung function that occur in asthmatic and some healthy persons following vigorous exercise. We focus attention on the initiating stimulus (i.e., airway dehydration) as the major determinant of occurrence and severity of EIA. We also consider the role of dehydration in the development of inflammation. Furthermore, we discuss successful interventions that may act to partly improve airway hydration and reduce loss of lung function in response to exercise.

II. POSSIBLE REASONS ASSOCIATED WITH EVAPORATIVE WATER LOSS THAT COULD CONTRIBUTE TO THE PATHOPHYSIOLOGY OF EIA OR EIB

A. Is the Source of Water Used to Humidify the Inspired Air During Exercise Adequate?

When air is inspired under most conditions it must be heated and humidified to body conditions (37°C and 100% RH, 44 mg H_2O/L) before it reaches the alveoli. In the process, some heat and some water will be lost from the airway mucosa. During expiration, some heat will be returned and some water will condense onto the cooled mucosa. The net effect is for some heat and water to be lost from the airways.

The surface liquid lining the lower airways is thought to provide a significant proportion of the water needed to humidify the inspired air during vigorous exercise [66,67]. The periciliary fluid is the primary component of the airway surface liquid (ASL), and the ultimate source of its water must be the bronchial circulation. The depth of the perciliary fluid is unknown, but is thought to be 3–5 μm—about 2 μm smaller than the length of the cilia. The fluid contains Na^+, Cl^-, K^+, and Ca^{2+} ions and is thought to have an osmolarity slightly greater than normal (300 miOsm/Liter) under resting conditions.

The source of the periciliary fluid is precisely known. There are two theories. One suggests that fluid is transported from the alveoli by the mucociliary escalator [69], and the other suggests that the epithelial cell absorbs and secretes water by the transport of Na^+ and Cl^- ions [70]. The airway epithelium of humans is absorptive under basal conditions [70]; however, it is unclear whether it can secrete water under the stress of dehydration. Under normal circumstances, the most dependable and continuous source of periciliary fluid could be the mucociliary escalator, with ion transport playing an important role in absorption and, occasionally, secretion. However, water transport by the mucociliary escalator is very slow, and it is unlikely to be the primary source of water during hyperpnea. Whatever the source of water for the airway surface liquid, it does appear that, under conditions of hyperpnea with dry air, the demand for water exceeds the supply, at least in the first 10–12 generations of airways.

B. Why Does Airway Dehydration Occur During Exercise?

1. Available Fluid and Extent of Respiratory Tract Involvement in Humidifying the Air

By taking into account the surface area, we have calculated the volume of the periciliary fluid to be less than 1.0 mL in the first 10–12 generations of airways [24,25,68] (Table 1). This is why only small losses of water by evaporation would be required to cause an increase in ion concentration and osmolarity of this fluid layer [24]. It appears that the volume of fluid in the first 10–12 generations of airways is insufficient to humidify air when the ventilation rate is more than 40 L min^{-1}, even if water is returned to the airway lumen at twice the normal resting rate [67]. The higher the ventilation and the drier and colder the air, the more generations that will need to be recruited into the humidifying process. Given the experimental data of intra-airway temperature in humans, the smaller airways would need to be recruited into the humidifying process within 3–4 min (Fig. 4). However, there is no evidence that more than 12 generations are involved in the conditioning of the air (Fig. 5). By the time the air reaches the 16th and 17th generation, there is ample water available to humidify the air (see Table 1). Thus, dehydration of the airways must be confined to earlier generations.

Table 1 Surface Area and Volume of Periciliary Fluid Layer Available in the Conducting Airways

Airway generation no.	Number of airways in generation	Diameter of airway (mm)	Surface area[a] (cm^2)	Periciliary fluid volume (μL) at depth of 7 μm	Cumulative no. of airways	Cumulative surface area (cm^2)	Cumulative volume (μL) of periciliary fluid at 7 μm
0	1	18	68	48	1	68	48
1	2	12.2	37	25	3	105	73
2	4	8.3	21	14	7	126	87
3	8	5.6	9	6	15	135	93
4	16	4.5	29	21	31	164	114
5	32	3.5	37	25	63	201	139
6	64	2.8	51	35	127	252	174
7	128	2.3	70	49	255	322	223
8	256	1.86	95	66	511	417	289
9	512	1.54	135	94	1023	552	383
10	1024	1.3	190	133	2047	742	516
11	2048	1.09	275	192	4095	1017	708
12	4096	0.95	397	277	8191	1414	985
13	8192	0.82	584	409	16383	1998	1394
14	16384	0.74	870	609	32767	2868	2003
15	32768	0.66	1312	918	65535	4180	2921
16	65536	0.6	1905	1330	131071	6085	4251

[a] Surface area was calculated using the data given by Weibel [75].

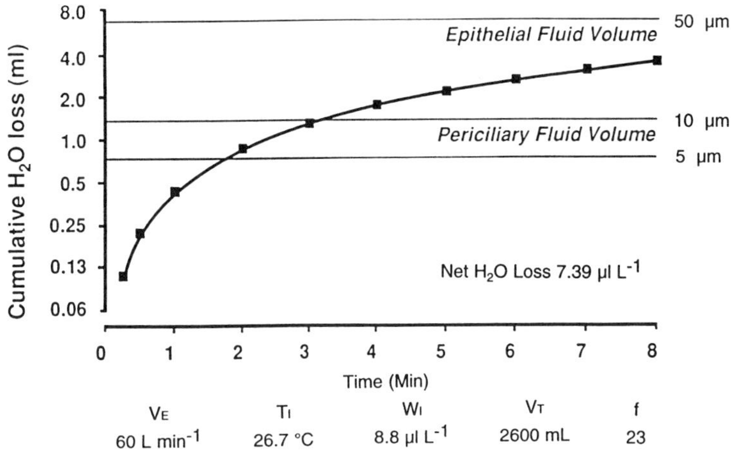

Fig. 4 Cumulative loss of water in relation to time predicted by the mathematical model of Daviskas [66,67]. The horizontal lines intercept the axis at the volume of periciliary fluid (assuming a depth of 5 or 10 μm) and epithelial cell fluid volume available (assuming depth of 50 μm) from the trachea to the 12th generation. For the ventilation (V_E) and inspired air conditions used in the model. A net loss of 7.39 μL H_2O is predicted to be lost per liter of air ventilated after accounting for predicted water return. Less than 2 min would be required to dehydrate the periciliary fluid if it had a depth of 5 μm. (From Ref. 25.)

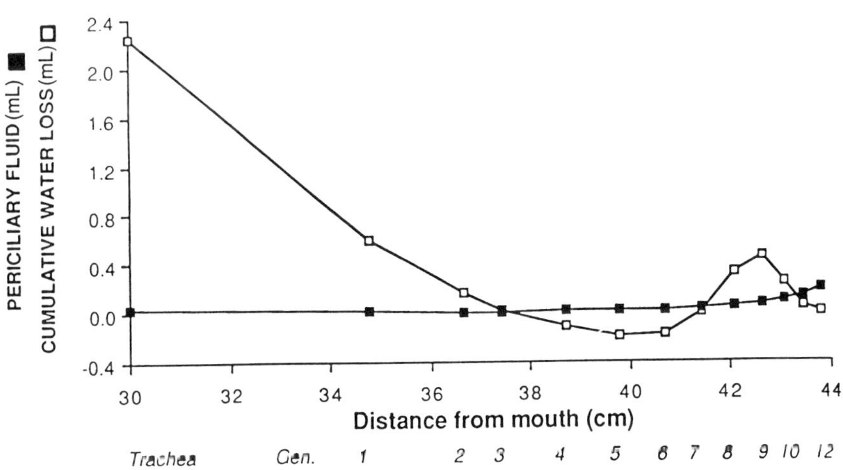

Fig. 5 Cumulative loss of water predicted for each generation from the model of Daviskas [66,67] under the same conditions as Fig. 4. The periciliary fluid volume available is also illustrated. The volume of water lost in 8 min exceeded the volume of periciliary fluid available in most generations. (From Ref. 25.)

A well-known example of demand exceeding supply of water in the airways is experienced during mechanical ventilation. During mechanical ventilation, the upper airways are bypassed, necessitating that the lower airways provide full humidification of the inspired air. Even though the air inspired is usually at temperate conditions (23°C and 50% RH) and the ventilation rates are less than 10 L min^{-1} the lower airways are unable to provide adequate hydration without pathological changes occurring. In recent times the need to humidify air, during treatment of sleep apnea, with continuous positive airway pressure through the nose has also been recognized. This suggests that the humidifying properties of the nose are also overwhelmed at relatively low-flow rates. Thus, despite the plexus of blood vessels, both in the lower and upper airways, they are unable to deliver water at a rate sufficient to cope with the humidification of large volumes of dry air.

2. Measurement of the Magnitude of Water Loss from the Airways During Hyperpnea

There have been few reports of measurements of expired water concentration, because of technical problems with accurately measuring water vapor pressure. These problems manifest themselves at the high frequencies of breathing that occur during exercise and at low inspired air temperatures, particularly those below freezing.

We have overcome many of these problems by: (a) using a gravimetric method; (b) using a rapidly responding relative humidity probe and thermistor; (c) keeping the frequency of breathing at less than 43 breaths per minute while using mass spectrometry and (d) using inspired air temperatures higher than 22°C [19,71,72]. When healthy subjects inspired air between 37° and 40°C containing between 12 and 13.5 mg of water per liter, the expired air contained 33.1 ± 1.4 mg of water per liter when measured gravimetrically [72]. We found similar values when we used a relative humidity probe and thermistor to measure expired water (32.8 ± 3 mgL^{-1}, n = 132) in adults exercising while inspiring hot dry air [72] (Fig. 6). A similar value was measured by mass spectrometry in children (33.2 ± 1.9 mg L^{-1}) exercising under similar inspired air conditions [71]. We found little variation in values for expired water concentration over a wide range of inspired air temperatures and ventilation rates when the inspired water was less than 13 mg L^{-1} (see Fig. 6). We have also measured the weight of expired water in normal subjects who performed isocapnic hyperventilation (not exercise) with dry air at 22–26°C at a ventilation rate of 50–65 L min^{-1} (28.9 ± 1.1 mg L^{-1}; expired temperature 31.2 ± 1.6°C) [73].

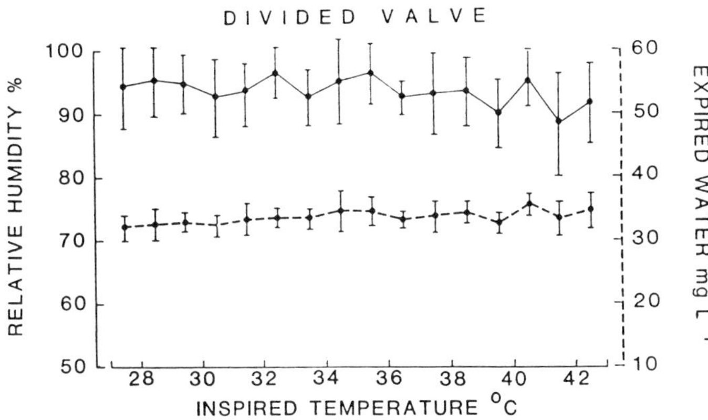

Fig. 6 Mean ± SD values for the relative humidity and expired water concentration in healthy adult subjects exercising for 15 min on a bicycle ergometer while inhaling air containing 4–6.5 mg H_2O per liter. The expired air temperature was measured using a Yellow Springs 520 thermistor and the relative humidity by a Vaisala 5121 probe. The standard equation relating relative humidity to water concentration was used. A total of 132 measurements were made. There was no significant difference between the expired water concentration between 27.5° and 42.5°C. (Data from Ref. 72.)

When using a value of 33 mg L^{-1}, the amount of water lost from the airways while breathing dry air, ranging in temperature from 26° to 43°C, is calculated to be 1.2, 1.8, and 2.4 mL min^{-1} breathing at ventilation rates of 40, 60, and 80 L min^{-1} respectively. Thus, over a period of 6–8 min the total loss of water during exercise at these ventilation rates is estimated to vary from 7 to 20 mL (Fig. 7).

We are unaware of any measurements of expired water concentration during exercise when the inspired temperature is below zero. Rather, water loss has been calculated by assuming that the expired air is fully saturated with water at the temperature measured at the mouth [27]. With this indirect technique, the calculation of water loss is critically determined by the accuracy of the expired temperature measurement. This measurement can be rendered difficult when breathing air of subzero temperatures. Because the thermocouples and thermistors can cool during inspiration, the water condensed on them during expiration can freeze. The consequence of this is a dampening of the response of the temperature sensor and an underestimate of expired temperature and expired water loss.

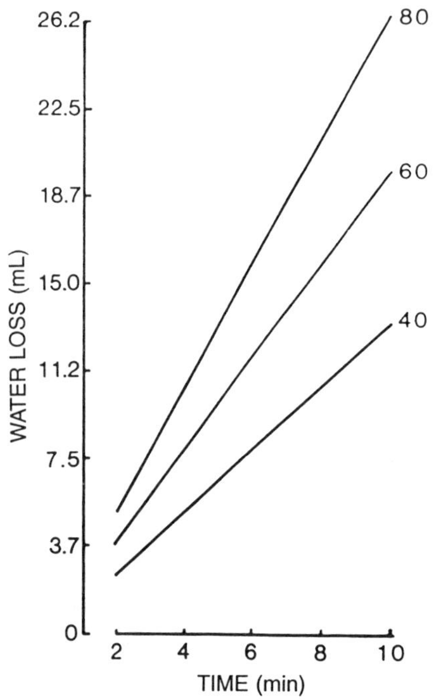

Fig. 7 Calculated water loss from the respiratory tract relative to time and level of ventilation in liters per minute (40, 60, or 80) when dry air is inhaled at temperatures between 26° and 42°C and the expired water concentration is 33 mgL^{-1}. (From Ref. 1.)

Measurements of absolute water loss at the mouth represent global losses from the mouth and lower airways. It is unknown what exact proportion of the expired water comes from the lower airways; but under conditions of exercise, breathing at 60 L min^{-1}, our computer model predicts about 40% [67]. However, computer models suggest that there are likely to be marked differences in the magnitude of water loss within the airway generations, particularly when there is a normal rate of return of water (see Fig. 5). Our model [66,67] predicts that the potential for water loss to exceed return under temperate conditions (inspired 26.7°C; inspired water 8.8 mg RH%) and moderate exercise can include up to generation 10 (see Fig. 5), which may increase to 12 with drier air or higher ventilation. Predictions using other models have been in keeping with this estimate [74].

Generations 10–12 include airways of 1.3–0.95 mm [75]. It is the recruitment of these smaller airways into the humidifying process that we consider may be the most important determinant for the severity of EIA.

C. Consequences of Water Loss from the Airways

In the process of losing water in humidifying the inspired air, it is thought that the airway surface liquid becomes hyperosmolar and that this may initiate the events that lead to EIA [19,24]. We think that the bronchoconstrictor response to exercise will be maximal only in asthmatics and may occur in healthy subjects only when airways of the 10th generation, or beyond, become dehydrated. Furthermore, we think that once the hyperosmolar stimulus reaches the 10th generation, or beyond, the cascade of events that results in narrowing of the airways occurs 5–10 mins later.

To compensate for the increased ion concentration of the airway surface liquid, water is likely to move from the epithelial cells causing a reduction in their volume [25,76,77]. Our dehydration theory incorporates epithelial cells' volume changes as a potentially important event in the pathogenesis of EIA [25,78]. Finally, as a result of the volume of the epithelial cells being restored by the movement of water across the basement membranes, the possibility of a small increase in osmolarity of the submucosa has been proposed [26]. This small increase in osmolarity may be the signal for bronchial blood flow to increase the rate of water return to restore normal osmolarity. The mediator for increasing blood flow is unknown but nitric oxide and neuropeptides are possible candidates [79,80].

The airways of patients with asthma narrow in response to an increase in osmolarity of the airway surface liquid [16,17]; however, there is no direct evidence in humans to show that hyperosmolarity of the airway surface liquid occurs during hyperpnea. It has been technically impossible to make accurate measurements of osmolarity during hyperpnea. This is because the extremely small volume of airway surface liquid is spread over a large surface area (see Table 1), and the potential for an increase in water flux to the airways when instruments are placed in them. Someday, as the instruments and their electronics are miniaturized, it may be technically possible to measure whether the predicted changes in osmolarity occur in the epithelial cells and submucosa.

However, there are studies that show a reduction in water content of expired air in asthmatic subjects, suggesting that the airway surface is hyperosmolar [81]. Furthermore, studies in animals and humans support hyperosmolarity of airway secretions as a result of evaporative water loss, even under resting conditions [82,83].

D. Experimental Evidence Supporting a Role for Recruitment of Small Airways into the Humidifying Process

There are many observations relating to EIA that support the concept that occurrence and severity of EIA or EIB may be related to the number of generations of airways becoming dehydrated.

The studies identifying that the importance of the intensity and duration of exercise, the inspired air conditions, and the ventilation rate, as determinants of the airway response, are in keeping with this [84–86]. The effect of duration on severity of EIA when breathing hot, dry air is well illustrated in Fig. 8. There is a marked and significant ($p < 0.025$)

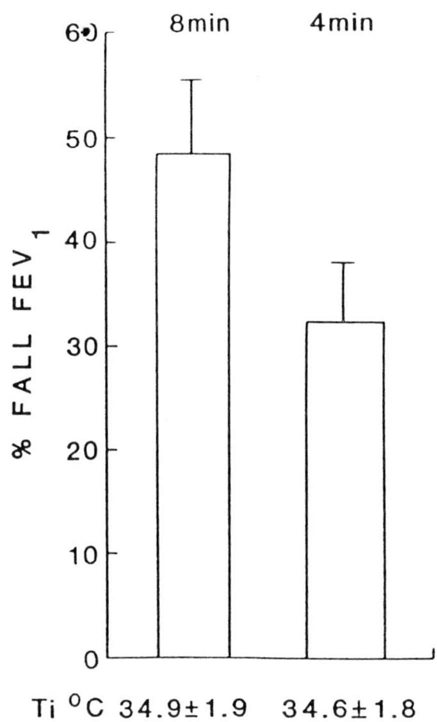

Fig. 8 Mean ± 1 SEM values for the reduction in FEV_1 expressed as a percentage of the prechallenge FEV_1 (% fall FEV_1) in nine asthmatic children who performed bicycle exercise for 8 min and 4 min while breathing hot air containing between 4 and 8 mg of water per liter. A period of 4 h separated the two tests. There was a significantly greater fall in FEV_1 ($p < 0.025$) after the 8-min exercise test. (From Ref. 25.)

difference in airway response between 4 and 8 min at the same intensity of exercise, at the same inspired air conditions, and at the same ventilation rate. High flow rates for 1–2 min may be insufficient to recruit airways beyond the 10th generation because, in that short time, sufficient fluid is available in the upper and lower airways. However, when ventilation rates in excess of 100 L min^{-1} were reached while breathing subfreezing air, O'Cain and colleagues [87] found that there was even a measurable reduction in FEV_1 and midexpiratory flow rates in healthy subjects.

If the severity of EIA depends on the number of generations that are recruited into the humidifying process, then this could also explain why similar values for the percentage fall in FEV_1 were observed over a wide range of temperatures when inspired water content and ventilation remained the same [27,88,89] (Fig. 9). However, when exercise was performed for 4 min, inspiring air of subfreezing temperature did enhance the response in some asthmatic subjects when the calculated loss of water was less than that breathing hot air [18,27] (see Fig. 9), suggesting additional factors contributed to the airway response. One factor may be that more generations of airways are recruited and are recruited faster into

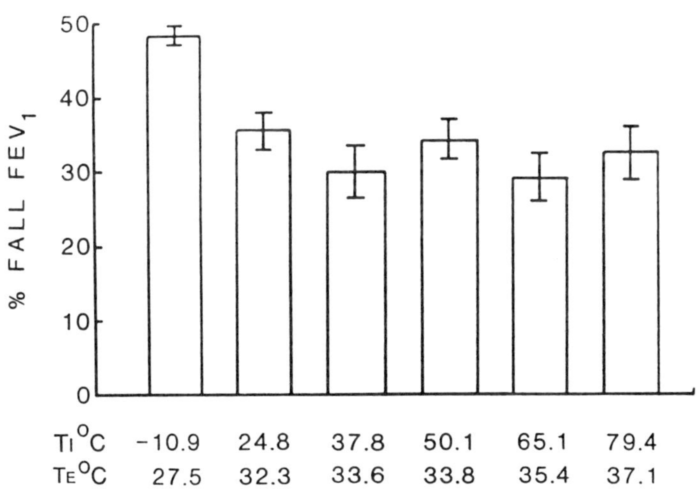

Fig. 9 Mean values for the percent fall in FEV_1 in 8 subjects with asthma who performed exhausting leg work on a bicycle while they were inspiring dry air at different temperatures (*T*I). The ventilation rate was similar on all occasions. The mean values recorded for expired air temperatures (*T*E) are also given and demonstrate that abnormal cooling of the airways was unlikely to have occurred during exercise at the highest inspired air temperatures. (From Ref. 27.)

the humidifying process during cold air breathing for the 4 min for which exercise was performed. As the more peripheral smaller airways are recruited, the airway response may be larger. Increasing the duration of exercise while breathing dry hot air, as illustrated in Fig. 8, would presumably have led to a greater airway response, perhaps equivalent to that observed during cold air breathing.

An analysis of many studies of EIA shows that the loss of water at a rate faster than 1.2 mL min^{-1} for 2–6 min is usually required for most patients with asthma to have a response [27,86,88,90]. Perhaps it is the duration of exercise, for 6–8 min or even longer, with this rate of water loss that also provokes airway narrowing in some otherwise healthy subjects.

The airway response is blunted when absolute water content exceeds 10 mg L^{-1} [19–22] (see Fig. 2). As the inspired water concentration increases, there is a smaller chance that airways beyond generation 10 will be recruited into the humidifying process. Even small increases in inspired water concentration appear to be effective in reducing the airway response. For example, masks that allow a small amount of water and heat to be inspired during exercise are successful in reducing the severity of EIA [90–93]. The severity of EIA is also reduced by breathing through the nose during exercise [94,95]. Again, this would act to reduce the amount of water needed to humidify the air below the pharynx.

Many patients with asthma are refractory to the effects of repeated exercise [96–98]. Furthermore, warm-up by submaximal exercise [99] or short-term sprints [100] may also reduce the severity of EIA. Some investigators [101,102], but not all [23,103], have found refractoriness to occur even when EIA is prevented by inhaling warm humid air. The mechanism for this is unknown, but exercise itself may improve rates of water return to the airways by a prostaglandin-sensitive pathway [104,105]. After dry air hyperpnea, mucociliary clearance rates increase, suggesting that airway surface liquid has been restored through some mechanism [106]. If water transport is enhanced by any of these means, then dehydration of the airways may be limited to fewer than 10 generations, so that on repeated challenge, refractoriness occurs.

III. PATHOLOGICAL CHANGES ASSOCIATED WITH AIRWAY DEHYDRATION

It has been recognized for many decades that significant pathological changes occur in the airways if the inspired air is not humidified during mechanical ventilation [77,107,108]. These changes are well described for the lower airways of humans and animals breathing under resting conditions for prolonged periods [107,108]. The pathological changes arising from breathing dry air for a short period have also been well studied in animals [76,77,109–111].

These studies on the effect of breathing dry air demonstrate denuded epithelium, mast cell degranulation, recruitment of eosinophils, and secretion of mucus by goblet cells [34,111]; the water content in the submucosa is also reduced [76].

The effects of dry air hyperpnea on the nasal mucosa of humans is also well described [112–114]. There are no known studies on the histological effect of dry air hyperpnea in the lower airways of humans. However, recent studies on mucociliary clearance demonstrate a marked reduction during dry air hyperpnea in subjects with asthma [106]. This finding is consistent with the concept of a reduction in the depth of the periciliary fluid layer from evaporative water loss. This reduction in mucociliary clearance also occurs in healthy subjects, but to a smaller extent (Fig. 10). Persons with asthma, compared with healthy subjects, may have a slower rate of delivery of water in the presence of the pathological changes (e.g., increased thickness of the basement membrane) associated with inflammation. The decrease in mucociliary clearance with dry air hyperpnea is followed by an increase in clearance [106]. This is thought to be due to mediators, released in response to hyperpnea, reestablishing the airway surface liquid and stimulating mucociliary clearance, by activation of Cl^- ion transport.

The finding that many animals have an increase in airway resistance to dry air breathing [115–117] associated with pathological changes demonstrates that these findings and their association are not unique to asthma. Furthermore, many of the findings in humans concerning the importance of dehydration rather than cooling, the role of mediators, and the effect of drugs have been reproduced in dogs [117]. In a recent review Freed [117] suggests that airway narrowing, and the pathological changes associated with it, may act as a protective mechanism in mammals to prevent further desiccation.

We think that EIA, in healthy subjects, occurs as a result of the pathological changes arising from dehydration of the airways as a result of inadequate water transport. This is likely to occur more readily in healthy subjects who exercise for long periods and who inhale large volumes of cold air. The airway narrowing in response to dehydration is exaggerated in persons with asthma because inflammation is part of the disease process. Asthmatics will have more inflammatory cells, a greater concentration of mediators, and a more responsive bronchial smooth-muscle, compared with healthy subjects. Thus, airways of persons with asthma would be expected to narrow more than the airways of normal subjects.

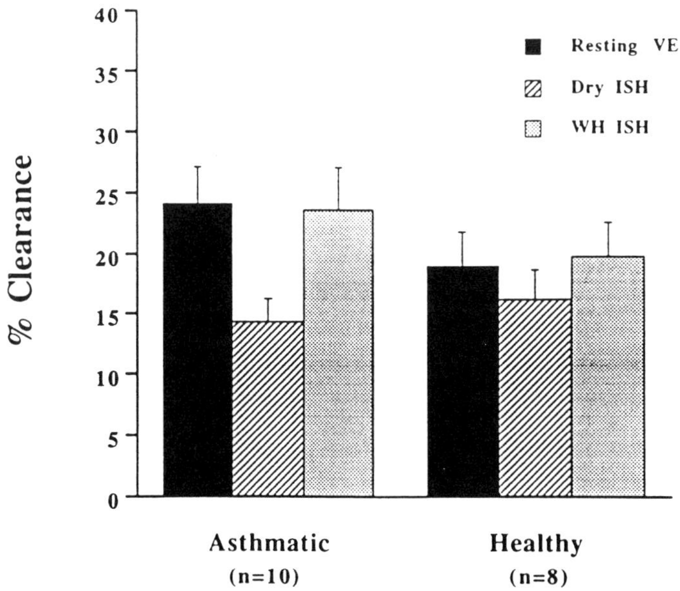

Fig. 10 Mean percentage clearance (±SEM) of the whole right lung during isocapnic hyperventilation (ISH) with dry and warm humid (WH) air and nasal resting-breathing (rest) over the same time interval in asthmatic and healthy subjects. Inhalation of dry air during ISH caused a significant reduction ($p < 0.002$) in mucociliary clearance when compared with warm humid air and nasal resting-breathing, both in asthmatic and healthy subjects. There was no difference between mucociliary clearance involving ISH with warm humid air and nasal resting-breathing. (From Ref. 106.)

In its early stages EIA may occur without abnormalities in lung function being detected at rest. As the inflammation increases, the pathological changes in the small airways will be reflected as a reduction of flow rates through the midportion of the vital capacity. These flow rates are known as the forced expiratory volume over 25–75% of the forced vital capacity (FEF_{25-75}) or the maximum midexpiratory flow rate (MMEFR).

In keeping with this concept, Mahler and Loke [118] have found an acute reduction in these flow rates in marathon runners inspiring air of subfreezing temperatures [118]. In the study by O'Cain [87], healthy subjects had a 14% reduction in the MMEFR breathing cold air at high flow rates. Haas and colleagues [119] also reported the unexpected and significant reductions in midexpiratory flow rates when asthmatic subjects were challenged with cold air repeatedly over days. Gradual reductions in the flow rates may also occur with intermittent breathing of dry air. There is a report showing that nonsmoking Eskimo hunters, older than 40 years of age, had marked reductions in midexpiratory flow rates. The authors suggested that the "frequent and lengthy exposure to extremely cold air during hard physical work" could have accounted for these findings [120].

IV. THE POTENTIAL FOR PHARMACOLOGICAL AGENTS TO IMPROVE WATER TRANSPORT

The beneficial effects of various medications on EIA [1] may be partly explained by their potential to improve water transport to the airways and to protect the airway submucosa from dehydration. For example, agents such as the calcium antagonists and isorbide nitrates, all give some benefit against EIA [1,121]. They may do so because they induce vasodilation, which is likely to increase water supply to the airways. β_2-adrenoceptor agonists and α-agonists stimulate Cl^- ion secretion on the apical membrane of the epithelial cell; accordingly, they have the potential to reduce the dehydrating and osmotic effects of evaporative water loss [122]. Although brief stimulation of Cl^- ion secretion could be beneficial in EIA, it may have detrimental effects if the stimulation is prolonged. It is possible that prolonged use of β_2-adrenoceptor agonists may lead to dehydration of the airway submucosa. This may be why the protective effect of long-acting β_2-agonists is reduced when these drugs are used daily [122].

Recently, it has been proposed that, in addition to their beneficial effects in protecting mast cells and nerves from effects on osmolarity, drugs such as cromolyn sodium, nedocromil sodium, furosemide (frusemide), and bumetanide may serve to block the Cl^- ion transport across the epithelial cell, thereby protecting it, and the submucosa, from dehydration [78].

Steroids increase the number of Na^+, K^+-ATPase pumps on the basolateral membrane of the epithelial cell [124]. This has the potential to enhance water absorption from the airway lumen, thereby reducing effects of dehydration in the submucosa while possibly enhancing the dehydration of the airway surface liquid. This may be why many asthmatics remain responsive to exercise while taking aerosol corticosteroids [3], but only need small doses of drugs to protect them [15].

The mediators released in response to initial dehydration (e.g., histamine, leukotrienes, or prostaglandins) whatever their cellular source, all have the potential to stimulate Cl^- ion secretion and to restore the balance of water in the airway lumen [70]. This may partly explain the refractory period after exercise that is prevented when prostaglandin production is inhibited by use of a nonsteroidal anti-inflammatory drug for 3 days [104,105].

V. CONCLUSION

In conclusion we think that the occurrence and severity of EIA or EIB could be linked to (a) the degree of airway inflammation; (b) the number of generations becoming dehydrated during exercise; (c) structural changes in the airway (e.g., thickening of the basement membrane); (d) bronchial smooth-muscle responsiveness; or (e) same combination thereof. We think that water transport to the airways in asthma is abnormal when demand is high during exercise. Under conditions of excessively high ventilation, low water content, or subfreezing temperatures, demand for water may exceed the supply, even in the healthy subjects. As smaller airways are recruited, the magnitude of the airway's response to exercise can be increased in persons with asthma and may occur for the first time in persons without asthma, but who exercise vigorously.

The pathological changes that occur in response to acute dehydration suggest that inflammation contributes to the airway response. Whether the inflammation persists is unknown. Whether inflammation from dehydration is similar to the inflammation that occurs in asthma is also unknown. What is known is that many otherwise healthy subjects do have a significant and abnormal reduction in lung function after vigorous exercise. Many of these persons exercise maximally in dry air for long periods. This reduction in lung function may represent an early manifestation of asthma. Whether or not this is true asthma should not discourage a trial of medication or the use of techniques to conserve water loss or improve water delivery to the airways.

It is possible that the cells resident in the airway and activated in response to the stress of dehydration, or cells attracted to the airway as a result of dehydration, are similar to those involved in the inflammatory changes of asthma. If this is true, then it would explain why so many persons involved in "cold" sport activities have respiratory problems. Perhaps it is most important to determine if spontaneous resolution of EIA or EIB occurs after a period of abstinence from exercise. In this way long-term deleterious effects on lung function from breathing dry air may be avoided.

REFERENCES

1. Anderson SD. Exercise-induced asthma. In: Middleton E, Reed C, Ellis E, Adkinson NF, Yunginger JW, eds. Allergy: principles and practice, Vol 2, 3rd ed. St Louis: CV Mosby, 1988; 1156–1175.
2. Haby MM, Anderson SD, Peat JK, Mellis CM, Toelle BG, Woolcock AJ. An exercise challenge protocol for epidemiological studies of asthma in children: comparison with histamine challenge. Eur Respir J 1994; 7:43–49.
3. Waalkans HJ, van Essen-Zandvliet EEM, Gerritsen J, Duiverman EJ, Kerrebijn KF, Knol K, the Dutch CNSLD Study Group. The effect of an inhaled corticosteroid (budesonide) on exercise-induced asthma in children. Eur Respir J 1993; 6:652–656.
4. Anderson SD, Mc Evoy JDS, Bianco S. Changes in lung volumes and airway resistance after exercise in asthmatic subjects. Am Rev Respir Dis 1972; 106:30–37.
5. Freedman S, Tattersfield AE, Pride NB. Changes in lung mechanics during asthma induced by exercise. J Appl Physiol 1975; 38:974–982.
6. Silverman M, Anderson SD, Walker SR. Metabolic changes preceding exercise-induced bronchoconstriction. Br Med J 1972; 1:207–209.
7. Bye PTP, Anderson SD, Daviskas E, Marty JJ, Sampson D. Plasma cyclic AMP levels in response to exercise and terbutaline sulphate aerosol in normal and asthmatic patients. Eur J Respir Dis 1980; 61:287–297.
8. Anderson SD, Seale JP, Rozea P, Bandler L, Theobald G, Lindsay DA. Inhaled and oral salbutamol in exercise-induced asthma. Am Rev Respir Dis 1976; 114:493–500.
9. Anderson SD, Seale JP, Ferris L, Schoeffel RE, Lindsay DA. An evaluation of pharmacotherapy for exercise-induced asthma. J Allergy Clin Immunol 1979; 64:612–624.
10. Anderson SD, Rodwell LT, Du Toit J, Young IH. Duration of protection of inhaled salmeterol in exercise-induced asthma. Chest 1991; 100:1254–1260.
11. Tullett WM, Tan KM, Wall RT, Patel KR. Dose–response effect of sodium cromoglycate pressurised aerosol in exercise induced asthma. Thorax 1985; 40:41–44.
12. Comis A, Valletta EA, Sette L, Andreoli A, Boner AL. Comparison of nedocromil sodium and sodium cromoglycate administered by pressurized aerosol, with and without a spacer device in exercise-induced asthma in children. Eur Respir J 1993; 6:523–526.
13. Albazzaz MK, Neale MG, Patel KR. Dose duration of nebulized nedocromil sodium in exercise-induced asthma. Eur Respir J 1992; 5:967–969.
14. Morton AR, Ogle SL, Fitch KD. Effects of nedocromil sodium, cromolyn sodium, and a placebo in exercise-induced asthma. Ann Allergy 1992; 68: 143–148.
15. Henriksen JM, Dahl R. Effects of inhaled budesonide alone and in combination with low dose terbutaline in children with exercise-induced asthma. Am Rev Respir Dis 1983; 128:993–997.

16. Anderson SD, du Toit JI, Rodwell LT, Jenkins CR. Acute effect of sodium cromoglycate on airway narrowing induced by 4.5 percent saline aerosol. Outcome before and during treatment with aerosol corticosteroids in patients with asthma. Chest 1994; 105:673–680.
17. Rodwell LT, Anderson SD, du Toit J, Seale JP. Nedocromil sodium inhibits the airway response to hyperosmolar challenge in patients with asthma. Am Rev Respir Dis 1992; 146:1149–1155.
18. Strauss RH, McFadden ER, Ingram RH, Deal EC, Jaegar JJ, Stearns D. Influence of heat and humidity on the airway obstruction induced by exercise in asthma. J Clin Invest 1978; 61:433–440.
19. Anderson SD, Schoeffel RE, Follet R, Perry CP, Daviskas E, Kendall M. Sensitivity to heat and water loss at rest and during exercise in asthmatic patients. Eur J Respir Dis 1982; 63:459–471.
20. Weinstein RE, Anderson JA, Kvale P, Sweet LC. Effects of humidification on exercise induced asthma (EIA). J Allergy Clin Immunol 1976; 57: A250–251.
21. Chen WY, Horton DJ. Heat and water loss from the airways and exercise-induced asthma. Respiration 1977; 34:305–313.
22. Bar-Or O, Neuman I, Dotan R. Effects of dry and humid climates on exercise-induced asthma in children and preadolescents. J Allergy Clin Immunol 1977; 60:163–168.
23. Anderson SD, Daviskas E, Schoeffel RE, Unger SF. Prevention of severe exercise-induced asthma with hot humid air. Lancet 1979; 2:629.
24. Anderson SD. Is there a unifying hypothesis for exercise-induced asthma. J Allergy Clin Immunol 1984; 73:660–665.
25. Anderson SD, Daviskas E, Smith CM. Exercise-induced asthma: a difference in opinion regarding the stimulus. Allergy Proc 1989; 10:215–226.
26. Anderson SD, Daviskas E. The airway microvasculature in exercise-induced asthma. Thorax 1992; 47:748–752.
27. Deal EC, McFadden ER, Ingram RH, Strauss RH, Jaeger JJ. Role of respiratory heat exchange in production of exercise-induced asthma. J Appl Physiol: Respir Environ Exerc Physiol 1979; 46:467–475.
28. McFadden ER, Lenner KA, Strohl KP. Postexertional airway rewarming and thermally induced asthma. J Clin Invest 1986; 78:18–25.
29. McFadden ER. Hypothesis: exercise-induced asthma as a vascular phenomenon. Lancet 1990; 1:880–883.
30. Anderson SD, Bye PTP, Schoeffel RE, Seale JP, Taylor KM, Ferris L. Arterial plasma histamine levels at rest, during and after exercise in patients with asthma: Effects of terbutaline aerosol. Allergy Proc 1981; 36:259–267.
31. Belcher NG, Murdoch RD, Dalton N, House FR, Clark TJH, Rees J, Lee TH. A comparison of mediator and catecholamine release between exercise- and hypertonic saline-induced asthma. Am Rev Respir Dis 1988; 137: 1026–1032.
32. Venge P, Henriksen J, Dahl R, Hakansson L. Exercise-induced asthma and the generation of neutrophil chemotactic activity. J Allergy Clin Immunol 1990; 85:498–504.

33. Pliss LB, Ingenito EP, Ingram RH, Pichurko B. Assessment of bronchoalveolar cell and mediator response to isocapnic hyperpnea in asthma. Am Rev Respir Dis 1990; 142:73–78.
34. Crimi E, Balbo A, Milanese M, Miadonna A, Rossi GA, Brusasco V. Airway inflammation and occurrence of delayed bronchoconstriction in exercise-induced asthma. Am Rev Respir Dis 1992; 146:507–512.
35. Solway J, Leff AR. Sensory neuropeptides and airway function. J Appl Physiol 1991; 71:2077–2087.
36. Hartley JPR, Charles TJ, Monie DH, Seaton A, Taylor WH, Westwood A, Williams JD. Arterial plasma histamine after exercise in normal individuals and in patients with exercise-induced asthma. Clin Sci 1981; 61:151–157.
37. Broide DH, Eisman S, Ramsdell JW, Ferguson P, Schwartz LB, Wasserman SI. Airway levels of mast cell-derived mediators in exercise-induced asthma. Am Rev Respir Dis 1990; 141:563–568.
38. Jarjour NN, Calhoun WJ. Exercise-induced asthma is not associated with mast cell activation or airway inflammation. J Allergy Clin Immunol 1992; 89:60–68.
39. Finnerty JP, Harvey A, Holgate ST. The relative contributions of histamine and prostanoids to bronchoconstriction provoked by isocapnic hyperventilation in asthma. Eur Respir J 1992; 5:323–330.
40. Manning PJ, Watson RM, Margolskee DJ, Williams VC, Schwartz JI, O'Byrne PM. Inhibition of exercise-induced bronchoconstriction by MK-571, a potent leukiotriene D_4-receptor antagonist. N Engl J Med 1990; 323: 1736–1739.
41. Israel E, Dermarkarian R, Rosenberg M, Sperling R, Taylor G, Rubin P, Drazen JM. The effects of a 5-lipoxygenase inhibitor on asthma induced by cold, dry air. N Engl J Med 1990; 323:1740–1744.
42. Robuschi M, Riva E, Fuccella LM, Vida E, Barnabae R, Rossi M, Gambaro G, Spagnotto S, Bianco S. Prevention of exercise-induced bronchoconstriction by a new leukotriene antagonist (SK&F 104353): a double-blind study versus disodium cromoglycate and placebo. Am Rev Respir Dis 1992; 145: 1285–1288.
43. Makker HK, Lau LC, Thomson HW, Binks SM, Holgate ST. The protective effect of inhaled leukotriene D_4 receptor antagonist ICI 204,219 against exercise-induced asthma. Am Rev Respir Dis 1993; 147:1413–1418.
44. Gilbert IA, McFadden ER. Airway cooling and rewarming. The second reaction sequence in exercise-induced asthma. J Clin Invest 1992; 90: 699–704.
45. Anderson SD, Daviskas E. An evaluation of the airway cooling and rewarming hypothesis as the mechanism for exercise induced asthma. In: Holgate S, Kay AB, Lichtenstein L, Austen F, eds. Asthma: physiology, immunopharmacology, and treatment, 4th International Symposium. London: Academic Press, 1993; 323–335.
46. Smith CM, Anderson SD, Walsh S, McElrea M. An investigation of the effects of heat and water exchange in the recovery period after exercise in children with asthma. Am Rev Respir Dis 1989; 140:598–605.

47. Ingenito E, Solway J, Lafleur J, Lombardo A, Drazen JM, Pichurko B. Dissociation of temperature-gradient and evaporative heat loss during cold gas hyperventilation in cold-induced asthma. Am Rev Respir Dis 1988; 138: 540–546.
48. Argyros GJ, Phillips YY, Rayburn DB, Rosenthal RR, Jaeger JJ. Water loss without heat flux in exercise-induced bronchospasm. Am Rev Respir Dis 1993; 147:1419–1424.
49. Godfrey S, Bar-Yishay E. Exercise-induced asthma revisited. Respir Med 1993; 87:331–344.
50. Souhrada JF, Souhrada M. Provocative challenge by exercise or hyperventilation. In: Spector SL, ed. Provocation testing in clinical practice. New York: Marcel Dekker, 1995; 425–450.
51. Tang GJ, Freed AN. The role of submucosal oedema in increased peripheral airway resistance by intravenous volume loading in dogs. Eur Respir J 1994; 7:311–317.
52. Blosser S, Mitzner W, Wagner EM. Effects of increased bronchial blood flow on airway morphometry, resistance and reactivity. J Appl Physiol 1994; 76:1624–1629.
53. Wagner EM, Mitzner W. Bronchial vascular engorgement and airway narrowing. Am J Respir Crit Care Med 1994; 149:A585.
54. Brown RH, Zerhouni EA, Mitzner W. Visualization of airway obstruction in vivo during pulmonary vascular engorgement and edema. J Appl Physiol 1995; 78:1070–1078.
55. Weiss ST, Tager IB, Weiss JW, Munoz A, Speizer FE, Ingram RH. Airways responsiveness in a population sample of adults and children. Am Rev Respir Dis 1984; 129:898–902.
56. Backer V, Ulrik CS. Bronchial responsiveness to exercise in a random sample of 494 children and adolescents from Copenhagen. Clin Exp Allergy 1992; 22:741–747.
57. Weiler JM, Metzger J, Donnelly AL, Crowley ET, Sharath MD. Prevalence of bronchial hyperresponsiveness in highly trained athletes. Chest 1986; 90: 23–28.
58. Drobnic F, Banquells M, Casan P, Miralda R, Sanchis J. Asthma, exercise induced asthma and bronchial reactivity in the elite athlete. Eur Respir J 1992; 5(suppl 15):456S.
59. Rupp NT, Brudno S, Guill MF. The value of screening for risk of exercise-induced asthma in high school athletes. Ann Allergy 1993; 70:339–332.
60. Burr ML, Butland BK, King S, Vaughan-Williams E. Changes in asthma prevalence: two surveys 15 years apart. Arch Dis Child 1989; 64:1452–1456.
61. Terblanche E, Stewart RI. The prevalence of exercise-induced bronchoconstriction in Cape Town schoolchildren S Afr Med J 1990; 78:744–747.
62. Haby MM, Peat JK, Mellis CM, Anderson SD, Woolcock AJ. An exercise challenge for epidemiological studies of childhood asthma: validity and repeatability. Eur Respir J 1995; 8:729–736.
63. Paul DW, Bogaard JM, Hop WC. The bronchoconstrictor effect of stren-

uous exercise at low temperatures in normal athletes. Int J Sports Med 1993; 14:433–436.
64. Nish WA, Schwietz LA. Underdiagnosis of asthma in young adults presenting for USAF basis training. Ann Allergy 1992; 69:239–242.
65. O'Donnell AE, Fling J. Exercise-induced airflow obstruction in a healthy military population. Chest 1993; 103:742–744.
66. Daviskas E, Gonda I, Anderson SD. Mathematical modelling of heat and water transport in human respiratory tract. J Appl Physiol 1990; 69:362–372.
67. Daviskas E, Gonda I, Anderson SD. Local airway heat and water vapour losses. Respir Physiol 1991; 84:115–132.
68. Anderson SD. Asthma provoked by exercise, hyperventilation, and the inhalation of non-isotonic aerosols. In: Barnes PJ, Rodger IW, Thomson NC, eds. Asthma: basic mechanisms and clinical management. 2nd ed. London: Academic Press, 1992; 473–490.
69. Kilburn KH. A hypothesis of pulmonary clearance and its implications. Am Rev Respir Dis 1968; 98:449–463.
70. Boucher RC. Human airway ion transport. Am J Respir Crit Care Med 1994; 150 (part 1): 271–281; (part 2):581–593.
71. Anderson SD, Schoeffel RE, Black JL, Daviskas E. Airway cooling as the stimulus to exercise-induced asthma—a re-evaluation. Eur J Respir Dis 1985; 67:20–30.
72. Anderson SD, Schoeffel RE, Gonda I, Daviskas E. Water concentration in the expired air of humans during exercise under arid conditions [abstract]. Am Rev Respir Dis 1984; 129:A260.
73. Smith CM, Anderson SD. Hyperosmolarity as the stimulus to asthma induced by hyperventilation? J Allergy Clin Immunol 1986; 77:729–736.
74. Hanna LM, Scherer PW. Regional control of local airway heat and water vapor losses. J Appl Physiol 1986; 61:624–632.
75. Weibel ER. Morphometry of the human lung. Berlin: Springer, 1963.
76. Van Oostdam JC, Walker DC, Knudson K, Dirks P, Dahlby RW, Hogg JC. Effect of breathing dry air on structure and function of airways. J Appl Physiol 1986; 61:312–317.
77. Tsuda T, Naguchi H, Tahkumi V, Aochi O. Optimal humidification of air administration to a tracheostomy in dogs. Scanning electron microscopy and surfactant studies. Br J Anaesth 1977; 49:965–977.
78. Anderson SD, Rodwell LT, Daviskas E, Spring JF, du Toit J. The protective effect of nedocromil sodium and other drugs on airway narrowing provoked by hyperosmolar stimuli: a role for the airway epithelium. J Allergy Clin Immunol 1996, 98:S124–S134.
79. Smith TL, Prazma J, Coleman CC, Drake AF, Boucher RC. Control of the mucosal microcirculation in the upper respiratory tract. Otolaryngol Head Neck Surg 1993; 109:646–652.
80. Umeno E, McDonald DM, Nadel JA. Hypertonic saline increases vascular permeability in the rat trachea by producing neurogenic inflammation. J Clin Invest 1990; 851:1905–1908.

81. Tabka Z, Ben Jebria A, Vergeret J, Guenard H. Effect of dry warm air on respiratory water loss in children with exercise-induced asthma. Chest 1988; 94:81–86.
82. Mann SFP, Adams GK, Proctor DF. Effects of temperature, relative humidity, and mode of breathing on canine airway secretions. J Appl Physiol 1979; 46:205–210.
83. Potter JL, LeRoy WM, Spector S, Lemm J. Studies on pulmonary secretions. Am Rev Respir Dis 1967; 96:83–87.
84. Silverman M, Anderson SD. Standardization of exercise tests in asthmatic children. Arch Dis Child 1972; 47:882–889.
85. Noviski N, Bar-Yishay E, Gur I, Godfrey S. Exercise intensity determines and climatic conditions modify the severity of exercise-induced asthma. Am Rev Respir Dis 1987; 136:592–594.
86. Deal EC, McFadden ER, Ingram RH, Jaeger JJ. Hyperpnea and heat flux: initial reaction sequence in exercise-induced asthma. J Appl Physiol Respir Environ Exerc Physiol 1979; 46:476–483.
87. O'Cain CF, Dowling NB, Slutsky AS, Hensley MJ, Strohl KP, McFadden ER, Ingram RH. Airway effects of respiratory heat loss in normal subjects. J Appl Physiol Respir Environ Exerc Physiol 1980; 49:875–880.
88. Hahn A, Anderson SD, Morton AR, Black JL, Fitch KD. A re-interpretation of the effect of temperature and water content of the inspired air in exercise-induced asthma. Am Rev Respir Dis 1984; 130:575–579.
89. Eschenbacher WL, Sheppard D. Respiratory heat loss is not the sole stimulus for bronchoconstriction induced by isocapnic hyperpnea with dry air. Am Rev Respir Dis 1985; 131:894–901.
90. Resnick AD, Deal EC, Ingram RH, Stearns D. A critical assessment of the mechanism by which hyperoxia attenuates exercise-induced asthma. J Clin Invest 1979; 64:541–549.
91. Brenner AM, Weiser PC, Krogh LA, Loren ML. Effectiveness of a portable face mask in attenuating exercise-induced asthma. JAMA 1980; 264: 2196–2198.
92. Eiken O, Kaiser P, Holmer I, Baer R. Physiological effects of a mouth-borne heat exchanger during heavy exercise in a cold environment. Ergonomics 1989; 32:645–653.
93. Nisar M, Spence DPS, West D, Haycock J, Jones Y, Walshaw MJ, Earis JE, Claverley PMA, Pearson MG. A mask to modify inspired air temperature and humidity and its effect on exercise induced asthma. Allergy Proc 1992; 47:446–450.
94. Shturman-Ellstein R, Zeballos RJ, Buckley JM, Souhrada JF. The beneficial effect of nasal breathing on exercise-induced bronchoconstriction. Am Rev Respir Dis 1978; 118:65–73.
95. Mangla PK, Menon MPS. Effect of nasal and oral breathing on exercise-induced asthma. Clin Allergy 1981; 11:433–439.
96. Edmunds A, Tooley M, Godfrey S. The refractory period after exercise-induced asthma: its duration and relation to the severity of exercise. Am Rev Respir Dis 1978; 117:247–254.

97. Schoeffel RE, Anderson SD, Gillam I, Lindsay DA. Multiple exercise and histamine challenge in asthmatic patients. Allergy Proc 1980; 35:164–170.
98. Anderson SD, Schoeffel RE. Respiratory heat and water loss during exercise in patients with asthma: effect of repeated exercise challenge. Eur J Respir Dis 1982; 63:472–480.
99. Reiff DB, Choudry NB, Pride NB, Ind PW. The effect of prolonged submaximal warm-up exercise on exercise-induced asthma. Am Rev Respir Dis 1989; 139:479–484.
100. Schnall RP, Landau LI. Protective effects of repeated short sprints in exercise-induced asthma. Allergy Proc 1980; 35:828–832.
101. Henriksen JM, Dahl R. Effects of inhaled budesonide alone and in combination with low-dose terbutaline in children with exercise-induced asthma. Am Rev Respir Dis 1983; 128:993–997.
102. Ben-Dov I, Bar-Yishay E, Godfrey S. Refractory period after exercise-induced asthma unexplained by respiratory heat loss. Am Rev Respir Dis 1982; 125:530–534.
103. Hahn AG, Nogrady SG, Burton GR, Morton AR. Absence of refractoriness in asthmatic subjects after exercise with warm, humid inspirate. Allergy Proc 1985; 40:418–421.
104. O'Byrne PM, Jones GL. The effect of indomethacin on exercise-induced bronchoconstriction and refractoriness after exercise. Am Rev Respir Dis 1986; 134:69–72.
105. Wilson BA, Bar-Or O, O'Byrne PM. The effects of indomethacin on refractoriness following exercise both with and without bronchoconstriction. Eur Respir J 1994; 12:2174–178.
106. Daviskas E, Anderson SD, Gonda I, Chan HK, Cook P, Fulton R. Changes in mucociliary clearance during and after isocapnic hyperventilation in asthmatic and healthy subjects. Eur Respir J 1995; 8:742–751.
107. Fonkalsrud EW, Sanchez M, Higashijima I, Arima E. A comparative study of the effects of dry vs humidified ventilation on canine lungs. Surgery 1975; 78:373–380.
108. Chalon J, Loew DAY, Malebranche J. Effects of dry anesthetic gases on tracheobronchial ciliated epithelium. Anesthesiology 1972; 37:338–342.
109. Barbet JP, Chauveau N, Labbe S, Lockhart A. Breathing dry air causes acute epithelial damage and inflammation of the guinea pig trachea. J Appl Physiol 1988; 64:1851–1857.
110. Freed AN, Omori C, Schofield BH, Mitzner W. Dry air-induced mucosal cell injury and bronchovascular leakage in canine peripheral airways. Am J Respir Cell Mol Biol 1994; 11:724–732.
111. Omori C, Schofield BH, Mitzner W, Freed AN. Hyperpnea with dry air causes time-dependent alterations in mucosal morphology and bronchovascular permeability. J Appl Physiol 1995; 78:1043–1051.
112. Togias AG, Lykens K, Kagey-Sobotka A, Eggleston PA, Proud D, Naclerio RM. Studies on the relationships between sensitivity to cold dry air, hyperosmolar solutions and histamine in the adult nose. Am Rev Respir Dis 1990; 141:1428–1433.

113. Anderson SD, Togias A. Dry air and hyperosmolar challenge in asthma and rhinitis. In: Busse W, Holgate S, eds. Asthma and rhinitis. Boston: Blackwell Scientific Publications, 1994:1178–1195.
114. Cruz AA, Togias AG, Lichtenstein LM, Kagey-Sobotka A, Proud D, Naclerio RM. Local application of atropine attenuates the upper airway reaction to cold, dry air. Am Rev Respir Dis 1992; 146:340–346.
115. Freed AN, Peters SP, Menkes HA. Airflow-induced bronchoconstriction: role of epithelium and eicosanoid mediators. J Appl Physiol 1987; 62: 574–58.
116. Ray DW, Garland A, Hernandez C, Eappen S, Alger L, Solway J. Time course of bronchoconstriction induced by dry gas hyperpnea in guinea pigs. J Appl Physiol 1991; 70:504–510.
117. Freed AN. Models and mechanisms of exercise-induced asthma. Eur Respir J 1995, 8:1770–1785.
118. Mahler DA, Loke J. Lung function after marathon running at warm and cold ambient temperatures. Am Rev Respir Dis 1981; 124:154–157.
119. Haas F, Pasierski S, Levine N, Bishop M, Axen K, Pineda H, Haas A. Effect of aerobic training on forced expiratory airflow in exercising asthmatic humans. J Appl Physiol 1987; 63:1230–1235.
120. Schaefer O, Eaton RDP, Timmermans FJW, Hildes JA. Respiratory function impairment and cardiopulmonary consequences in long-term residents of the Canadian Arctic. Can Med Assoc J 1980; 123:997–1004.
121. Anderson SD. Exercise-induced asthma. In: Middleton E, Reed C, Ellis E, Adkinson NF, Yunginger JW, eds). Allergy: principles and practice, vol 2. 4th ed. St. Louis: CV Mosby, 1993:1343–1367.
122. Wang D, Chen HI, Chou CL, Hsu K, Freed AN. Terbutaline acts at multiple sites to inhibit bronchoconstriction induced by dry air in canine peripheral airways. Am Rev Respir Dis 1992; 145:1295–1300.
123. Ramage L, Lipworth BJ, Ingram CG, Cree IA, Dhillon DP. Reduced protection against exercise induced bronchoconstriction after chronic dosing with salmeterol. Respir Med 1994; 88:363–368.
124. Rechkemmer GR. The molecular biology of chloride secretion in epithelia. Am Rev Respir Dis 1988; 138:S7–S9.

6

Pathophysiology: Role of Mediators in Exercise-Induced Asthma

Himender K. Makker and Stephen T. Holgate
Southampton General Hospital, Southampton, United Kingdom

I. INTRODUCTION

Exercise causes various cardiorespiratory and neurohormonal adaptive changes to meet an increase in the metabolic demands of exercising muscles. It is believed that an increase in minute ventilation during exercise provides the essential stimulus for exercise-induced bronchoconstriction (EIB) in asthma. During hyperventilation, conditioning of high volumes of inspired air to body temperature and humidity results in loss of heat and water from the airways, causing cooling and drying of airway lining. It is thought that it is these physical changes in the presence of airway inflammation that cause bronchoconstriction. Exercise induces bronchoconstriction in most persons with asthma, provided sufficient workload is given during the exercise, whereas no such response is observed in normal subjects (Fig. 1). Asthmatic airways contain greater numbers of activated inflammatory cells—mast cells, eosinophils, and neutrophils—than are present in normal airways. These inflammatory cells are the source of highly potent constrictor mediators, some preformed and others newly generated, that can be released by appropriate stimulation. It is proposed that physical changes in the airway lining, induced by exercise, cause release of constrictor mediators from airway inflammatory cells, leading to exercise-induced bronchoconstriction.

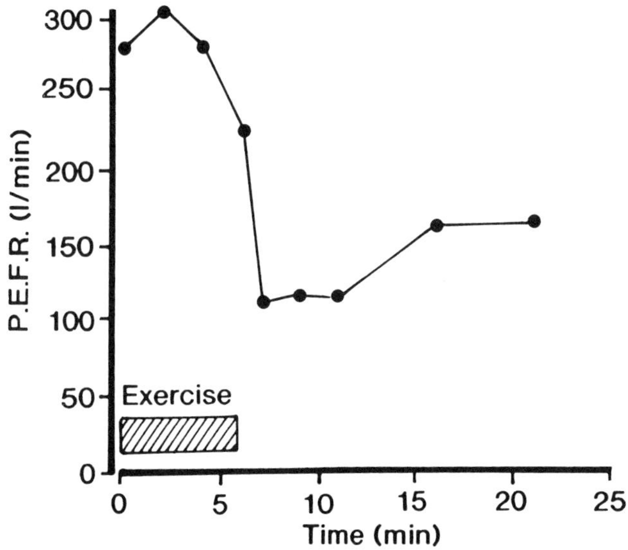

Fig. 1 The response of asthmatic airway to exercise showing initial bronchodilation during the exercise, followed by bronchoconstriction.

The role of mediator release in exercise-induced asthma (EIA) has been investigated by detecting the mediators in body fluids following exercise challenge, and by determining the effect of specific antagonists or inhibitors of synthesis on the exercise-induced airway response. The pharmacological approach provides indirect, but conclusive, evidence for the mediator release, whereas detection of mediators in body fluids, although direct, provides only circumstantial evidence for specific exercise-related release.

II. CONTRIBUTION OF MEDIATOR RELEASE TO EXERCISE-INDUCED BRONCHOCONSTRICTION

A. Histamine

Histamine is stored preformed in the secretory granules of mast cells and basophils. In EIA, hypertonicity of the airway lining fluid, owing to evaporative water loss during exercise, is thought to provide stimulus for mast cell degranulation and histamine release [1]. In vitro studies have demonstrated that hypertonic solutions induce dose-dependent mast cell histamine release that peaks between 1 and 5 min after challenge, similar to the timing of peak bronchoconstriction following exercise [2,3]. Moreover, temperature and osmolarity for optimal histamine release are similar to directly recorded airway temperature and osmolarity of airway lining fluid during the hyperventilation of exercise [4,5]. In asthma, inhalation of histamine induces bronchonconstriction by acting on H_1-receptors present on airway smooth muscle and on the microvascular bed. The time course of histamine-induced bronchoconstriction, which peaks within 1–4 min and on average lasts for 20 min, is similar to that of exercise-induced bronchoconstriction.

The role of histamine release in EIA was first suggested in 1968 by Davies, when it was shown that sodium cromoglycate (a drug known to be an inhibitor of mast cell-mediator release) given before exercise inhibited EIA [6]. Because histamine was thought to be the main preformed constrictor mediator released from mast cells, histamine H_1-receptor antagonists have been employed to examine further the role of histamine in EIA. Eiser [7] observed a 40–50% protection after intravenous chlorpheniramine administration, whereas Hartley and Norgrady [8] found 50% protection with inhaled clemastine. In these studies, the maximum dose of H_1-receptor blockade could not be achieved because of the sedating effect of the antihistamines. Furthermore, bronchodilation caused by an anticholinergic effect made it difficult to assess the protection given by histamine H_1-receptor blockade alone.

With the development of highly selective and potent histamine H_1-receptor antagonists, such as terfenadine, it became possible to assess the effect of more complete H_1-receptor blockade on EIA. Different studies have found a consistent protection of about 30% with terfenadine (Fig. 2); higher doses of terfenadine provided no further increase in protection [9–11]. Moreover, cetirizine, a more potent H_1-receptor antagonist, provided no more protection than that observed with terfenadine [12]. However, when cetirizine was given by inhalation a much greater dose-dependent protection was observed; 40% with 5 mg and 60% with 10 mg (Table 1). This suggests that local tissue concentrations of the antihistamine are most relevant to its protective efficacy against EIA. It is possible that, with the inhaled route, higher tissue concentrations of the drug are achieved at the site where histamine produces its H_1-receptor-mediated smooth-muscle constriction and increased microvascular permeability.

In addition to providing pharmacological probes, histamine H_1-receptor antagonists have helped in determining the contribution of stimulus provided by hypertonicity of airway lining fluid and hyperventilation to bronchoconstriction in EIA. Finnerty and co-workers compared the protective effect of terfenadine at a single 120-mg dose against exercise-,

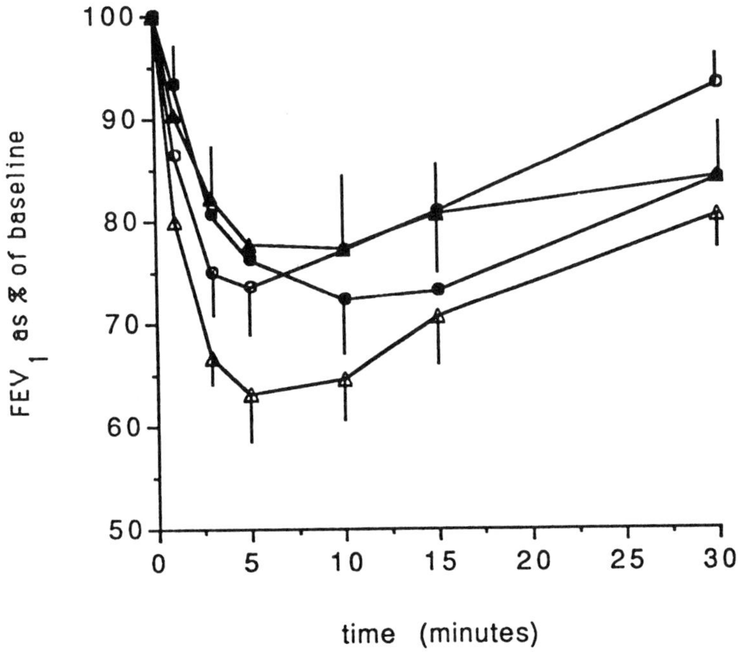

Fig. 2 Percentage fall in FEV_1 over 30 min from baseline values before exercise; following exercise challenge for each of the drug treatments; placebo (△—△); terfenadine (▲—▲); flurbiprofen (○—○); and flurbiprofen plus terfenadine (●—●).

hyperventilation-, and hypertonic saline-induced bronchoconstriction and found 23.8, 43.7, and 56.4% protection, respectively [11,13,14]. These findings suggest that the stimulus provided by hypertonicity and hyperventilation can only partly explain EIA.

Although studies with histamine H_1-receptor antagonists provided useful evidence in support of a contributory role of histamine release in EIA, it has proved difficult to demonstrate direct evidence for such release. In earlier studies blood histamine levels were measured only in asthmatics, with no controls [15]. Moreover, not all asthmatics developed exercise-induced bronchoconstriction following exercise. Some studies did find a rise in blood histamine levels in relation to EIA, but a similar rise was also observed in normal subjects [16,17]. The rise in histamine appeared to be related more to an increase in circulating basophils than to mast cell activation. Anderson and co-workers reported a rise in arterial

Table 1 Effect of Mediator Receptor Antagonists on Exercise-Induced Bronchoconstriction

Mediator	Dose and route	Average protection (range; %)	Refs.
Histamine H_1 receptor antagonists			
Clemastine	0.5 mg inhaled	40	17
Chlorpheniramine	20 mg intravenously	40–50	7
Terfenadine	60 mg orally		9,10,11
	60–180 mg orally	30	
	180 mg orally		
Cetirizine	10 mg orally bid × 1 week	No	
	5 mg inhaled	40	12
	10 mg inhaled	60	
Prostaglandin inhibition			
Indomethacin	50 mg orally bid × 3 days	None	39
Flurbiprofen	150 mg orally	30	11
Thromboxane receptor antagonists			
GR 32191 (vapiprost)	120 mg orally	None	41
BAYu 3405 (ramatroban)	20 mg orally	None	42
Leukotriene D_4 receptor antagonists			
MK-571	160 mg intravenously	69.5	30
ICI 204,219 (zafirlukast)	20 mg orally	44	31
SKF 104353 (pobilukast)	800 μg inhaled	31	32
ICI 204,219 (zafirlukast)	400 μg inhaled	48	33

plasma histamine in five asthmatic subjects with bronchoconstriction provoked by exercise, with the level of increase corresponding to the degree of bronchoconstriction achieved [18]. However, no similar rise was seen in a further four asthmatics with exercise-induced bronchoconstriction who had lower baseline plasma histamine levels. Similarly, by using an improved assay for histamine measurement, Barnes and Brown [19] were able to demonstrate a significant rise in venous plasma histamine during exercise in subjects with exercise-induced bronchoconstriction. However, results of these studies could not be confirmed by others [20]. When the same group repeated their earlier study and care was taken with sample handling to exclude basophil degranulation, the exercise-induced bronchoconstriction was not associated with a rise in plasma histamine [21]. Furthermore, higher baseline plasma histamine levels observed in the asthmatics were due to increase in spontaneous basophil release or "leaky basophils" [22]. Thus, because of various methodological problems with measurement of blood histamine, one must conclude that, altogether, the various studies have failed to provide any conclusive evidence in support of histamine release in EIA.

It was felt that plasma histamine levels may not reflect local airway levels of histamine, and local airway, rather than peripheral blood, levels of histamine are likely to be more relevant to the causation of airway narrowing. To address this issue, fiber-optic bronchoscopy has been employed to obtain bronchoalveolar lavage (BAL) fluid for the measurement of airway levels of mediators. Following hyperventilation-induced bronchoconstriction Pliss and colleagues [23] found an increase in the levels of histamine in the BAL fluid; in contrast Brodie and co-workers [24] compared histamine levels in BAL pre- and postexercise, in seven subjects with EIA, and found no significant rise. Similar results have been obtained by Jarjour and co-workers [25]. However, these studies received criticism for the methods employed, because there was an appreciable delay in obtaining the lavage fluid after completing the exercise task. In addition, the lavage was performed in the presence of β_2-agonists. Because of the short half-life of histamine, and delay in obtaining lavage fluid after providing the exercise stimulus, histamine concentrations measured in BAL fluid are most unlikely to accurately reflect the airway levels of histamine pertinent to the onset of exercise-induced bronchoconstriction, especially because β_2-agonists are potent inhibitors of mast cell histamine release [26]. With the technique of isolated airway segment lavage, Jarjour et al. also failed to demonstrate any rise in local airway levels of histamine in EIA [27]. Similarly, we have performed local airway challenge with hypertonic saline in asthmatics with a history of EIA and obtained BAL fluid and biopsy samples immediately following the observed hypertonic saline-induced bronchoconstriction, without premedication with β_2-agonist [28]. However, even with these modifications and improvements in methods, we failed to find an increase in histamine levels or evidence of increased mast cell degranulation over those present at baseline in EIA. In the face of these antihistamine studies, we are left to conclude that BAL lacks sufficient sensitivity for the detection of small changes in histamine levels.

B. Leukotriene Release

The sulfidopeptide leukotrienes (LTs) are generated by 5-lipoxygenase modification of arachidonic acid, followed by conjugation with the tripeptide glutathione. The initial product is LTC_4, followed by LTD_4 and LTE_4, resulting from the sequential cleavage of the terminal amino acid. Leukotrienes are all bronchoconstrictors in asthma, being 100–1000 times more potent than histamine, and have a relative activity of $LTD_4 > LTC_4 > LTE_4$ [29]. The bronchoconstrictor effect of sulfidopeptide leukotrienes results from the activation of specific cell surface receptors. Their physiological affects can be modulated either through the inhibition of formation by 5-lipoxygenase or by high-affinity, specific LTD_4-receptor antagonists. Several studies have clearly shown attenuation of exercise-induced bronchoconstriction with selective LTD_4-receptor antagonists [30–33]. Among these, Manning and co-workers [30] have reported significant attenuation of exercise-induced bronchoconstriction with the leukotriene antagonist MK-571, given intravenously 20 min before to exercise. The mean percentage inhibition for the group was 69.5%, with almost complete inhibition in four subjects and partial inhibition in the remainder. Further studies have confirmed the protective effect of other LTD_4-receptor antagonists, including zafirlukast (ICI 204,219; Accolate) and pobilukast (SKF 104353) [31–33]. In our studies a single dose of oral or inhaled zafirlukast (ICI 204,219) given before exercise, produced an overall 50% protection against exercise-induced asthma [31,33] (Fig. 3). Together, these studies provide convincing evidence for a role of leukotriene release in EIA. When comparing H_1-antagonist with LTD_4 antagonists, it appears that the former are active on the early component of the exercise-provoked narrowing, whereas the latter have a greater effect on the terminal phase of airway narrowing, suggesting a different time course of release of the two mediator classes.

However, as with histamine, it has been difficult to demonstrate leukotriene release in the lavage fluid or the presence of appropriate metabolites in the urine with conventional assays [24,25,34]. This does not mean that leukotrienes are not generated after exercise, but as with histamine, once released, their recovery and measurement is particularly difficult. With an improved method for urinary leukotriene assay, Kikawa and co-workers found increased levels of urinary LTE_4, the chief metabolite of LTD_4 after an exercise challenge in asthmatic children [35].

Although, leukotrienes undoubtedly contribute to EIA, their cellular provenance is unknown. The most likely source is mast cells, the mediator release threshold of which is reduced in asthma, possibly because of prim-

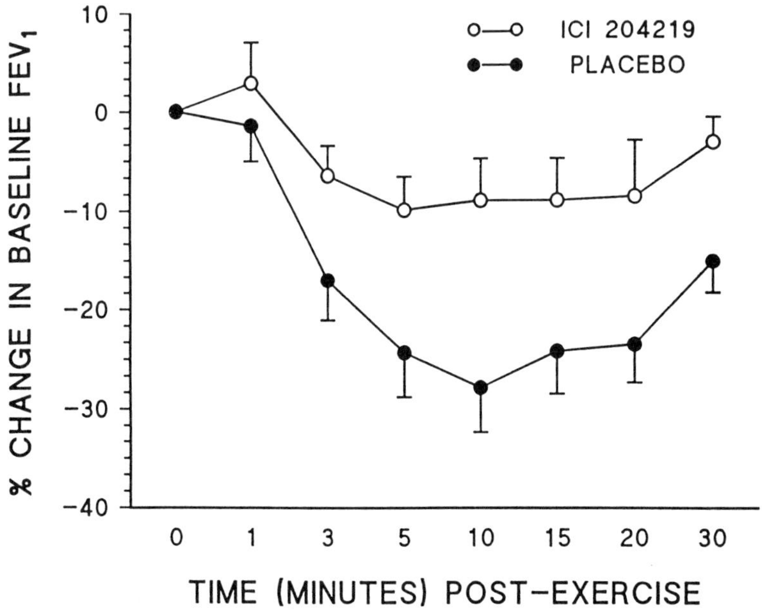

Fig. 3 Mean (±SEM) change in the baseline FEV_1 expressed as percentage of the baseline at each time point after exercise challenge following inhaled leukotriene D_4-antagonist zafirlukast (ICI 204,219; 400 μg) (○—○) and placebo (●—●).

ing by cytokines, such as interleukin-4 (IL-4), tumor necrosis factor-α (TNF-α), and mast cell growth factor (MCGF) itself (stem cell factor; SCF). Monocytes, macrophages, and eosinophils are also important sources of leukotrienes, but any mechanisms for their activation with exercise are unknown.

C. Prostanoid Release

Prostanoids are derived from the cyclooxygenation of arachidonic acid and comprise the biologically active prostaglandins (PGs) and thromboxane (Tx)A_2. Some of the cyclooxygenase products, such as PGD_2, $PGF_{2\alpha}$, and TxA_2 are potent bronchoconstrictors, whereas other prostaglandins—PDE_2 and PGI_2—possess bronchodilator and antibronchoconstrictor properties [36].

Asthmatic airways contain higher levels of constrictor prostanoids such as PGD_2 when compared with airways of normal subjects. Inhalation of PGD_2 aerosol induces a dose-dependent bronchoconstriction in asthmatics by acting through the thromboxane TP_1 receptor on airway smooth muscle. Prostaglandin D_2 is the major cyclooxygenase product of human mast cells, and mast cells are likely to be its major source. However, because of chemical instability in body fluid and limited specificity and sensitivity of the PGD_2 assay, it has proved difficult to demonstrate any rise in the plasma or BAL levels of this mediator or its metabolite in EIA [24,37]. One problem associated with measurement of circulating prostanoids is their short half-life. Thromboxane A_2 release has also been implicated in the pathogenesis of EIA, but it is difficult to measure in the body fluid because it is highly unstable and rapidly metabolized into its inactive metabolite TxB_2. However, it is possible to measure TxB_2, and increased urinary excretion has been reported by Morris and co-workers [38] in exercise-induced asthma. If endogenously released prostanoids contribute to EIA, it should be possible to prevent or attenuate exercise-induced bronchoconstriction by either inhibiting their synthesis or antagonizing their target receptors. This has been examined with cyclooxygenase inhibitors by determining the effect of thromboxane receptor antagonists and modulation of prostaglandin synthesis on exercise-induced bronchoconstriction. No protection was observed when the cyclooxygenase inhibitor indomethacin was used, but flurbiprofen (which is ten times more potent than indomethacin) did provide 30% protection against EIA [31,39] (see Fig. 2). Similarly, the TxA_2 synthase inhibitor ozagrel (OKY-046) inhibited EIA in 7 of 11 subjects studied [40]. However, no protection could be demonstrated with the thromboxane (TP_1) receptor antagonist vapiprost (GR32191), whereas this inhibitor showed good inhibition of PGD_2-induced bronchoconstriction [41]. Another highly potent thromboxane-receptor antagonist, ramatroban (BAY u 3405), has also been ineffective in attenuating exercise-induced bronchoconstriction [42]. These conflicting results showing attenuation of exercise-induced bronchoconstriction with cyclooxygenase inhibitors, but not with thromboxane-receptor antagonists, may be due to the difference in the contribution of different types of constrictor prostanoids to EIA, with $PGF_{2\alpha}$ probably more important than PGD_2.

III. ROLE OF BRONCHODILATOR PROSTANOIDS AND HEPARIN RELEASE IN MODULATION OF EXERCISE-INDUCED BRONCHOCONSTRICTION

A. Prostaglandin E_2

Inhalation of PGE_2 causes bronchodilation in asthmatics and antagonizes the effect of constrictor prostaglandins [43]. Prostaglandin E_2 is present in the airways in much higher concentration than in blood [44]. Because smooth-muscle contraction itself can generate PGE_2, it is possible that bronchoconstriction during exercise induces PGE_2 release, which can modulate the bronchoconstrictor effect of constrictor prostanoids. Cyclooxygenase inhibitors are likely to inhibit the synthesis of both constrictor and bronchodilator prostanoids, and their net protective effect in EIA would depend on the relative amount of constrictor and dilator prostanoids present at a given moment in the airways. It has been further proposed that PGE_2 release contributes to the refractoriness following EIA, because this phenomenon is inhibited by cyclooxygenase inhibitors [39,45].

Alteration in the generation of PGE_2 may also contribute to exercise-induced bronchoconstriction. The protective effect of inhaled furosemide in EIA is thought to be mediated by PGE_2 generation, because treatment with cyclooxygenase inhibitor before furosemide inhalation abolishes its protective effect [46]. Furthermore, inhalation of PGE_2 before exercise markedly attenuates exercise-induced bronchoconstriction [47]. These studies provide at least some evidence of a role for bronchodilator prostanoids in EIA. Thus, it is plausible that an alteration in the ratio of constrictor and bronchodilator prostanoids generated during exercise partly accounts for exercise-induced bronchoconstriction.

B. Heparin

Mast cell degranulation and mediator release occur through a series of cellular events involving generation of inositol triphosphate and intracellular calcium mobilization. Heparin is one of the many preformed mediators present in the secretory granules of human mast cells and released during mast cell degranulation [48]. Heparin is a selective inositol receptor antagonist and blocks inositol triphosphate-mediated calcium mobilization [49]. Thus, it is possible that heparin release during mast cell degranulation interferes with signal transduction and further mast cell degranulation and mediator release. It has been proposed that failure of this self-regulatory function of heparin may be a cause of exercise-induced asthma. The view has been supported by a study by Ahmed and co-workers demonstrating inhibition of exercise-induced bronchoconstriction with inhaled heparin given before exercise [50]. Inhaled heparin reduced exercise-provoked bronchoconstriction by 70% and had no significant effect on coagulation. Furthermore, heparin was more effective in preventing exercise-induced bronchoconstriction than an established agent, cromolyn sodium.

IV. ROLE OF INFLAMMATORY CELL ACTIVATION IN THE PATHOGENESIS OF EIA

It is believed that an essential stimulus for exercise-induced bronchoconstriction is provided by the cooling and drying of the airways caused by evaporative water loss during hyperventilation. However, there is increasing evidence to suggest that exercise itself can lead to the activation of proinflammatory cells, such as mast cells, eosinophils, and neutrophils. The mechanism(s) of bronchoconstriction in relation to the inflammatory cell activation in EIA is speculative. Nevertheless, observations point to an important link between airway inflammatory changes in asthma and development of exercise-induced bronchoconstriction.

A. Mast Cell Activation

An increase in the activity of neutrophil chemotactic factor (NCF) is associated with mast cell activation and mediator release; therefore, NCF has been used as a marker for mast cell activation in EIA [51]. The exact molecular nature of NCF has not been characterized, but its heat stability and high molecular weight suggest that it is a member of the chemokine family (e.g., IL-8) and a serum protein (possibly fibronectin or α_2-macroglobulin). An increase in serum levels of NCF occurs in EIA, although this is not reproduced by isocapnic hyperventilation [52]. This suggests a direct influence of exercise on NCF release, possibly from mast cells. Crimi and co-workers have provided direct evidence for mast cell activation in EIA by demonstrating that the percentage of mast cell degranulation in bronchial biopsies after EIA is greater than after methacholine challenge [53]. However, we have been unable to confirm this, suggesting that if mast cells are important, it is those at the very surface of the airways that are involved in mediator release [28].

B. Neutrophil Activation

Neutrophil activation occurs in EIA, as suggested by an increase in the expression of neutrophil complement receptors [54]. Activated neutrophils have enhanced cytotoxicity and LTB_4 generation [55,56]. These changes in neutrophil activation and cytotoxicity are preceded by an increase in the NCF activity and further suggest that mediator release contributes to the pathogenesis of EIA.

C. Eosinophil Activation

There is some recent evidence to suggest eosinophil activation in EIA. Venge and colleagues examined eosinophil activation in EIA by measuring the eosinophilic cationic protein (ECP) in the serum; they found a rise in ECP levels in subjects with exercise-induced bronchoconstriction [57]. Baseline ECP levels in subjects with EIA were higher than in subjects without EIA, and correlated with the fall in peak flow rate. The exact mechanism by which eosinophilic activation contributes to exercise-induced bronchoconstriction is unknown. It is possible that an increase in ECP release from activated eosinophils during EIA is associated with increased generation of sulfidopeptide leukotrienes and platelet-activating factor (PAF).

D. Platelet Activation

There have been some attempts to link platelet activation and release of platelet factors to the development of exercise-induced bronchoconstriction. Johnson and co-workers examined the role of platelet activation in EIA by measuring the plasma levels of platelet factor 4 and β-thromboglobulin [58]. They found an increase in platelet factors' release in subjects with exercise-induced bronchoconstriction, but no change in normal subjects. The attenuation of exercise-induced bronchoconstriction by prior treatment with albuterol (salbutamol) or sodium cromoglycate was also associated with inhibition of the rise in platelet factors. The stimulus for platelet activation and the mechanism(s) of bronchoconstriction caused by platelet activation remain to be defined. However, it has been suggested that release of PAF from airway inflammatory cells may provide the necessary stimulus for platelet activation. Prior treatment with a PAF antagonist inhibits the rise in release of platelet factors and of bronchoconstriction caused by exercise [59].

E. T Lymphocytes

The T lymphocytes have been proposed as the orchestrating cell in the pathogenesis of asthma, and exercise can alter the immune response. Therefore, Bury and co-workers examined the effect of exercise challenge on T-lymphocyte proliferation in patients with EIA [60]. T lymphocytes in the peripheral blood significantly reduced spontaneous and phytohemagglutinin (PHA)-induced proliferation, whereas no such abnormality was observed in the normal subjects.

V. CONTRIBUTION OF NEUROHORMONAL CHANGES IN EIA

A. Catecholamine Release

Although human airways are not innervated by adrenergic supply, circulating catecholamines can stimulate airway β_2-adrenoreceptors and cause bronchodilation. Furthermore, stimulation of pulmonary mast cells by β_2-adrenoreceptors inhibits mediator release [61]. Thus, it is possible that in asthma an impaired sympathoadrenal response to exercise may facilitate mast cell mediator release and contribute to exercise-induced bronchoconstriction. A reduced sympathoadrenal response has been reported in EIA by some investigators [62,63]. However, in these studies there was no standardization of the work load administered; asthmatics received less work load than normal subjects. When the work load was carefully matched, the reduced sympathoadrenal response to exercise could not be confirmed [64–66]. Nevertheless, Tsuda and co-workers [67] found that those patients with asthma who developed exercise-induced bronchoconstriction had a smaller rise in circulating norepinephrine than those who failed to exhibit an airway constrictor response (1.5-fold versus 4-fold increase from baseline) [67].

Whether reduced sympathoadrenal response contributes to EIA remains controversial, but there is convincing evidence to support the idea that catecholamine release *during* the exercise contributes to initial bronchodilation after the exercise challenge, as well as to modulating exercise-induced bronchoconstriction [66]. Catecholamine release during the exercise is related to the level of muscle activity because there is no rise in circulating levels during isocapnic hyperventilation [62]. Plasma catecholamines levels exactly mirror the fluctuation in airway size in EIA, rising with bronchodilation and falling with bronchoconstriction. An increase in the sympathoadrenal activity with repetitive exercise modifies the severity of postexercise bronchoconstriction [68].

B. Atrial Natriuretic Peptide

Atrial natriuretic peptide (ANP), a smooth-muscle relaxant, was originally discovered in the cardiac granules in atrial muscle and released in response to atrial stretch [69]. Its synthesis has also been detected in the lung, and it reduces bronchomotor tone in normal subjects and causes bronchodilation in patients with asthma [70–72]. Exercise induces a rise in the circulating levels of ANP both in asthmatic and normal subjects, but no similar rise has been observed following isocapnic hyperventilation [73]. This suggests that the stimulus for ANP release is provided by exercise alone, possibly owing to an associated increase in adrenergic response and heart rate, or to an increase in central blood volume. It has also been suggested that bronchoconstriction itself might induce ANP release. Whatever the reason, the levels of circulating ANP with exercise are similar to those able to cause bronchodilatation and to reduce nonspecific bronchial hyperresponsiveness [74]. It is possible that ANP's release reduces the airway response to exercise and, in this negative way, protects against EIA.

C. Neuropeptide Release

Broncho- and vasoactive neuropeptides are released from sensory, parasympathetic, and sympathetic neurons in the respiratory tract. These nonmyelinated C fibers are sensitized to a range of inflammatory mediators. For example, bronchoconstriction caused by kinins (bradykinin) in asthma is mediated by release of substance P, neurokinin A, and calcitonin gene-related peptide (CGRP) [75]. The possible association between the activity of the kinin system and EIA has been examined by Neuman and colleagues [76]. They have suggested that provocation of EIA is associated with a certain threshold level of kallikrein, below which no symptoms occur, EIA being triggered when this threshold is exceeded. Havidsten and co-workers [77] measured plasma concentrations of various gastrointestinal regulatory peptides in relation to EIA, and found a significant rise in plasma vasoactive intestinal polypeptide (VIP) and cholecystokinin. It has also been suggested that hypertonicity of airway-lining fluid during exercise causes local airways release of neuropeptides from exposed nerve endings present in the asthmatic airways. Umeno and co-workers have shown that hypertonic saline induces neurogenic inflammation in the rat trachea and inhibition of neutral endopeptidase, an enzyme that cleaves and inactivates the neuropeptides and potentiates the neurogenic inflammatory response [78].

D. Release of Endogenous Opioids

Exercise induces an increase in endogenous opioids, including β-endorphin and met-enkephalin, in addition to corticotropin (adrenocorticotropic hormone; ACTH). Endogenous opioids have been reported to cause mast cell degranulation, and speculation has arisen that their release may have a role in EIA. If this is true, then opiate antagonism should attenuate the bronchoconstrictor response to exercise. However, when given intravenously or orally, opiate receptor antagonists failed to provide any protection against exercise-induced bronchoconstriction, but when naloxone was locally delivered by inhalation to the airways, the bronchoconstrictor response was attenuated [79–81]. Furthermore, inhibition of EIA with naloxone was not the result of the bronchodilator effect or some influence on ventilation. Thus, it remains possible that the endogenous opioid release during exercise may contribute to the pathogenesis of EIA.

VI. SUMMARY

There is sufficient evidence to suggest that release of constrictor mediators, histamine, sulfidopeptide leukotrienes, and prostaglandins provides an important contribution to exercise-induced bronchoconstriction. The bronchoconstrictor response cannot be explained by release of any single mediator, and the relative contribution of different constrictor mediators is likely to vary among subjects. In some, the response may be mediated by leukotrienes, whereas in others, by histamine. In most, however, it is likely to be the result of a combined effect of different constrictor mediators. Difficulty in demonstrating systemic or local mediator release in EIA is probably because of technical problems. Measurement of small quantities of mediator in BAL is probably insufficiently sensitive to detect a transient rise in the mediators that occurs in EIA. The dilution of mediators from a small area of the airways with a large amount of fluid renders the detection of small changes difficult. Inhibition of exercise-induced bronchoconstriction with histamine H_1-receptor antagonists, cylcooxygenase inhibitors, lipoxygenase inhibitors, and LTD_4-receptor antagonists, when mediator release could not be detected in blood or BAL fluid, suggests that relative concentrations of mediators in biological fluids may not necessarily reflect their clinical importance. It is also possible that, with exercise, mediators are released as a short pulse into the airways, but do not achieve concentrations that are detectable in body fluids, or that their peaks are not at the time of sampling.

Studies investigating the role of mediator release in EIA, so far, have taken a simplistic view of EIA. It was believed that physical changes of airway cooling and drying caused by hyperventilation, induce the release of constrictor mediators and cause bronchoconstriction. Effects of exercise itself on inflammatory cell activation, neurohormonal release, and cardiovascular system were largely ignored. This led investigators to substitute hyperventilation and hypertonic saline challenge for exercise to study the role of mediator release. However, it is now clear that hyperventilation and hypertonicity of airway-lining fluid provide only a part of the stimulus for EIA. Thus, it is not surprising that, despite a large number of studies investigating the mechanisms of EIA over the last 25 years, there is no consensus on the exact stimulus for the exercise-induced bronchoconstriction.

It is clear that release of constrictor mediators alone cannot fully explain the complex phenomenon of EIA. There is accumulating evidence to suggest the role of regulatory mechanisms, such as release of bronchodilating prostanoids and heparin, in modifying the bronchoconstrictor response to exercise. Furthermore, neurohormonal changes during exercise, such as the increase in catecholamines, atrial natriuretric peptide, neuropeptides, and endogenous opioids, can affect bronchomotor tone and airway reactivity, and are likely to have an important role in further modulating of the bronchoconstrictor response to exercise. Exercise-induced bronchoconstriction probably represents dynamic equilibrium between the release of constrictor and bronchodilator mediators and the mechanisms that modulate the release and effect of these mediators. The relevance of inflammatory cell activation to the pathogenesis of exercise-induced bronchoconstriction is as yet unclear, but it reaffirms the multifaceted and complex natures of changes in EIA (Fig. 4). Fortunately, a simple approach of treatment with the inhaled bronchodilator sodium

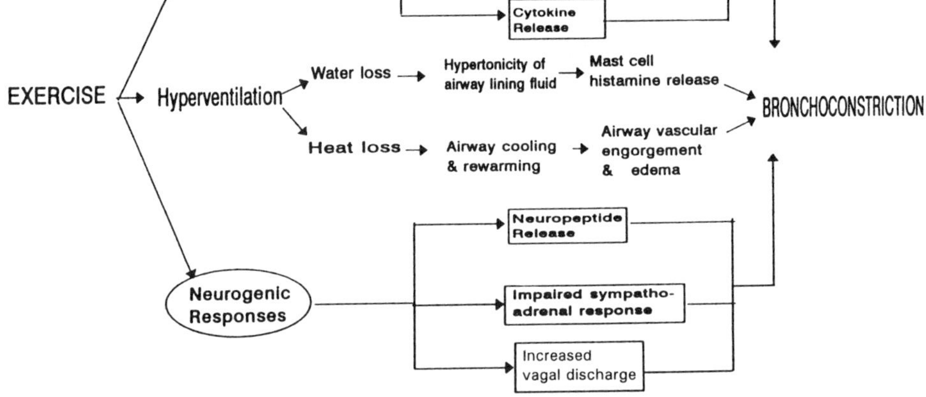

Fig. 4 Schematic representation of physiological mechanisms proposed for exercise-induced bronchoconstriction.

cromoglycate and, over the longer term, topical corticosteroids is successful in preventing exercise-induced bronchoconstriction in most subjects with asthma.

REFERENCES

1. Anderson SD. Is there a unifying hypothesis for exercise-induced asthma? J Allergy Clin Immunol 1984; 73:660–665.
2. Eggleston PA, Kagey-Sobotka A, Schleimer RB, Lichenstein LM. Interaction between IgE-mediated histamine release from basophils and mast cells. Am Rev Respir Dis 1984; 130:86–91.
3. Eggleston PA, Kagey-Sobotka A, Lichenstein LM. A comparison of the osmotic activation of basophils and human lung mast cells. Am Rev Respir Dis 1987; 135:1043–1048.
4. Smith CM, Anderson SD. Hyperosmolarity as the stimulus to asthma induced by hyperventilation. J Allergy Clin Immunol 1986; 77:729–736.
5. Gilbert IA, Fouke JM, McFadden ER Jr. Heat and water flux in intrathoracic airways and exercise-induced asthma. J Appl Physiol 1987; 63:1681–1691.
6. Davies SE. The effect of disodium cromoglycate on exercise-induced asthma. Br Med J 1968; 3:593–594.
7. Eiser NM. Histamine antagonists and asthma. Pharmacol Ther 1982; 17: 239–250.
8. Hartley JPR, Norgrady SG. Effect of inhaled antihistamine on exercise-induced asthma. Thorax 1980; 35:675–679.
9. Patel KR. Terfenadine in exercise-induced asthma. Br Med J 1987; 288: 1496–1497.
10. McFarlane PI, Heaf DP. Selective histamine blockade in childhood asthma: the effect of terfenadine on resting bronchial tone and exercise-induced bronchoconstriction. Respir Med 1989; 83:19–24.
11. Finnerty JP, Twentyman OP, Harris A, Palmer JBD, Holgate ST. Effect of GR 32191, a potent thromboxane receptor antagonist, on exercise induced bronchoconstriction in asthma. Thorax 1991; 46:190–192.
12. Ghosh SK, DeVos C, McIlory I, Patel KR. Effect of cetirizine on exercise-induced asthma. Thorax 1991; 46:242–244.
13. Finnerty JP, Wilmot C, Holgate ST. Inhibition of hypertonic saline-bronchoconstriction by terfenadine and flurbiprofen. Am Rev Respir Dis 1989; 140: 593–597.
14. Finnerty JP, Holgate ST. Evidence of the role of histamine and prostaglandins as mediators in exercise-induced asthma: the inhibitory effect of terfenadine and flurbiprofen alone and in combination. Eur Respir J 1990; 3:540–557.
15. Karr RM, Brach BB, Wilson MR, Anicetti V, Salvaggio JE. Changes in levels of arterial blood histamine during exercise-induced asthma. J Allergy Clin Immunol 1979; 63:154.

16. Harries MG, Burge PS, O'Brien I, Cromwell O, Pepys J. Blood histamine levels after exercise testing. J Allergy Clin Immunol 1979; 9:437–441.
17. Hartley JPR, Charles TJ, Monie DH, Seaton A, Taylor WH, Westwood A, Williams JD. Arterial plasma histmine after exercise in normal individuals and in patients with exercise-induced asthma. Clin Sci 1981; 61:151–157.
18. Anderson SD, Bye PTP, Schoeffel RE, Seale JP, Taylor KM. Arterial plasma histamine level at rest, and during and after exercise in patients with asthma: effects of terbutaline aerosol. Thorax 1981; 36:259–267.
19. Barnes PJ, Brown MJ. Plasma venous histamine in exercise and hyperventilation-induced asthma. Clin Sci 1981; 61:661–665.
20. Morgan DJR, Phillips MJ, Moodley I, Elliott EV, Davies RJ. Histamine, neutrophil chemotactic factor and circulating basophils levels following exercise in asthmatic and control subjects. Clin Allergy 1982; 12(suppl):29–27.
21. Ind PW, Barnes PJ, Brown MJ, Causon R, Dollery CT. Measurement of plasma histamine in asthma. Clin Allergy 1983; 13:61–67.
22. Howarth PH, Pao GJK, Church MK, Holgate ST. Exercise and isocapnic hyperventilation-induced bronchoconstriction in asthma: relevance of circulating basophils to measurements of plasma histamine. J Allergy Clin Immunol 1984; 73:391–399.
23. Pliss LB, Ingentio EP, Ingram RH Jr, Pichurko B. Assessment of bronchoalveolar cell and mediator response to isocapnic hyperpnea in asthma. Am Rev Respir Dis 1990; 142:73–78.
24. Brodie DH, Eisman S, Ramsdell JW, Fergusson P, Schwartz LB, Wasserman SI. Airway levels of mast cell-derived mediators in exercise-induced asthma. Am Rev Respir Dis 1990; 141:563–568.
25. Jarjour NN, Calhoun WJ, Stevens CA, Salisbury BS. Exercise-induced asthma is not associated with mast cell activation or airway inflammation. J Allergy Clin Immunol 1992; 89:60–68.
26. Church MK, Young KD. The characteristics of inhibition of histamine release from human lung fragments by sodium cromoglycate, salbutamol, and chlorpromazine. Br J Pharmacol 1983; 68:671–679.
27. Jarjour NN, Calhoun WJ, Reed HE, Murphy K, Stevens CA, Swenson CA. The use of double lumen balloon catheter for serial sampling of airway secretions in exercise induced asthma [abstract]. Am Rev Respir Dis 1992; 145: A23.
28. Makker HK, Walls AF, Goulding D, Montefort S, Varley JG, Carroll M, Howarth P, Holgate ST. Airways effects of local challenge with hypertonic saline in exercise-induced asthma. Am J Respir Crit Care Med 1994; 149: 1012–1019.
29. Drazen JM, Austen KF. Leukotrienes and airway responses. Am Rev Respir Dis 1987; 136:985–988.
30. Manning PJ, Watson RM, Margolskee DJ, Williams VC, Schwartz JI, O'Byrne PM. Inhibition of exercise-induced bronchoconstriction by MK-571, a potent leukotriene D_4-receptor antagonist. N Engl J Med 1990; 323: 1736–1739.

31. Finnerty JP, Wood-Baker R, Thomson H, Holgate ST. Role of leukotrienes in exercise-induced asthma: inhibitory effect of ICI 204, 219, a potent leukotriene D_4-receptor antagonist. Am Rev Respir Dis 1992; 145:746–749.
32. Robushi M, Riva E, Fuccella LM, Vida E, Barnabe R, Rossi M, Gambaro G, Spagnotto S, Bianco S. Prevention of exercise-induced bronchoconstriction by a new leukotriene antagonist (SKF 104353): a double-blind study versus disodium cromoglycate and placebo. Am Rev Respir Dis 1992; 145: 1285–1288.
33. Makker HK, Lau LC, Thomson HW, Binks SM, Holgate ST. The protective effect of inhaled leukotriene D_4-receptor antagonist ICI 204,219 against exercise-induced asthma. Am Rev Respir Med 1993; 147:1413–1418.
33. Field J, Allergra J, Trautelin J, Demers L, Gillin M, Zelis R. Measurement of plasma prostaglandins during exercise-induced bronchospasm. J Allergy Clin Immunol 1976; 58:581–585.
34. Taylor JK, Welling R, Taylor GW, Fuller RW. Urinary leukotriene E_4 (LTE_4) excretion in exercise-induced bronchoconstriction. Am Rev Respir Dis 1992; 145:A15.
35. Kikawa Y, Miyanomae T, Inoue Y, Saito M, Nakai A, Shigematsu Y, Hosoi S, Sudo M. Urinary leukotriene E_4 after exercise challenge in children with asthma. J Allergy Clin Immunol 1992; 89:1111–1119.
36. Robinson C, Holgate ST. The synthesis, release and effects of prostaglandins in lung. In: Kay AB, ed. Asthma, clinical pharmacology and therapeutic progress. Oxford: Blackwell 1986; 221–225.
38. Morris HG, Sherman NA, Sheppardson FT. Effect of aspirin on plasma and urinary thromboxane in patients with EIA [abstract]. J Allergy Clin Immunol 1981; 67:45.
39. O'Byrne P, Jones G. The effect of indomethacin on exercise-induced bronchoconstriction and refractoriness after exercise. Am Rev Respir Dis 1986; 134:69–72.
40. Hoshino M, Fukushima Y. Effect of OKY-046 (thromboxane A_2 synthetase inhibitor) on exercise-induced asthma. J Asthma 1991; 28:19–29.
41. Finnerty JP, Harvey A, Holgate ST. The relative contribution of histamine and prostanoids to bronchoconstriction provoked by isocapnic hyperventilation in asthma. Eur Respir J 1992; 5:323–530.
42. Magnussen H, Boerger S, Templin K, Baunack AR. Effects of thromboxane-receptor antagonist BAY u 3405, on prostaglandin D_2- and exercise-induced bronchoconstriction. J Allergy Clin Immunol 1992; 89:1119–1126.
43. Smith AP, Cuthbert MF, Dunlop LS. Effects of inhaled prostaglandin E_1, E_2 and $F_{2\alpha}$ on the airways of healthy and asthmatic man. Clin Sci Med 1975; 48:421.
44. Ozaki T, Rennard SI, Crystal RG. Cyclo-oxygenase metabolities are compartmentalized in the human lower respiratory tract. J App Physiol 1987; 62: 219–212.
45. Margolskee DJ, Bigby BG, Boushey HA. Indomethacin blocks airway toler-

ance to repetitive exercise but not to eucapnic hyperpnea in asthmatic subjects. Am Rev Respir Dis 1988; 137:842–846.
46. Pavord A, Wisniewski A, Tattersfield AE. Inhaled frusemide and exercise induced asthma: evidence for a role of inhibitory prostanoids. Thorax 1992; 47:797–800.
47. Melillo E, Woolly KL, Manning PJ, Watson RM, O'Byrne PM. Effect of inhaled PGE_2 on exercise-induced bronchoconstriction in asthmatic subjects. Am J Respir Crit Care Med 1994; 149:1138–1141.
48. Lane DA, Adams L. Non-anticoagulant uses of heparin. N Engl J Med 1993; 329:129–130.
49. Ghosh TK, Eis PS, Mullaney JM, Ebert CL, Gill DL. Competitive, reversible, and potent antagonism of inositol 1,4,5-triphosphate-activated calcium release by heparin. J Biol Chem 1988; 263:11074–11079.
50. Ahmed T, Garrigo J, Danta I. Preventing bronchoconstriction in exercise-induced asthma with inhaled heparin. N Engl J Med 1993; 329:90–95.
51. Lee TH, Nagy L, Nagakura T, Walport MJ, Kay AB. Identification and partial characterisation of an exercise-induced chemotatic factor in atopic asthmatics. J Allergy Clin Immunol 1982; 70:73–81.
52. Nagakura T, Lee TH, Assoufi BK, Denison DM, Newman-Taylor AJ, Kay AB. Neutrophil chemotactic factor in exercise and hyperventilation induced asthma. Am Rev Respir Dis 1983; 128:294–296.
53. Crimi E, Balbo A, Milanese M, Miadonna A, Rossi GA, Brusasco V. Airway inflammation and delayed bronchoconstriction in exercise-induced asthma. Am Rev Respir Dis 1992; 146:507–512.
54. Papaeorgiou N, Carroll M, Durham SR, Lee TH, Walsh GM, Kay AB. Complement receptor enhancement as evidence of neutrophil activation following exercise-induced asthma. Lancet 1983; 2:1220–1222.
55. Moqbel R, Durham SR, Shaw RJ, et al. Enhancement of leukocyte cytotoxicity after exercise-induced asthma. Am Rev Respir Dis 1986; 133:609–613.
56. Arm JP, Horton CE, Lee TH. Enhanced leukotriene B_4 generation by circulating neutrophils following exercise-induced asthma. J Allergy Clin Immunol 1987; 79:129.
57. Venge P, Henriksen J, Dahl R. Eosinophils in exercise-induced asthma. J Allergy Clin Immunol 1991; 88:699–704.
58. Johnson CE, Belfield PW, Davies S, Cooke NJ, Spencer A, Davies JA. Platelet activation during exercise-induced asthma: effect of prophylaxis with cromoglycate and salbutamol. Thorax 1986; 41:290–294.
59. Wilkens JH, Wilkens H, Uffmann J, Bovers J, Fabel H, Frolich JC. Effects of a PAF-antagonist (BN 52063) on bronchoconstriction and platelet activation during exercise-induced asthma. Br J Clin Pharmacol 1990; 29:85–91.
60. Bury TB, Corhay JL, Louis R, Radermecker MF. Decrease of T-lymphocyte proliferation in exercise-induced asthma. Eur J Allergy Clin Immunol 1994; 49:605–610.
61. Barnes PJ. Neural control of airway smooth muscle. In: Crystal RJ, West JB, et al., eds. The lung: scientific foundations. New York: Raven Press, 1991; 903–915.

62. Barnes PJ, Brown MJ, Silverman M, Dollery CT. Circulating catecholamines in exercise and hyperventilation-induced asthma. Thorax 1981; 36:435–440.
63. Warren JB, Keynes RJ, Brown MJ, Jenner DA, McNicol NW. Blunted sympathoadrenal response to exercise in asthmatic subjects. Br J Dis Chest 1982; 76:147–50.
64. Larsson K, Hijemdahl P, Martisson A. Sympathoadrenal reactivity in exercise-induced asthma. Chest 1982; 82:560–567.
65. Berkin KE, Walker G, Inglis GC, Ball SG, Thomson NC. Circulating adrenaline and noradrenaline concentrations during exercise in patients with exercise-induced asthma and normal subjects. Thorax 1988; 43:295–299.
66. Gilbert IA, Lenner KA, McFadden ER. Sympatho-adrenal response to repetitive exercise in normal and asthmatic subjects. J Appl Physiol 1988; 64: 2667–2674.
67. Tsuda H, Tsuda A, Ito M, Nambu M, Mayumi M, Mikawa H. Roles of eosinophils and catecholamines in the pathophysiology of exercise-induced asthma. Pediatr Allergy Immunol 1993; 4:221–225.
68. Pichurko BM, Sullvian B, Porcelli RJ, McFadden ER. Endogenous adrenergic modification of exercise-induced asthma. J Allergy Clin Immunol 1986; 77:796–801.
69. Rubinstein I, Reiss TF, Gardner DG, Liu J, Bigby BG, Boushey HA Jr. Effect of exercise, hyperpnea, and bronchoconstriction on plasma atrial natreiuretic peptide. J Appl Physiol 1989; 67:2565–2570.
70. Gutkowska J, Nemer M. Structure, expression, and function of atrial factor in extratrial tissues. Endocrinol Rev 1989; 10:519–536.
71. Hulks G, Jardine AG, Connell JMC, Thomson NC. Bronchodilator effect of atrial natriuretic peptide in asthma. Br Med J 1989; 299:1081–1082.
72. Hulks G, Jardine AG, Connell JMC, Thomson NC. Effect of atrial natriuretic peptide factor on bronchomotor tone in the normal human airway. Clin Sci 1990; 79:51–55.
73. Hulks G, Mohammed AF, Jardine AG, Connell JMC, Thomson NC. Circulating plasma concentrations of atrial natriuretic peptide and catecholamines in response to maximal exercise in normal and asthmatic subjects. Thorax 1991; 46:824–828.
74. Hulks G, Jardine AG, Connell JMC, Thomson NC. The influence of elevated plasma levels of atrial natriuretic factor on bronchial reactivity in asthma. Am Rev Respir Dis 1991; 143:778–782.
75. Fuller RW, Dixon CMS, Cuss FMC, Barnes PJ. Bradykinin-induced bronchoconstriction in humans; mode of action. Am Rev Respir Dis 1987; 135: 176–180.
76. Neuman I, Inbar O, Creter D. The kinin system in exercise-induced asthma. Ann Allergy 1984; 53:351–354.
77. Havidsten D, Jenssen TG, Bolle R, Burhol PG. Plasma gastrointestinal regulatory peptides in exercise-induced asthma. Eur J Respir Dis 1986; 68: 326–331.
78. Umeno E, McDonald DM, Nadel JA. Hypertonic saline increases vascular

permeability in rat trachea by producing neurogenic inflammation. J Clin Invest 1990; 85:1905–1908.

79. Gaillard RC, Bachman M, Rochat T, et al. Exercise induced asthma and opioids. Thorax 1986; 41:350–354.
80. Christopher MA, Wyzan D, Harman E, Hendeles L. The effects of nalmefene, a potent oral opiate antagoinst, on exercise-induced bronchospasm. J Allery Clin Immunol 1988; 82:1037–1041.
81. Popa V, Reints P. The effect of inhaled naloxone on the resting bronchial tone and exercise-induced asthma. Am Rev Respir Dis 1989; 139:702–709.

7

Is There a Late Response After Exercise-Induced Asthma?

Noe Zamel
University of Toronto, Toronto, Canada

The induction or exacerbation of asthmatic symptoms following exercise in patients with established asthma has been recognized for about 30 years [1,2]. There are several recent review articles on this topic and one, in particular [3], addresses the pathogenesis in great detail. In fact, to emphasize the underlying pathogenesis of this condition, the term *thermally induced asthma* has been proposed.

It appears that the pathogenesis of exercise-induced asthma is due to fluxes in heat and water that develop in the airways during conditioning of large volumes of air. Exercise is often the first precipitant of asthma, and other precipitants follow with time. Initially, all studies on exercise-induced asthma were limited to the first few hours following the exercise challenge. The airflow limitation starts soon after stopping the exercise, making its peak in 5–10 min, with a virtually complete recovery within 30–60 min. In 1980 Bierman et al. [4] reported for the first time a late response as well. These authors describe a fall in expiratory flows in nine adult asthmatics within 10 min following a 6-min treadmill exercise challenge and during this period, the flows were density-dependent. All patients then recovered spontaneously within 2.5 h, but eight of the nine patients had a secondary fall 3.5–6 h following exercise, and during this period, the flows were density-independent.

This study not only indicated a dual response to exercise, but also suggested a different site of airflow limitation so that the early response was predominantly at the level of the central airway, and the late response was at the level of the peripheral airways. Several other reports followed, suggesting that a biphasic asthmatic reaction to exercise occurred in 30–60% of patients with asthma, particularly among children [5–11]. Simson [12] was the first to question this high prevalence of a late response to exercise and even questioned its existence altogether. In 1987, Rubinstein et al. [13] studied 53 persons with asthma (37 adults and 16 children) and found that only 8 had a delayed asthmatic response. However, similar delayed responses were observed on control days when an exercise challenge had not been performed. They concluded that in patients who have immediate asthmatic response to exercise, a second asthmatic response occurring later, after the exercise, was uncommon. Therefore, a controversy was evident concerning the presence of a late asthmatic response following exercise. To establish the absence of a phenomenon is much harder than to establish its presence. The studies of Rubenstein et al. [13] have at least shown the low prevalence of the late asthmatic response after exercise. There are many reasons for the discordance of results. In the reports of Lee et al. [5] and Iikura et al. [6], the protocol was a 3-day study so that the control day always preceded the exercise day. All bronchodilation medication was stopped in the first 24 h, and no further ventilation tests were done. During the following 24 h, control measurements of FEV_1 and maximum expiration flows were done during a 12-h period. On the third day (48 h after stopping all medication) the exercise challenge was performed, and the patients were followed for an additional 12 h. The late asthmatic response following exercise was observed to occur between 4 and 10 h after the completion of the exercise challenge (52–58 h after the patient had last taken their bronchodilator medication).

The other four studies [4,7,8,10] did not include a nonexercise control day as part of their protocol. One study [9] that included a control nonexercise day did not specify the details of medication administration. The late asthmatic responses observed in these studies could be attributed to a worsening of the asthmatic condition related to the interruption of bronchodilator for a prolonged period.

Another factor that could explain the discordance in results may be related to the way that the delayed asthmatic response to exercise was defined. A 14% fall in FEV_1 has been used by most studies, based on a study of Cartier et al. [14] on the late asthmatic response to allergens. Rubinstein et al. [13] used a 20% fall in FEV_1 to define the delayed asthmatic response, but even when the results were based on a 14% fall in FEV_1, the prevalence of the late asthmatic response following exercise continued to be uncommon. Finally, another reason for the discrepancies in the results could be the type of asthmatic patient who was studied. Lee et al. [5] and Bierman et al. [10] have suggested that the delayed asthmatic responses occurred in patients having a severe early asthmatic response to exercise (greater than 40% fall in FEV_1 from control values), and these patients did not have a complete return to control FEV_1 values within 3 h following the completion of the exercise challenge. They [5,10] suggested that hormonal factors associated with the early asthmatic response may sustain the initial airflow limitations in susceptible asthmatics and result in the delayed asthmatic reactions.

Rubenstein et al. [13] had sufficient numbers of asthmatic patients with severity similar to those in the studies by Bierman et al. [10], but these patients failed to have the delayed asthmatic response to exercise. All these arguments support the view that the major reason for the different results is the withdrawal from bronchodilation medication.

Many other studies [15–17] followed the initial study of Rubinstein et al. [13], confirming the rarity of the occurrence of a delayed asthmatic response to exercise. In addition, Varga et al. [18] could not find a late asthmatic reaction to cold air challenge in asthmatic children. In conclusion, if there is a late response after exercise-induced asthma, this response is at least a very rare phenomenon.

REFERENCES

1. Jones RS, Buston MH, Wharton MJ. The effects of exercise on ventilatory function in the child of asthma. Br J Dis Chest 1962; 56:78–86.
2. McNeill RS, Nairn JR, Miller JS, Ingram CG. Exercise induced asthma. Q J Med 1966; 35:55–67.
3. McFadden ER JR, Gilbert IA. Exercise-induced asthma. N Engl J Med 1994; 330:1362–1366.
4. Bierman CW, Spiro SG, Petheram I. Late response in exercise-induced asthma [abstract]. Allergy Clin Immunol 1980; 65:206.
5. Lee TH, Nagakura T, Papageorgiou N, Iikura Y, Kay AB. Exercise-induced late asthmatic reactions with neutrophil chemotactic activity. N Engl J Med 1983; 308:1502–1505.
6. Iikura Y, Inui H, Nagakura T, Lee TH. Factors predisposing to exercise-induced late asthmatic responses. J Allergy Clin Immunol 1985; 75:285–289.
7. Feldman CH, Fox J, Kraut E, Feldman BR, Davis WJ. Exercise induced asthma: treatment for early and late responses [abstract]. Am Rev Respir Dis 1982; 125(suppl):195.
8. Horw CR, Jones RM, Lee D, Brennan SR. Late response in exercise-induced asthma. Clin Allergy 1984; 14:307–309.
9. Boner A, Niero E, Antolini I, Warner JO. Biphasic (early and late) asthmatic responses to exercise in children with severe asthma, resident at high altitude. Eur J Pediatr 1985; 144:164–166.

10. Bierman CW, Spiro SG, Petheram I. Characterization of the late response in exercise-induced asthma. J Allergy Clin Immunol 1984; 74:701–706.
11. Speelberg B, Verhoeff NPLG, VanderBerg NJ, Oosthoek CHA, Herwaarden CLA, Bruijnzeel PLB. Nedocromil sodium inhibits the early and late asthmatic response to exercise. Eur Respir J 1992; 5:430–437.
12. Godfrey S. Late response to exercise-induced asthma. J Allergy Clin Immunol 1985; 76:876.
13. Rubinstein I, Sevison H, Slutsky AS, Hak H, Wells J, Zamel N, Rebuck AS. Immediate and delayed bronchoconstriction after exercise in patients with asthma. N Engl J Med 1987; 317:482–485.
14. Cartier A, Thomson NC, Frith PA, Roberts R, Hargreave FE. Allergen-induced increase in bronchial responsiveness to histamine: relationship to the asthmatic response and change in airway caliber. J Allergy Clin Immunol 1982; 70:170–177.
15. Zawadski DK, Lenner KA, McFadden ER Jr. Re-examination of the late asthmatic response to exercise. Am Rev Respir Dis 1988; 137:837–841.
16. Boner AL, Vallone G, Chiesa M, Spegia E, Fambri L, Sette L. Reproducibility of late phase pulmonary response to exercise and its relationship to bronchial hyperreactivity in children with chronic asthma. Pediatr Pulmonol 1992; 14:156–159.
17. Pujol J-L, Varray A, Savy-Pacaud A-M, Godard P, Midrel F-B, Prefaut C. Evolution de l'hyperreativite bronquique au cours de l'asthme post-exercise. Rev Mal Respir 1992; 9:517–523.
18. Varga E-M, Eber E, Zach MS. Cold air challenge for measuring airway reactivity in children: lack of a late asthmatic reaction. Lung 1990; 168: 267–272.

8

Treatment of Exercise-Induced Asthma: β-Agonists

Nancy K. Ostrom
Allergy and Asthma Medical Group and Research Center, San Diego, California

I. INTRODUCTION

Exercise has long been recognized as a potent stimulus to bronchoconstriction since its description in the second century AD by Aretaeus the Cappadocian, as follows: "If from running, gymnastic exercise, or any other work, the breathing becomes difficult, it is called Asthma" [1]. As discussed in this volume, several different mechanisms have been proposed as causes of exercise-induced bronchospasm. Pharmacological attenuation of this effect has been achieved through the use of medications operative on different phases of the response [2–4]. These include, with variable clinical effect, β-adrenergic agonists, mast cell stabilizers (blocking both the early and late phase of the bimodal response), parasympathetic blockers, theophylline, and far less commonly, calcium channel blockers and inhaled diuretics [5–7].

Although there are multiple purported mechanisms underlying exercise-induced bronchospasm (EIB), treatment with β-adrenergic agents (β-agonists) is considered the most effective therapy for prevention of symptoms occurring during the early-phase bronchoconstrictive response [8,9]. Agents currently available are protective in 80–90% of cases. Proposed mechanisms for this therapeutic effect include (a) direct bronchodilation of the airways through the smooth-muscle β-receptor, (b) partial inhibition of mediator release, and (c) possible improvement in water transport across the epithelial cell and in mucociliary clearance [3]. Standardized procedures have been developed to provoke exercise-induced bronchospasm in a controlled setting for clinical diagnosis as well as for investigation of the therapeutic effect of pharmacological agents [10,11]. This generally involves a 6 to 8-min run on a treadmill at 80–90% of predicted maximal heart rate. Spirometric assessment of pulmonary function is done before and after medication administrations and at 5 to 10-min intervals following the exercise challenge [12–15]. Using standardized methods for exercise challenge with appropriate EIB subjects, several β-agonists have been studied in comparison with placebo, as well as with other medications, to evaluate potential clinical benefit. Such studies have corroborated the protective effect against exercise-induced bronchospasm of short-acting agents delivered by metered-dose inhaler (MDI), including procaterol, fenoterol, and rimiterol (available for clinical use outside the United States) [16–19], and metaproterenol, albuterol, bitolterol, and terbutaline (available in the United States) [20–23]. Of interest is that oral β-agonist medications that provide clinically therapeutic bronchodilation have a shorter duration of action and are generally much less effective in preventing the bronchoconstrictive effect of an exercise challenge [3,24,25].

An example of this difference is shown in Fig. 1 from a study by Konig and colleagues comparing oral and inhaled metaproterenol for prevention of exercise-induced asthma in 24 adults with asthma [25]. Comparable bronchodilation was achieved when either the metaproterenol tablet or inhaler was given 1 h before exercise. However, when subjects performed an exercise challenge at 1 h after treatment, there was significantly less reduction in pulmonary function (1-S forced expiratory volume; FEV_1) after exercise in the group receiving the medication in the inhaled form. Protection from EIB was even greater when the inhaler was given 10 min before exercise in a crossover trial with the same group of patients.

β-Adrenergic agents given by metered-dose inhalers are, therefore, the drugs of choice for treatment of exercise-induced bronchospasm. Such agents currently available in the United States as "press-and-breathe" MDI units include metaproterenol, terbutaline, albuterol, bitolterol, and pirbuterol. Albuterol is also available as a breath-actuated dry powder inhaler, and pirbuterol is also available as a breath-actuated MDI. Clinical trials documenting the protective effect of pirbuterol against exercise-induced bronchospasm have not been published. Short-acting β-agonists generally provide 3–6 h of bronchodilation, but only 2–4 h of protection against EIB, perhaps owing to increased metabolism through enhanced pulmonary circulation during exercise [26,27]. Differences have been identified between these agents in their β-selectivity, duration of action, and effectiveness in preventing the bronchoconstrictive effect of exercise. Terbutaline, albuterol, and pirbuterol are considered to have the highest

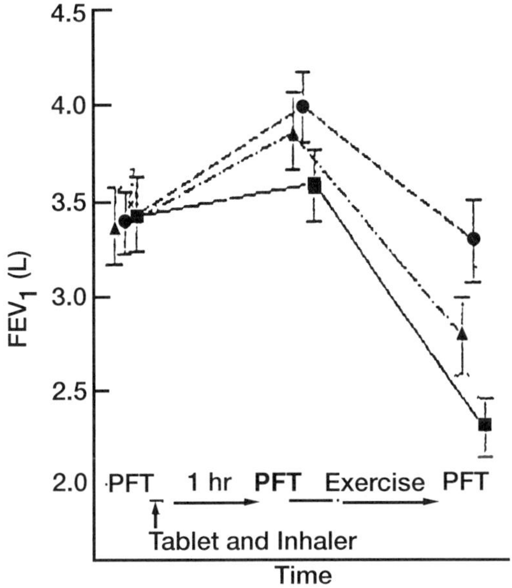

Fig. 1 Group means of FEV_1 with oral vs. inhaled metaproterenol followed by exercise challenger: The bars represent ± 1 SEM. PFT, pulmonary function tests. ▲, tablet active; ●, inhaler active; ■, placebo (Ref. 25).

β_2/β_1-selectivity ratio of the short-acting agents available in the United States. The more β_2-selective agents tend to be the most effective in this clinical area [28,29]. For example, bitolterol has longer protective effect than albuterol when the agents are given 45 min before exercise [23]. Albuterol (salbutamol) is superior in its protection against EIB as well as the duration of that effect when compared with metaproterenol sulfate [22]. Treatment with short-acting agents at least 15 min before the onset of exercise will result in onset of action within 5–15 min and peak bronchodilation in 15–60 min, providing adequate protection from the bronchoconstrictive effect of aerobic activities for approximately 2–3 h in most patients [21,22,30].

Other classes of pharmacological agents, as described elsewhere in this volume, are useful in the prophylaxis of exercise-induced bronchospasm (see Chap. 9). However, β_2-adrenergic agents are superior to other medications in protecting against EIB. The β-adrenergic agonist, salbutamol (albuterol) had a protective effect superior to other agents, including cromolyn and atropine, when studied in crossover fashion in a single group

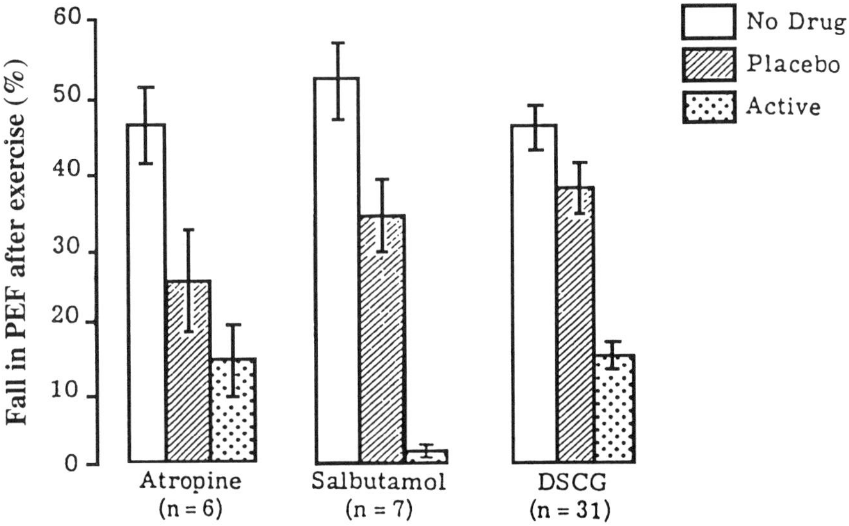

Fig. 2 Demonstration of the effect of placebo and active drugs on the severity of postexercise fall in PEFR in groups of asthmatic children. In the atropine study, the drug and its placebo were both given intravenously, in the salbutamol (albuterol) study the drug and its placebo were given by aerosol, and in the cromolyn study (DSCG) the drug and its placebo were given through a spinhaler (Ref. 31).

of 15 children aged 5–14 years [31] (Fig. 2). Salbutamol (albuterol) showed similar superiority to ipratropium and cromolyn in the prevention of bronchospasm induced by exercise and hyperosmolar challenges [30]. Albuterol showed superiority to cromolyn in a randomized, parallel group study of 80 subjects, in spite of 4 weeks of *daily* cromolyn therapy in that study group [32].

Cromolyn sodium and nedocromil sodium both have some protective effect against both the early and late phase EIB responses, thought to be due to reduced mediator release from mast cells, as discussed elsewhere in this volume (see Chap. 6). They have shown similar quality and duration of effect in several research trials [33–36]. β_2-agonists generally have a superior protective effect with longer duration than cromolyn and nedocromil against EIB. However, some patients, who do not achieve protection from EIB with β-agonist medication alone, may benefit from combination therapy with these agents. An interesting study compared the duration of protective effect of terbutaline sulfate and cromolyn sodium alone and in combination on exercise-induced asthma in adult subjects. Both agents significantly reduced EIB for up to 2 h. However, the duration of that protective effect was *doubled* with the combination of terbutaline and cromolyn before exercise [37].

Patient education on appropriate use of β_2-adrenergic agents is important for maximal effectiveness in preventing exercise-induced bronchospasm. Documentation of the appropriate technique for use of the MDI is critical to ensure optimal drug deposition in the airways. The use of breath-activated devices may be helpful for patients who are unable to coordinate the press-and-breathe technique. Spacer devices may also be helpful in such patients [38]. Of note is the need to warm the inhaler when used in cold ambient environments to ensure maximal deposition of aerosol medications in the airways [39].

In summary, β_2-selective agonists provide the most effective protection against EIB in the research setting. This has been corroborated in clinical experience with most patients achieving satisfactory exercise tolerance when using these medications before aerobic activities. When breakthrough symptoms occur in spite of this treatment regimen, the addition of inhaled cromolyn or nedocromil will generally offer successful prophylaxis against EIB.

II. LONG-ACTING β-ADRENERGIC AGENTS: USEFULNESS FOR PREVENTION OF EXERCISE-INDUCED BRONCHOSPASM

A long-acting bronchodilator in this clinical setting may produce sustained baseline bronchodilation as well as protection from the bronchoconstrictive effect of exercise at any time during the day. Formoterol and salmeterol are two long-acting β-adrenergic agents that have been effective for prevention of EIB, the latter of the two being available for use in the United States.

Formoterol is a lipophilic drug with a high affinity for β-receptors, which are characteristics contributing to its prolonged bronchodilatory effect (up to 12 h). In spite of this long duration of action, its use has not been associated with significant cardiovascular side effects [40,41]. In a crossover study of 15 children with EIB, this agent provided protection from exercise-induced bronchospasm at 3 and 12 h after administration, in comparison with salbutamol (albuterol), which did not show that protective effect [42]. In another study comparing these same medications, 12 patients with atopic asthma showed similar bronchodilation at 4 h after administration. However, protection from EIB at this time point occurred only in patients who had received baseline treatment with formoterol [43]. These findings were confirmed in other trials involving subjects with EIB

[44,45]. However, this agent is not yet available for clinical use in the United States.

Recent availability of salmeterol xinafoate in the United States for treatment of asthma has focused a great deal of attention on its safety and efficacy in patients with varying clinical presentations. In light of the unique mechanism of action through an "exoreceptor" site affording a sustained clinical effect, its study in EIB will be discussed in greater detail here [46].

III. SALMETEROL IN PATIENTS WITH EXERCISE-INDUCED ASTHMA

The newest of the β_2-agonists to be approved in the United States for the prevention of exercise-induced bronchospasm is salmeterol xinafoate (Serevent). This long-acting asthma drug has bronchodilator effects that may exceed 12 h [47] (Fig. 3).

Salmeterol is administered by inhalation from a metered-dose inhaler or, in some countries, from a breath-activated dry powder device, at a dose of 50 μg every 12 h for maintenance bronchodilation. Long-term

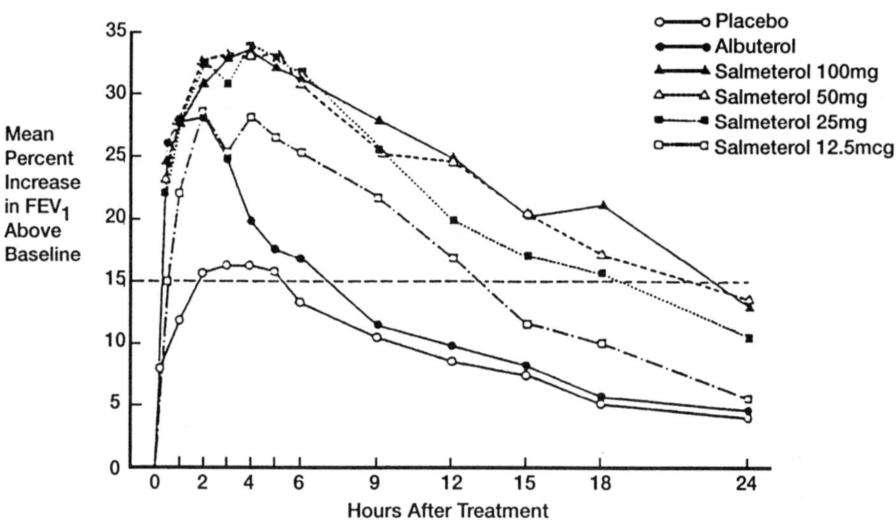

Fig. 3 Mean percentage change in FEV_1 above baseline at each evaluation time after treatment (n = 24) (Ref. 47).

studies, usually of 3-months duration, have yet to show drug-related adverse effects, increase in asthma severity, a failure to respond to rescue therapy such as the additional use of β_2-agonist, or the development of clinically significant tolerance [48–50]. Salmeterol is also an effective drug for the treatment of patients who have nocturnal asthma, because it generally decreases the number of awakenings from asthma. Its use at bedtime results in higher morning peak expiratory flow values compared with patients taking placebo or albuterol [48]. Salmeterol has a prolonged protective effect against the bronchial spasmogen histamine [51]. Such a drug, with prolonged bronchodilator effects and protection against inhaled bronchoconstrictive substances, should have clinical benefit in patients with exercise-induced asthma.

The first published study [52] of the effects of salmeterol in patients with exercise-induced asthma evaluated the effects of albuterol (200 μg) and salmeterol (50 μg) when delivered from a metered-dose inhaler with a Volamatic spacer. The 17 subjects in this study exercised for 8 min on a bicycle ergometer breathing compressed, dry air. Of the 17 subjects, 10 were also taking either inhaled beclomethasone or cromolyn. Patients were exercised 30 min, 2.5, 4.5, and 6.5 h after treatment on different days with salmeterol or albuterol. Both drugs showed an equal peak bronchodilatory effect at 0.5 and 2.5 h after treatment but, as would be expected, by 4.5 and also at 6.5 h salmeterol showed a greater improvement in FEV_1. The mean percentage fall in FEV_1 following exercise was approximately 36% during screening and with placebo treatment, whereas salmeterol was able to attenuate this effect for 6.5 h with only a 20% fall in FEV_1 seen at this time point. The protective effect of albuterol had mostly subsided by 2.5 h (Fig. 4). Because therapeutically similar bronchodilator and bronchoprotective effects were not seen at 2.5 h after administration, this study further confirms the belief that protection by β_2-agonists against the effects of exercise is not just a function of the presence of the agonist on the smooth-muscle β_2-receptor [53–56].

The next reported study evaluating salmeterol in subjects with exercise-induced asthma was a much larger clinical trial involving 161 adolescent and young adult subjects (12–35 years), who exercised on a treadmill for 6 min, at 80% of maximum predicted heart rate, breathing dry (0% humidity) compressed air [57]. These subjects were not taking inhaled corticosteroids or cromolyn sodium. Exercise tests were performed at 0.5, 5.5, and 11.5 h following salmeterol (50 μg), albuterol (200 μg), or placebo administration. Both active drugs blocked the effects of exercise at 0.5 h following treatment, but only salmeterol had a protective effect at 5.5 and 11.5 h (Fig. 5). If a decrease in FEV_1 less than 20% below baseline FEV_1 is used as a criterion for protection against exercise, then

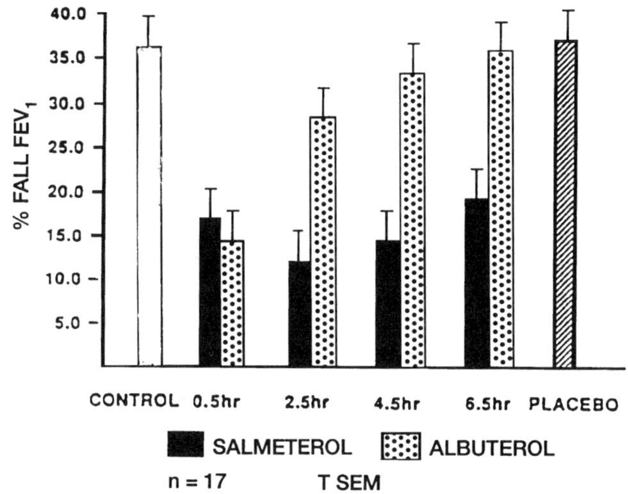

Fig. 4 Mean values = 1 SEM for percentage fall in FEV_1 following exercise challenge recorded on the control and placebo days, and at various times after treatment (Ref. 52).

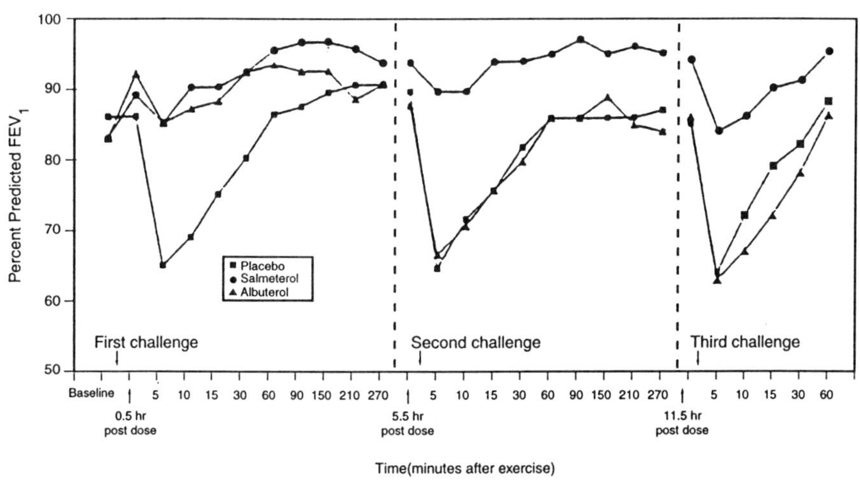

Fig. 5 Mean FEV_1 in the treatment groups as a percentage of the predicted normal value following serial exercise challenge (Ref. 57).

89, 89, and 78% of subjects who received salmeterol were protected at 0.5, 5.5, and 11.5 h after treatment, respectively.

Both of these studies used single doses of salmeterol, which raises the question: Is there the possibility of the development of tolerance with repeated use of salmeterol? Ramage et al. [58] addressed this question in 12 subjects who participated in a placebo-controlled, double-blind crossover study lasting 4 weeks. In this study, much of the protective effect of salmeterol against exercise was lost after 4 weeks of repeated dosing. However, this apparent development of tolerance was not seen with the

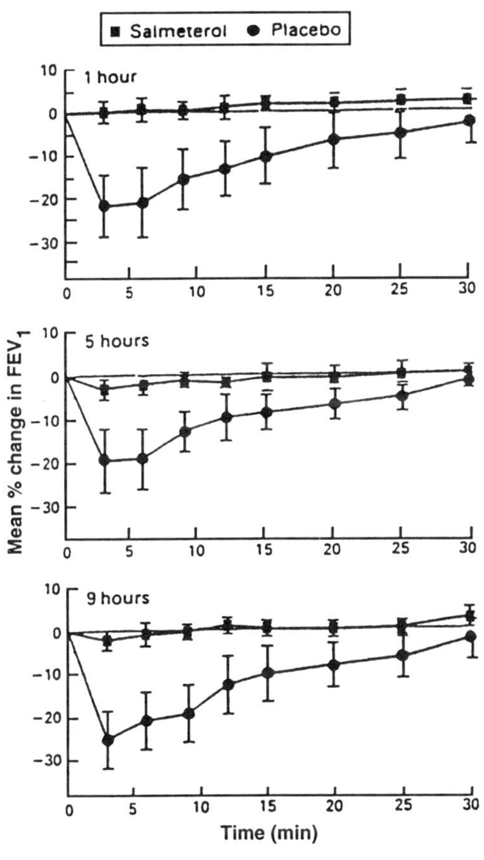

Fig. 6 Change in FEV_1 after exercise. Bars show 95% CI (Ref. 59).

bronchodilator effects of salmeterol, which were maintained for the 4 weeks of the study. Also, this decrease in protective effect with continued dosing has not been apparent in my clinical experience. Further study is needed to clarify this issue.

In the only published study of the effects of salmeterol in children with exercise-induced bronchospasm, Green and Price [59] found that 50 μg of salmeterol in children 8–15 years of age (mean 12) prevented EIB (2.7–5.3% fall in FEV_1) for 9 h when exercised on a treadmill, compared with decreases of 20–25% in FEV_1 in the placebo group. This was a single-dose study and should be confirmed by a multidose study similar to that reported by Ramage et al. [58] in adults (Fig. 6).

Given the reported studies evaluating the effects of salmeterol, it appears to be a very useful drug for the protection of exercise-induced asthma, even before the peak bronchodilator effect that is seen between 2 and 3 h. All studies show a maximal effect as early as 30 mins postdose and protective effects in most patients for at least 12 h. The long protective effect against EIB is a potential benefit for many children and adults who exercise at repeated times throughout the day. It may eliminate the need for the school-aged child to visit a school nurse for asthma medication before recess or physical education class. Further research and clinical experience should help define the effectiveness of this medication alone or in combination with other therapeutic agents.

IV. SAFETY OF β-AGONISTS

β-Adrenergic agents carry an inherent risk of side effects based on cardioactive effects (e.g., increases in heart rate and blood pressure) mediated through the β_1-receptor as well as direct β_2-effects on the skeletal muscle and vascular smooth muscle (vasodilation and reflex tachycardia) [60]. Development of agents with greater β_2/β_1-selectivity has reduced the cardiac side effect profile of these agents, resulting in improved safety and tolerance, without loss of efficacy [28,29]. The long-acting β_2-receptor agonist salmeterol has a safety profile similar to that of albuterol in clinical trials of up to 12 weeks [61]. A recent review and critical analysis of the safety of β-adrenergic agonists in general concluded that this class of medications does not lead to a significant incidence of major adverse reactions [62]. Studies evaluating safety and efficacy of these agents when used to ameliorate exercise-induced bronchospasm have supported the lack of general adverse effects in otherwise healthy individuals.

V. THE USE OF β-AGONISTS IN COMPETITIVE ATHLETIC AND SCHOOL PROGRAMS

The incidence of exercise-induced bronchospasm in high-level competitive athletes is relatively high, as noted in 67 of the 597 American athletes (11.2%) at the 1984 Summer Olympics. With proper treatment, 41 of these athletes won medals (including 15 gold) in 14 different sports [63] (Table 1).

Table 1 Number of Medals Won in the 1984 Summer Olympics by Athletes with Exercise-Induced Bronchospasm

Sport	Athletes with a positive history of EIB
Baseball	1
Men's basketball	2
Women's basketball	2
Canoe/kayaking	2
Cycling	13
Equestrian	5
Fencing	1
Men's field hockey	1
Women's field hockey	2
Men's team handball	1
Women's team handball	1
Modern pentathlon	2
Men's rowing	2
Women's rowing	5
Shooting	1
Men's swimming	2
Women's swimming	1
Men's tennis	3
Men's track and field	5
Women's track and field	5
Women's volleyball	3
Waterpolo	4
Weightlifting	1
Wrestling	1
Yachting	1
Total	67

Source: Ref. 63.

Concern about the possible ergogenic (performance-enhancing) effects of β-adrenergic agents has been raised by the National Collegiate Athletic Association (NCAA) and the United States Olympic Committee (USOC) and is discussed in Chapter 21. However, the increase in ventilatory capacity produced with the use of bronchodilating β-agonists (e.g., albuterol) in athletes with exercise-induced bronchospasm has not enhanced performance during aerobic activity in nonasthmatic individuals [64,65]. Animal studies with clenbuterol (a β-adrenergic agent available in the United States only for veterinary use), revealed some anabolic activity. Protein deposition in muscle tissue of rats and cattle has resulted in both muscular hypertrophy and strength at β-agonist doses of up to 100 times what humans can tolerate [66]. Continuous exposure to constantly high blood concentrations of β-agonists appears to produce growth-promoting effects. The *illicit* use of clenbuterol, ($t_{1/2}$ of 34 h) for potential anabolic effect, has been banned by both the NCAA and the USOC [67]. Two American athletes (hammer throw and shot put) were disqualified in the 1992 Summer Olympics for testing positive for clenbuterol.

Revocation of a gold medal for United States swimmer Rich DeMont because of his use of an antiasthma medication (Marax) during the 1972 Summer Olympics highlighted concern for the allowance of appropriate medical treatment during competitive events [68–71]. Both the NCAA and the USOC have developed policies on the use of β-adrenergic agents in their respective competitive athletic events. The USOC allows the use of only inhaled albuterol or terbutaline by asthmatic athletes, whereas the NCAA allows all inhaled β-agonists. Oral β_2 agents are disallowed by both organizations [72,73] (Table 2). Further updated information on banned

Table 2 Asthma Medications Allowed and Banned by the USOC

Allowed	Banned
Albuterol[a] (Proventil Ventolin)	Bitolterol (Tornalate)
Terbutaline[a] (Brethaire)	Metaproterenol (Alupent)
Salmeterol (Serevent)	Orciprenaline
	Rimiterol
	Pirbuterol (Maxair)

[a] Permitted in inhalant form only, and only with written notification from physician on file with the USOC before competition.
Source: Ref. 72.

medications is available from the United States Olympic Committee (telephone 1-800-233-0393).

Screening for unrecognized EIB in high school and college athletes has revealed a 12–23% incidence of this condition [74,75]. General screening of school children for exercise-induced asthma through the use of peak flow meters has been suggested [76]. School officials, teachers, and coaches should be aware of expert recommendations for exercise in students with asthma in light of the potential effect on their ability to enjoy aerobic sports and achieve appropriate conditioning when this problem is recognized and treated appropriately [77].

Conflict may exist between school officials and students over the ready availability of the β-agonist MDI for use before or after exercise if acute wheezing occurs in this setting. The student is often expected to visit the nurse's or administrative office to receive treatment. This creates unnecessary inconvenience for the student that may defer preventative therapy or, at worst, delay treatment for acute bronchospasm. The American Academy of Pediatrics Committee on Sports Medicine and Fitness, therefore has, written a position statement supporting the personal use of the MDI for the appropriate application in the school setting [78]. This group supports the participation of children with asthma in school sports without penalty because of appropriate treatment. They have produced a policy statement with the following recommendation:

> Asthmatic children should be encouraged, not discouraged, from participating in all athletic endeavors. They should pursue their athletic goals with the knowledge that various (antiasthma) drugs may be taken without being considered "doping" [79].

In summary, treatment with β-adrenergic agents, 15–30 min before aerobic activity, provides relatively rapid bronchodilation and protection against exercise-induced bronchospasm. Short-acting agents with favorable β_2/β_1-selectivity are more protective against the early bronchoconstrictive response than are other classes of medications used in this clinical application. Long-acting β-agonists provide the additional benefit of long-term baseline bronchodilation and longer duration of protection without redosing. Cummulative experience with β-agonists in both research trials and clinical settings supports the accepted clinical practice of their use in both amateur and high-level competitive athletic endeavors.

REFERENCES

1. Adams F. The extant works of Aretaeus the Cappadocian. London: The Sydenhan Society, 1856. Cited in: Samter M. Excerpts from classics in allergy. Columbus, OH: Ross Laboratories, 1969; 3.

2. McFadden ER, Gilbert IA. Current concepts: exercise-induced asthma. N Engl J Med 1994;330:1362–1367.
3. Anderson SD. Exercise-induced asthma. In: Middleton E Jr, Reed CE, Ellis EF, Adkinson NK, Yunginger JW, Busse WW, eds. Allergy: principles and practice. St Louis: Mosby-Year Book, 1993; 1343–1367.
4. Virant FS. Exercise-induced bronchospasm: epidemiology, pathophysiology, and therapy. Med Sci Sports Exerc 1992; 24:851–5.
5. Feather IR, Olson LG. Frusemide antagonises exercise-induced but not histamine-induced bronchospasm. Aust NZ J Med 1991; 21:7–10.
6. Fanta CH. Calcium-channel blockers in prophylaxis and treatment of asthma. Am J Cardiol 1985; 55:202–9.
7. Patel KR, Peers E. Felopidine, a new calcium antagonist, modifies exercise-induced asthma. Am Rev Respir Dis 1988; 138:54–6.
8. Morton AR, Fitch KD. Asthmatic drugs and competitive sport: an update. Sports Med 1992; 14:228–242.
9. Lemanske RF Jr, Henke KG. Exercise-induced asthma. In: Gisolfi CV, Lamb DR, eds. Perspectives in exercise science and sports medicine. vol 2. Indianapolis: Benchmark Press, 1989; 465–511.
10. Sprenkle AC, Van Arsdel PP Jr, Bierman CW. New drug evaluation using exercise-induced bronchospasm. Pediatrics 1974; 56:937–9.
11. Anderson SD, Seale JP, Ferris L, et al. An evaluation of pharmacotherapy for exercise-induced asthma. J Allergy Clin Immunol 1979; 64:612–24.
12. Konig P. Exercise challenge: indications and techniques. Allergy Proc 1989; 10:345–8.
13. Eggleston PA, Rosenthal RR, Anderson SA, et al. Guidelines for the methodology of exercise challenge testing of asthmatics: Study Group on Exercise Challenge, Bronchoprovocation Committee, American Academy of Allergy. J Allergy Clin Immunol 1987; 64:642.
14. Eggleston PA, Guerrant JL. A standardized method of evaluating exercise-induced asthma. J Allergy Clin Immunol 1976; 58:414–25.
15. Godfrey S, Silverman M, Anderson SD. The use of the treadmill for assessing exercise-induced asthma and the effect of varying the severity and duration of exercise. Pediatrics 1975; 56(suppl):893–8.
16. Magnussen H, Rabe KF. The protective effect of low-dose inhaled fenoterol against methacholine and exercise-induced bronchoconstriction in asthma; a dose response study. J Allergy Clin Immunol 1992; 90:846–851.
17. Morton AR, Scott CA, Fitch KD. Rimiterol and the prevention of exercise-induced asthma. J Allergy Clin Immunol 1989; 83:61–65.
18. Rabe KF, Jorres R, Magnussen H. The effect of 10, 50 and 200 micrograms inhaled fenoterol on exercise induced asthma. Clin Exp Allergy 1993; 23: 440–5.
19. Shapiro GG, Kemp JP, DeJong R, Chapko M, Bierman CW, Altman LC, Furukawa CT, Meltzer EO, Orgel HA, Pierson WE, Welch MJ. Effects of albuterol and procaterol on exercise-induced asthma. Ann Allergy 1990; 65: 273–6.

20. Sly RM. beta-Adrenergic drugs in the management of asthma in athletes. J Allergy Clin Immunol 1984; 73:680–5.
21. Afrasiabi R, Spector SL. Exercise-induced asthma. It needn't sideline your patients. Phys Sportsmed 1991; 19:49–62.
22. Berkowitz R, Schwartz D, Bukstein D, Grunstein M, Chai H. Albuterol protects against exercise-induced asthma longer than metaproterenol sulfate. Pediatrics 1986; 77:173–86.
23. Bierman CW. Exercise-induced asthma. Acta Paediatr Jpn 1987; 29:686–691.
24. Fuglsang G, Hertz B, Holm EB. No protection by oral terbutaline against exercise-induced asthma in children: a dose response study. Eur Respir J 1993; 6:527–30.
25. Konig P, Eggleston PA, Serby CW. Comparison of oral and inhaled metaproterenol for prevention of exercise-induced asthma. Clin Allergy 1981; 11: 597–604.
26. Lemanske RF, Joad JP. Uses of β_2-agonists in asthma: a comparison. J Respir Dis 1989; June (suppl):101–109.
27. Anderson SD. Drugs and the control of exercise-induced asthma. Eur Respir J 1993; 6:1090–92.
28. McFadden ER Jr. beta Receptor agonist: metabolism and pharmacology. J Allergy Clin Immunol 1981; 68:91–7.
29. Reed CE. Adrenergic bronchodilators: pharmacology and toxicology. J Allergy Clin Immunol 1985; 76:335–41.
30. Boulet L-P, Turcotte H, Tennina S. Comparative efficacy of salbutamol, ipratropium and cromoglycate in the prevention of bronchospasm induced by exercise and hyperosmolar challenges. J Allergy Clin Immunol 1989; 83: 882–7.
31. Godfrey S, Konig P. Suppression of exercise-induced asthma by salbutamol, theophylline, atropine, cromolyn, and placebo in a group of asthmatic children. Pediatrics 1975; 56(suppl):930–4.
32. Rohr AS, Siegel SC, Katz RM, Rachelefsky GS, Spector SL, Lanier R. A comparison of inhaled albuterol and cromolyn in the prophylaxis of exercise-induced bronchospasm. Ann Allergy 1987; 59:107–9.
33. Morton AR, Ogle SL, Fitch KD. Effects of nedocromil sodium, cromolyn sodium, and a placebo in exercise-induced asthma. Ann Allergy 1992; 68: 143–8.
34. Konig P, Hordvik NI, Kreutz C. The preventive effect and duration of action of nedocromil sodium and cromolyn sodium on exercise-induced asthma (EIA) in adults. J Allergy Clin Immunol 1987; 79:64–8.
35. Comis A, Valleta EA, Sette L, Andreoli A, Boner AL. Comparison of nedocromil sodium and sodium cromoglycate administered by pressurized aerosol, with and without a spacer device in exercise-induced asthma in children. Eur Respir J 1993; 6:523–6.
36. de Benedictis FM, Tuteri G, Bertotto A, Bruni L, Vaccaro R. Comparison of the protective effects of cromolyn sodium and nedocromil sodium in the treatment of exercise-induced asthma in children. J Allergy Clin Immunol 1994; 94:684–8.

37. Woolley M, Anderson SD, Quigley BM. Duration of protective effect of terbutaline sulfate and cromolyn sodium alone and in combination on exercise-induced asthma. Chest 1990; 97:39–45.
38. McFadden ER. Improper patient techniques with metered dose inhalers: clinical consequences and solutions to misuse. J Allergy Clin Immunol 1995; 96:278–83.
39. Wilson AF, Mukai DS, Ahdout JJ. Effect of canister temperature on performance of metered-dose inhalers. Am Rev Respir Dis 1991; 143:1034–1037.
40. Lofdahl CG, Svedmyr N. Formoterol fumarate, a new beta-2 adrenoceptor agonist. Allergy 1989; 44:264–71.
41. Arvidsson P, Larsson S, Lofdahl G, Melander L, Wahlander L, Svedmyr N. Formoterol, a new long-acting bronchodilator for inhalation. Eur Respir J 1989; 2:325–30.
42. Boner AL, Spezia E, Piovesan P, Chiocca E, Maiocchi G. Inhaled formoterol in the prevention of exercise-induced bronchoconstriction in asthmatic children. Am J Respir Crit Care Med 1994; 149:935–9.
43. McAlpine LG, Thomson NC. Prophylaxis of exercise-induced asthma with inhaled formoterol, a long-acting β_2-adrenergic agonist. Respir Med 1990; 84:293–5.
44. Patessio A, Podda A, Carone M, Trombetta N, Donner CF. Protective effect and duration of action of formoterol aerosol of exercise-induced asthma. Eur Respir J 1991; 4:296–300.
45. Henriksen JM, Agertoft L, Pedersen S. Protective effect and duration of action of inhaled formoterol and salbutamol on exercise-induced asthma in children. J Allergy Clin Immunol 1992; 89:1176–82.
46. Bradshaw J, Brittain RT, Coleman RA, et al. The design of salmeterol. A long-acting selective β_2-adrenoceptor agonist. Br J Pharmacol 1987; 92:590P.
47. Kemp JP, Bierman CS, Cocchetto DM. Dose-response study of inhaled salmeterol in asthmatic patients with 24-hour spirometry and Holter monitoring. Ann Allergy 1993; 70:316–22.
48. Pearlman D, Chervinsky P, LaForce C, et al. A comparison of salmeterol with albuterol in the treatment of mild-to-moderate asthma. N Engl J Med 1992; 327:1420–5.
49. Britton MG, Earnshaw JS, Palmer JBD. A twelve month comparison of salmeterol with salbutamol in asthmatic patients. Eur Respir J 1992; 5: 1062–7.
50. Castle W, Fuller R, Hall J, Palmer J. Serevent nationwide surveillance study: comparison of salmeterol with salbutamol in asthmatic patients who require regular bronchodilator treatment. Br J Med 1993; 306:1034–7.
51. Maconochie JG, Forster JK, Fowler P, Thomas M. An initial comparison of salmeterol and salbutamol against histamine-induced bronchoconstriction in healthy subjects. Br J Clin Pharmacol 1988; 25:115P.
52. Anderson SD, Rodwell LT, Du Toit J, Young IH. Duration of protection by inhaled salmeterol in exercise-induced asthma. Chest 1991; 100:1254–1260.
53. Anderson SD, Seale JP, Rozea P, Bandler L, Theobald G, Lindsay DA.

Inhaled and oral salbutamol in exercise-induced asthma. Am Rev Respir Dis 1976; 114:493–500.
54. Anderson SD, Rozea PJ, Dolton R, Lindsay DA. Inhaled and oral bronchodilator therapy in exercise-induced asthma. Aust NZ J Med 1975; 5:544–50.
55. Anderson SD, Bye PTP, Shoeffel RE, Seale JP, Taylor KM, Ferris L. Arterial plasma histamine levels at rest, during and after exercise in patients with asthma: effects of terbutaline aerosol. Thorax 1981; 36:259–67.
56. Howarth PH, Durham SR, Lee TH, Kay AB, Church MK, Holgate ST. Influence of albuterol, cromolyn sodium and ipratropium bromide on the airway and circulating mediator responses to allergen bronchial provocation in asthma. Am Rev Respir Dis 1985; 132:986–92.
57. Kemp JP, Dockhorn RJ, Busse WW, Bleecker ER, van As A. Prolonged effect of inhaled salmeterol against exercise-induced bronchospasm. Am J Respir Crit Care Med 1994; 150:1612–5.
58. Ramage L, Lipworth BJ, Ingram CG, Cree IA, Dhillon DP. Reduced protection against exercise induced bronchoconstriction after chronic dosing with salmeterol. Respir Med 1994; 88:363–8.
59. Green CP, Price JF. Prevention of exercise induced asthma by inhaled salmeterol xinafoate. Arch Dis Child 1992; 67:1014–7.
60. Nelson HS. β-Adrenergic bronchodilators. N Engl J Med 1995; 333:499–506.
61. Nathan RA, Seltzer JM, Kemp JP, Chervinsky P, Alexander WJ, Liddle R, Mills R. Safety of salmeterol in the maintenance treatment of asthma. Ann Allergy 1995; 75:243–8.
62. McFadden ER. Perspectives in β_2-agonist therapy: vox clamantis in deserto vel lux in tenebris? J Allergy Clin Immunol 1995; 95:641–51.
63. Pierson WE, Voy RO. Exercise-induced bronchospasm in the XXIII summer Olympic games. N Engl Reg Allergy Proc 1988; 9:209–13.
64. Morton A, et al. Is salbutamol ergogenic? The effects of salbutamol on physical performance in high-performance nonasthmatic athletes. Clin J Sports Med 1992; 2:93–7.
65. Meeuwisse WH, McKenzie DC, Hopkins SR, Road JD. The effect of salbutamol on performance in elite nonasthmatic athletes. Med Sci Sports Exerc 1992; 24:1161–6.
66. DiPasquale G. Clenbuterol: a new anabolic drug. Drugs Sports 1992; 1:8–10.
67. White J. Doping at the Olympics: clenbuterol. Phys Sportsmed 1992; 20: 19–20.
68. Pierson WE, Voy RO. Exercise-induced bronchospasm in the XXIII summer Olympic games. N Engl Reg Allergy Proc 1988; 9:209–13.
69. Fitch KD. Management of allergic Olympic athletes. J Allergy Clin Immunol 1984; 73:722–7.
70. Godfrey S. Symposium on special problems and management of allergic athletes. J Allergy Clin Immunol 1984; 73:630–3.
71. Oseid S. Doping and athletes—prevention and counseling. J Allergy Clin Immunol 1984; 73:735–9.
72. Nastasi KJ, Heinly TL, Blaiss MS. Exercise-induced asthma and the athlete. J Asthma 1995; 32:249–57.

73. United States Olympic Committee, Division of Sports Medicine, Drug Education and Doping Control Program. Guide to banned medications. Colorado Springs CO, 1993;1–15.
74. Rupp NT, et al. The value of screening for risk of exercise-induced asthma in high school athletes. Ann Allergy 1993; 70:339–42.
75. Shield S, Wang-Dohlman A. Incidence of exercise-induced bronchospasm in high school football players [abstract]. J Allergy Clin Immunol 1991; 87: 166.
76. Kyle JM, Walker RB, Hanshaw SL, Leaman JR, Frobase JK. Exercise-induced bronchospasm in the young athlete: guidelines for routine screening and initial management. Med Sci Sports Exerc 1992; 24:856–9.
77. American Academy of Pediatrics (Section on Allergy and Immunology, Section on Diseases of the Chest). Exercise and the asthmatic child. Pediatrics 1989; 84:392–3.
78. American Academy of Pediatrics (Committee on Sports Medicine and Fitness). Metered-dose inhalers for young athletes with exercise-induced asthma. Pediatrics 1994; 94:129–30.
79. American Academy of Pediatrics. Exercise and the asthmatic child. Pediatrics 1989; 84:392–3.

9

Treatments of Exercise-Induced Asthma Other Than β-Agonists

Sheldon L. Spector
University of California—Los Angeles, and
Allergy Research Foundation, Los Angeles, California

I. INTRODUCTION

Treatment of exercise-induced asthma with β-agonists is discussed in Chapter 8 of this book. This chapter describes various treatments other than β-agonists, including nedocromil and cromolyn, antihistamines, calcium channel blockers, theophylline, corticosteroids, anticholinergic agents, antileukotrienes, and heparin.

II. NEDOCROMIL AND CROMOLYN IN THE TREATMENT OF EXERCISE-INDUCED ASTHMA

Nedocromil has been compared with placebo in many studies for its ability to block exercise-induced asthma [EIA] in both adult [1] and pediatric aged groups [2–4]. In some studies, nedocromil was compared with cromolyn. For example, in one study of nine asthmatics, nedocromil (2 mg) was compared with cromolyn sodium by metered-dose inhaler 30 min before two successive exercises challenges, separated by a 2-h–rest period. Both compounds decreased the severity of EIA, with a residual blocking effect that lasted through the second exercise challenge, although smaller than with the initial blockage [5].

In another study of 12 patients, nedocromil sodium (4 mg) was compared with sodium cromolyn (20 mg) and placebo. Although both active medications provided some protection from EIA at 20 min, by 2 h after drug administration, only cromolyn was significantly different from placebo, implying that the latter compound had the longer duration of action [6]. In a study of 17 children, de Benedictis [7] found comparable protection from EIA with both 4 mg nedocromil sodium and 10 mg cromolyn sodium, using a 6-min treadmill run to 85% maximum heart rate. This represents the recommended dose of nedocromil and five times the recommended dose of cromolyn.

Morton and co-workers [8] compared nedocromil (8 mg) versus cromolyn (4 mg) in their study of 19 patients, age 13–30 with EIA, employing an 8-min treadmill run at 70% of the patient's $\dot{V}O_2max$. More subjects were completely protected after treatment with nedocromil (62.5%) than after treatment with cromolyn (25%). This study used twice the recommended dose of both cromolyn and nedocromil. The dose–response characteristics of nedocromil were assessed in a study for which placebo, or 1, 4, or 8 mg nedocromil was given 60 min before the exercise challenge [9]. Pretreatment with nedocromil sodium reduced the fall in peak expiratory flow rate compared with placebo, and the 4- and 8-mg doses gave greater protection than the 1-mg dose. When increasing doses of nedocromil sodium were given by a nebulizer in concentrations of 0.5, 5, 10, and 20 mg/mL versus placebo 15 min before exercise, there were no significant differences among any of the doses administered [10]. Protection with all doses was about 50%, which is similar to that afforded by 4 mg of nedocromil from a metered-dose inhaler. Controversy surrounds the existence of (or incidence of) the late-phase reaction following exercise-induced asthma. A Dutch study [11] examined the inhibition of both the early- and late-phase asthmatic response; 12 of 19 subjects had early responses to exercise, and 8 of these 12 had inhibition of the early reaction by nedocromil sodium; 9 of the 19 patients with the late reaction after exercise, were clearly protected by pretreatment with nedocromil sodium, 4 showing protection equal to placebo, and 6 had no protection. Nedocromil has also been compared with other agents, such as minocromil. Both 2- and 4-mg nedocromil pretreatment in nine patients, and 4-mg minocromil in eight patients gave significant protection compared with placebo, as assessed by the reduction in the maximal percentage of forced expiratory volume in 15 (FEV_1) [12]. There were no significant differences in the inhibitory effect among the active agents versus placebo. An interesting Italian study [13] looked at inhaled furosemide (30 mg) compared with inhaled nedocromil, and the combination of these two medications versus placebo, in preventing exercise-induced asthma. Medication was given 20 min before an exercise challenge in a double-blind fashion. The patients were then followed at 2, 4, 6, 8, 10, 15, 20, and 30 min after the exercise challenge. Nedocromil and furosemide provided a comparable protective effect and had a statistically significant additive effect [13]. Nedocromil has not been approved as a preventative agent for exercise-induced bronchospasm, despite the numerous studies cited to support its use for that purpose.

III. BLOCKING EFFECTS OF ANTIHISTAMINES AND ANTIHISTAMINE-LIKE COMPOUNDS

In most studies, antihistamines are administered by the oral route, but occasionally are also given by aerosolization. It is interesting that a military study recently compared a single oral dose of a sedating and nonsedating H_1-receptor antagonist on exercise performance in a double-blind, randomized study. Performance measures included oxygen uptake, heart rate, rectal temperature, and postexercise plasma lactate concentration. Neither diphenhydramine (50 mg) nor terfenadine (60 mg) compromised nor improved aerobic or glycolytic work performance under these exercise conditions [14].

A. Antihistamines by the Oral Route

In one study, terfenadine blocked treadmill-induced EIA in a dose-dependent fashion [15]. In another study, a relatively large dose of terfenadine (180 mg po) was compared with ipratropium bromide (0.5 mg by nebulization) versus the combination, in ten asthmatic subjects with EIA in a randomized double-blind study [16] (Table 1). The mean maximum percentage fall in FEV_1 after exercise following placebo therapy was 33.6 ± 3.8%, compared with 27.2 ± 3.6% after terfenadine; 21.8% ± 3.9% after ipratropium; and 15.1 ± 4.1% after the combination of both drugs. Thus, the addition of ipratropium bromide to terfenadine improved the protection provided by terfenadine alone. It would appear that both histamine release and vagal stimulation contributed independently and additively to EIA [16]. Terfenadine also attenuates hyperventilation-induced bronchospasm [17].

Theoretically, ketotifen should be a good candidate for blocking EIA because it blocks mediator release from mast cells [18] and release of neutrophil chemotactic factor during exercise [19]. However, most investigators have found little, if any, blocking effect of ketotifen [20–22]. In the study by Tan et al. [20], ten asthmatics were exercised on a treadmill before and after treatment for 1 week with placebo or ketotifen (1 mg) twice daily. Cromolyn sodium (10 mg four times a day) was used as a

Table 1 Effect of Terfenedine, Ipratropium and Combination on Exercise-Induced Asthma[a]

Drug	Decreased FEV_1 (%)
Placebo	34
IB (0.5 mg) nebulized	27
Terfenedine (180 mg po)	21
Combination	15

[a] Ten Asthmatic Subjects with EIA on Treadmill
Source: Ref. 3.

positive control. Cromolyn, but not ketotifen, protected against EIA. This study should be contrasted with one in which ketotifen was given by inhalation at 0.25 and 0.5 g/Liter [21]. Although the authors concluded that there was no effect with inhaled ketotifen, two patients did not have EIA after inhalation of either ketotifen concentrations [21]. Petheram and co-workers studied 12 asthmatic subjects with exercise-induced asthma and, in a random, double-blind order, administered placebo or 1, 2, and 4 mg of ketotifen 2 h before exercise [22]. There was no difference in the mean decreases in lung function from preexercise baseline values after three doses of ketotifen, compared with placebo. Thus, single doses before exercise did not seem to modify EIA. Moreno and co-workers [23] looked at a subgroup of asthmatic patients, and found that in the seasonal asthma group, ketotifen was effective in protecting against asthma provoked by exercise. By contrast, in the perennial asthma group (patients with bacterial or mite triggers), ketotifen had no effect. The dose of ketotifen was 1 mg every 12 h for 15 days.

In another study, a standard treadmill protocol, with running for 8 min, was performed in seven atopic adult asthmatics. A double-dummy technique was employed with placebo, oral ketotifen, inhaled clemastine, ipratropium, and cromolyn given in a random single-blind fashion on different days. The mean postexercise percentage fall in FEV_1 ($\pm$SEM) was 47 ($\pm$6.95), 39 ($\pm$8.35), 27 ($\pm$7.17), 23 ($\pm$7.69), and 7.0 ($\pm$4.62%), respectively. There was significantly less bronchoconstriction with cromolyn, ipratropium, and clemastine; six of seven individuals had significant protection against EIA with cromolyn, four with ipratropium, three with clemastine, but only one with ketotifen [24]. However, it would appear that patient selection is important, because McClean and co-workers [18] studied four patients with both cholinergic urticaria and EIA, whereby plasma histamine rose 6- to 20-fold above baseline values after exercise. All four patients were refractory to conventional antihistamine therapy. Ketotifen, in doses ranging from 3 to 8 mg/day resulted in symptomatic improvement. In three subjects, exercise challenge with ketotifen pretreatment demonstrated blockade of mast cell-mediated release. In the fourth patient, histamine rose to about half the level observed before ketotifen therapy. This study has interesting implications. Perhaps histamine must be demonstrated in the plasma of individuals with exercise-induced asthma to predict the subgroup of patients who will respond to antihistamine treatment [18].

Azelastine is a compound that antagonizes histamine as well as leukotrienes in animal models. It was given as a single oral dose of 4.4 mg in ten known asthmatic subjects during the breathing of cold air. Placebo had no effect on baseline pulmonary function or postexercise obstruction of the airway. By contrast, azelastine was associated with a small, but significant bronchodilation and significant attenuation of bronchoconstriction [25]. In another study, azelastine was compared with diphenhydramine and placebo after exercise on the treadmill [26]. The maximum percentage fall in FEV_1 without medication with diphenhydramine and with azelastine was 38.9 ± 5, 20.1 ± 3.8, and 11.3 ± 3.1%, respectively. Significant differences were found among each group ($p < 10.05$).

Cetirizine, a low-sedating antihistamine and metabolic product of hydroxyzine, was examined in EIA; 12 patients received oral placebo or cetirizine, 10 mg twice daily for 1 week, in a double-blind randomized order [27]. Subjects were exercised on a treadmill for 6–8 min at a submaximal workload 2 h after a final dose. Cetirizine failed to inhibit exercise-induced bronchoconstriction with this oral dose. Another 8 patients received 1 mL of cetirizine at 5 and 10 mg/mL, administered through a Wright nebulizer in a double-blind placebo-controlled trial. The fall in FEV_1 after exercise was 23.7% after placebo, and 15.2% after 5 mg of cetirizine and 10.2% after 10 mg. There were 2 patients who had no effect with cetirizine.

B. By Inhalation

The H_2-receptor blocker ranitidine, when given by oral inhalation, blocks exercise-induced asthma [28]. In another study, chlorpheniramine (10 mg) by aerosol or a saline placebo was administered 40 min before a submaximal exercise challenge (cycloergometer) in a double-blind randomized fashion [29]. The authors concluded that chlorpheniramine promoted mild bronchodilation, but probably did not have a clinically meaningful effect on EIA. Manning and co-workers [30] attempted to examine the phenomenon of exercise refractoriness, as it relates to the reduced magnitude of a subsequent exercise, compared with the original exercise. These workers had previously been able to inhibit tachyphylaxis of inhaled histamine with an H_2-blocker such as cimetidine [31], but were unable to affect exercise-induced bronchospasm or the refractoriness that develops with ranitidine or cimetidine [30].

IV. EFFECTS OF CALCIUM CHANNEL BLOCKERS ON EXERCISE-INDUCED ASTHMA

Many studies have investigated the protective effect of calcium antagonists using various bronchoconstrictor challenges, including exercise-induced asthma. In one of the first reports on the effects of calcium antagonists on EIA, nifedipine (20 mg sublingually) completely prevented exercise-induced asthma in ten patients with mild asthma [32]. Each subject performed 10 min of steady-state exercise on a bicycle ergometer on three separate occasions: once on a control day without any premedication, and then again on 2 additional days, 30 min after premedication with either placebo or nifedipine, in a single-blind fashion. Airflow obstruction was assessed by measuring peak expiratory flow rate (PEFR) and flow after exhalation of 50 and 75% of the vital capacity ($\dot{V}max_{50}$ and $\dot{V}max_{25}$). All three parameters demonstrated a mean decrease of approximately 40% from baseline values after exercise on the control and the placebo premedication days, but no change from the normal range when exercise was preceded by nifedipine administration. Nifedipine completely protected asthmatic subjects from exercise-induced bronchoconstriction. At the same time, sublingual nifedipine (20 mg) failed to alter resting lung function in another group of ten asthmatic patients.

Subsequent studies found less complete protection with nifedipine. Barnes and co-workers [33] studied eight extrinsic asthmatic subjects, ages 16–38 years, who underwent a treadmill exercise test performed 30 min after nifedipine (20 mg sublingually). The maximum fall in PEF after exercise was $36.0 \pm 5.3\%$ SEM compared with a maximum fall of $56.5 \pm 4.1\%$ after placebo capsules when given in a double-blind, randomized manner on separate days. This reduction was statistically significant ($p < 0.01$). Other investigators also studied the blocking effect of nifedipine in EIA [34,35]. Gordon et al. studied only four patients after pretreatment with 20 mg nifedipine, and found no significant protection [35]. Olive and co-workers found that 30 mg of nifedipine was associated with a mild bronchodilation before exercise, but did not significantly protect against exercise-induced asthma 2 h after the drug [36]. In this same study, the investigators also compared darodipine (PY 108/068) at 75 and 150 mg. Only the 150-mg dose and the 150-mg dose compared with placebo significantly attenuated EIA.

In a related study published elsewhere, some of the same investigators commented that darodipine not only attenuated EIA, but also caused resting bronchodilation, which is a rather unique finding for calcium channel blockers [37]. With careful scrutiny of the literature, however, if measurements are done for a relatively long period (i.e., at 1–2 h after nifedipine) bronchodilation has also been reported [38] or suggested by the data [39,40]. Verapamil also has a mild-blocking effect on EIA [41,42].

Boner et al. reported a negative study on the effectiveness of inhaled verapamil [42]. In the first phase they studied 15 children with EIA and compared verapamil with cromolyn sodium and ipratropium using saline as a control. After exercise, the maximum percentage fall in FEV_1 was 40.9 ± 17.2 after inhalation of saline; 15.3 ± 11.7 after cromolyn; 36.2 ± 21.4 after verapamil; and 21.7 ± 17.7 after ipratropium. The inhibitory effects of cromolyn and ipratropium were significant, whereas verapamil had no significant effect. To ascertain if a double dose of verapamil was more effective, nine different children with EIA were provoked with the same standardized treadmill running, after a placebo (4 mL of saline), and after verapamil, 10 mg and 4 mL, and again verapamil was ineffective. Gordon and co-workers studied a new calcium channel blocker, flordipine in doses of 25 and 50 mg versus placebo, and in the four patients they studied, there was no significant protection from EIA [35]. Another calcium antagonist called flordipine was also studied for its effect on EIA in a double-blind randomized manner in a trial in nine patients. The 10-mg flordipine dose in oral solution was compared with placebo on separate days using an exercise challenge consisting of a steady-state running at submaximal workloads for 6–8 min, starting at 30 min after the treatments. The FEV_1 was measured at 1, 2, 5, 10, 15, and 30 min after the end of the exercise [41]. In another study, felodipine had no effect on resting lung function, but the mean percentage fall in FEV_1 after exercise with placebo was 27.0 ± 4.5%, and with felodipine it was 13.5 ± 3.7%, which was statistically significant [43]. Additionally, seven patients on the felodipine and one on placebo had a transient headache [43]. Other calcium channel blockers, such as gallopamil and diltiazem have provided only modest protection against EIA, at best, with a short duration of action [44].

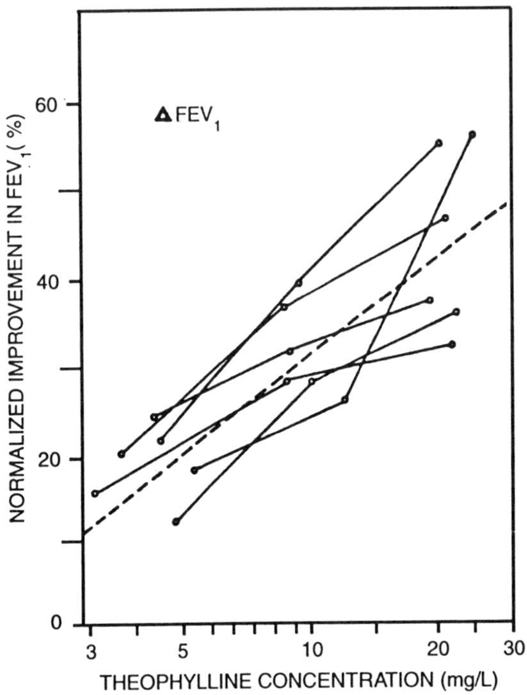

ΔFEV$_1$
NORMALIZED IMPROVEMENT IN FEV$_1$ (%)
60
40
20
0
3
5
10
20
30
THEOPHYLLINE CONCENTRATION (mg/L)

A

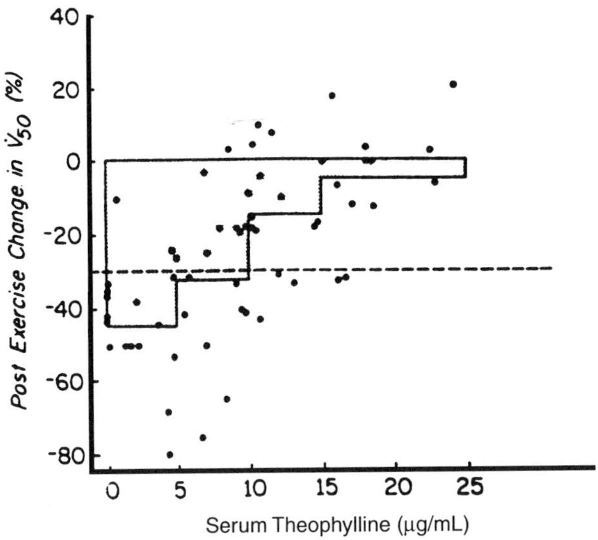

Post Exercise Change in $\dot{V}_{50}$ (%)
40
20
0
-20
-40
-60
-80
0
5
10
15
20
25
Serum Theophylline (μg/mL)

B

V. THEOPHYLLINE AND ITS EFFECT ON EXERCISE-INDUCED BRONCHOSPASM

Theophylline has demonstrated a blocking effect on exercise-induced bronchoconstriction according to various investigators [45–47]. The blocking effect seems to be dose-related, with the greatest effect occurring at concentrations higher than 15 μg/mL [47]. Figure 1 shows the relation between the serum theophylline concentration and exercise-induced bronchospasm following a standardized treadmill exercise.

The challenge was performed on 12 children before and at 2, 4, and 6 h following a 7.5-mg/kg dose of a rapidly absorbed theophylline formulation. The $\dot{V}_{50}$ is the flow rate at 50% of vital capacity during a maximal forced expiration. The shaded area represents mean flow rate changes for the data points at each 5-μg/mL serum concentration interval. The dashed line indicates a 30% decrease in pulmonary function, which many investigators feel is the accepted decrement that is clinically important. The mean Spearman rank correlation coefficient was 0.75 ($p < 0.01$) [48]. Magnusson and co-workers studied the attenuation of EIA in 11 mild asthmatic subjects, using an intravenous infusion of theophylline dissolved in various diluents. The diluents had no effect, whereas theophylline attenuated EIA in a dose-dependent fashion, with significant protection at serum concentrations beginning at 6 mg/L [49]. The effects of enprofylline (1.5 mg/kg), were compared with those of theophylline (5 mg/kg) versus placebo, administered intravenously in a double-blind crossover comparison in eight asthmatic subjects with EIA [50]. Theophylline produced a significantly better protection against EIA compared with enprofylline and placebo. Enprofylline produced only a slight protection from EIA, which was not significant.

Recently, there has been a revived interest in the blocking effect of theophylline in EIA, to assess equivalency of a generic slow-release

---

Fig. 1 (A) Dose-response relation for changes in forced expiratory volume in the first second (ΔFEV_1) against the plasma theophylline concentration plotted semilogarithmically. Plots for each subject are presented individually (●—●—●), as well as the unweighted least squares regression line for the whole group (—). For each subject the ΔFEV_1 is normalized by division of the mean difference from the placebo value at each drug concentration plateau by the predicted value minus the placebo value. (B) Relation between maximal postexercise change in $\dot{V}_{50}$ and corresponding serum theophylline measurement. Superimposed bar graph represents mean postexercise changes in $\dot{V}_{50}$ for serum theophylline intervals indicated. Dotted line at 30% identifies response to exercise conventionally accepted as clinically important. (From Ref. 47.)

theophylline tablet with the proprietary theophylline tablet. Attenuation of exercise-induced asthma was included as an efficacy parameter. In one study, 14 adults with asthma received a generic slow-release theophylline tablet or Theo-Dur at bedtime for 4 nights, in a double-blind crossover design. Neither product effectively attenuated EIA because mean serum concentrations during the exercise challenges were unexpectedly below 10 μg/mL for both products [51].

In another study of 38 children, ages 6–16, Theo-Dur was compared with another generic tablet given every 12 h for 5 days, and a standardized exercise stress test was performed at 24 h (i.e., at the trough serum concentration) [52]. Again, neither formulation effectively blocked the response to exercise, but the trough serum concentration was less than 10 μg/mL in 15 subjects after administration of Theo-Dur, and in 20 subjects after the administration of the generic product.

VI. CORTICOSTEROIDS AND THEIR EFFECT ON EXERCISE-INDUCED BRONCHOSPASM

Steroids can be given by various routes and doses in an attempt to block EIA. Steroids are generally used for long-term treatment, rather than for immediate prophylaxis for EIA. Oral steroids are typically thought to "stabilize" the patient with asthma as an integral part of a total therapy to control inflammation in the moderate to severely afflicted patient. Investigators have examined the ability of steroids to eliminate EIA, reduce its severity, and possibly block the late-phase response after exercise. For the latter, there is controversy over the existence or incidence of a late-phase response. In one study, involving 11 children with a known dual response to exercise, pretreatment of 11 asthmatics with prednisolone and 5 asthmatics with beclomethasone inhibited only the late response and not the early response [53]. By contrast, pretreatment with cromolyn sodium totally inhibited the dual reaction and albuterol (salbutamol) inhibited primarily the early-phase reaction.

Inhaled corticosteroids usually must be given for a relatively long period to have any effect on EIA. Dutch investigators studied 55 children, ages 7–18, in a multicenter study and compared albuterol at 600 μg/day, plus the inhaled corticosteroid budesonide, 600 μg/day, versus albuterol plus placebo before and after 2–8 months of treatment [54]. Eighteen of 22 children (82%) who were treated with the placebo–steroid aerosol had EIA, compared with 18 of 33 children (65%) who were treated with the albuterol–steroid aerosol combination. When the placebo groups were switched to active aerosol and studied 2–8 months later, only about 59% (about the same percentage as those originally receiving albuterol plus the steroid aerosol) demonstrated EIA [54].

In a study employing another design, Vathenen and co-workers demonstrated that steroid aerosols could reduce the mean fall in FEV_1 not only to exercise, but also to other stimuli, compared with placebo [55]. After 6 weeks of treatment with inhaled budesonide (800 μg twice daily), 40 asthmatic subjects underwent various challenges of bronchoreactivity, including histamine, exercise, and eucapnic dry air hyperventilation. The mean percentage fall in FEV_1 in response to eucapnic hyperventilation, exercise, and histamine, was similar before budesonide (25.5, 26.6, and 24.5%), and the reduction in the percentage fall in FEV_1 with budesonide after 6 weeks of therapy was similar for the three challenges (18.9, 17.5, and 16.6%), all of which differed significantly from placebo. The authors suggested that corticosteroids act by similar mechanisms to protect against these three different challenges [55]. Even a smaller dose of budesonide, given for a shorter time, has ability to block EIA, as shown in the study by Henriksen et al. [56]. These investigators studied 14 children with EIA before and during a 4-week–treatment period with aerosolized budesonide (400 μg/day), accompanied by either aerosolized terbutaline, in a dose of 32.5 μg, or placebo. Terbutaline alone, budesonide plus placebo, and budesonide plus terbutaline, reduced the exercise-induced fall in FEV_1 by 30, 51, and 84%, respectfully. Thus, the combination therapy proved best in blocking EIA, confirming that 1–4 weeks of therapy with inhaled steroid decreases the severity of EIA. The dose–response characteristics of budesonide were further clarified in a double-blind crossover study of 19 children, for whom there was a 2 week placebo run-in, followed by three 4-week treatments of either 100, 200, or 400 μg/day of budesonide in randomized order [57]. There was a significant dose–response effect, whereby 200 μg of budesonide was significantly better than 100 μg, and 400 μg was significantly better than 200 μg. In fact, 100 μg produced 53% of the maximum protection, and 400 μg produced 83% of the maximum protection [57].

Oral corticosteroids are reported by some investigators to affect exercise responses. The length of time that they are administered is probably an important variable. Prednisone, administered at a dose of 5 mg four times a day for an average of 3.3 days before exercise, reduces by half the increase in airway obstruction that followed treadmill exercise in asthmatic children [58]. Jones reported no effect of oral steroids on the lability index [59]. Konig and co-workers reported inhibition of exercise-induced asthma in three of nine asthmatic subjects treated with oral prednisone daily for 1 week. Interestingly, he also reported that 3 of 11 subjects who inhaled beclomethasone dipropionate (100 μg) 20–30 mins before exercise also had a blocking effect of EIA [60].

The intranasal administration of corticosteroid can also influence EIA. In a double-blind study of 37 asthmatic children who were allocated randomly to 4 weeks of intranasal budesonide (400 μg/day) or placebo spray, the children not only had improved nasal symptoms, but also demonstrated less exercise-induced asthma, along with decreased cough and decreased asthma severity [61]. Welsh and co-workers also noted a decrease in asthma symptoms with treatment of the upper airways [62]. Watson et al. also reported that treatment of the upper airways produced decreased hyperreactivity as measured by methacholine challenge [63]. Similarly Corren et al. found that nasal beclomethasone prevented seasonal increases in bronchial responsiveness, as measured by methacholine, in patients with both allergic rhinitis and asthma [64].

VII. EFFECTS OF ANTICHOLINERGIC AGENTS ON EXERCISE-INDUCED BRONCHOSPASM

There is considerable variability in the degree of protection afforded by anticholinergic agents against EIA. Early studies with atropine showed inhibition of EIA in only a small proportion of subjects [65–67]. Some individuals experience good protection, whereas others experience little, if any. This variability does not appear to be due to the anticholinergic agent employed, because almost all adult and pediatric population have shown a blocking effect to some degree or another.

The failure of some studies to show an effect of ipratropium on EIA may have been due to the dose employed. Hartley and Davies reported that an aerosol of 100 μg ipratropium bromide by ultrasonic nebulizer (Devilbiss 42) failed to block EIA in seven of ten adult patients. They increased the dose to 1000 μg on a separate occasion, and showed a significant block in EIA in all but three of the patients [68].

On the other hand, Boner et al. did not find a dose-related protection of EIA [69], using 125, 250, 500, or 750 mg of ipratropium bromide in 12 subjects ages 7–13 years. Poppius and co-workers administered ipratropium powder to ten adult patients with mild asthma [70]. In doses of ipratropium up to 20–50 times higher than those known to have a marked effect on resting bronchomotor tone, they did not block the bronchoconstriction response following exercise with cold air breathing. Perhaps, if the mechanism for EIA were better understood, we might be better able to differentiate responder groups from nonresponder groups. Finnerty and Holgate studied the blocking effect of nebulized ipratropium bromide (0.5 mg) versus terfenedine (180 mg po) versus the combination, compared with placebo in ten stable asthmatic subjects in a randomized, double-blind study [71]. The mean percentage fall after placebo was 33.6 ± 3.8% compared with 27.2 ± 3.6% after terfenedine, 21.8 ± 3.9% after ipratropium bromide, and 15.1 ± 4.1% after the combination. These data suggest that both histamine release and vagal stimulation contributed independently and additively to EIA.

Thomson et al. postulated that ipratropium bromide might have an effect only in those patients in whom the main site of airflow obstruction was the large central airway [72]. They studied 13 subjects and compared cromolyn sodium versus ipratropium bromide versus the combination and tried to characterize responder and nonresponder groups.

Svenonius et al. reported that cromolyn and ipratropium bromide prevented EIA, mainly in the large airways (i.e., FEV_1 to 95%), but only to about 50% in small airways (i.e., measured by VTG) [73].

Singh and co-workers characterized patients as better responders to ipratropium than to albuterol who were more than 40 years of age and who had eosinophilia [74]. By contrast, those who responded best to albuterol were smokers, patients with family history of bronchial asthma, and younger patients. Others have postulated that anticholinergic agents are more likely to be effective in patients with marked receptor reactivity in cold air, or who are reactivity to air pollutants [75].

Despite the larger intersubject differences in protection, anticholinergics generally do not protect against EIA as well as β-agonists [72,76]. When Boulet et al. studied the inhibitory effects of albuterol (100 μg), ipratropium (80 μg), and cromolyn (4 mg) in 11 subjects, albuterol had a greater effect than ipratropium, and ipratropium had a greater effect than cromolyn [76].

VIII. EFFECTS OF ANTILEUKOTRIENES ON EXERCISE-INDUCED ASTHMA

Many studies have demonstrated inhibition of EIA by leukotriene antagonists administered by various routes. When MK-571 (a Merck compound) was administered intravenously, there was a mean drop in FEV_1 of only 9.2%, compared with 25.2% with placebo ($p < 0.001$) [77]. This represents 65% inhibition. In addition, there was a mean time to recovery after exercise of 8.4 min in the active treatment group, compared to 33.4 min in the placebo group. When zafirlukast (Accolate; ICI 204,219) was given orally to eight asthmatic patients, 20 mg of the active compound before exercise reduced the maximum percentage fall in FEV_1 to 21.6%, compared with 36.0% following placebo [78]. When 400 μg zafirlukast was given to eight patients by inhalation 30 min before a cycle ergometry challenge, the maximal percentage fall in FEV_1 was 14.5% after active medication, compared with 30.2% after placebo, and the median time to recovery after zafirlukast was 20 min versus 60 min with placebo ($p = 0.0018$) [79].

When the leukotriene antagonist pobilukast (SKF-104353) was given by the oral route to 18 asthmatic subjects, there was approximately a 40% inhibition of the EIA response to cycle ergometry; 20 mg of nebulized sodium cromolyn was given as a positive control and the effects of the antileukotriene exceeded those of the cromolyn [80]. One of the older 5-lipoxygenase inhibitors, piriprost, given by the inhaled route, failed to block exercise-induced bronchoconstriction in humans [81].

IX. HEPARIN

Ahmed and co-workers studied the effect of inhaled heparin on preventing EIA in 12 subjects [82]. Heparin (4 mL at 1000 U/kg), cromolyn sodium (20 mg), or placebo were administered 45 min before the exercise. Although inhaled heparin and cromolyn sodium had no effect on specific airway conductance at baseline, both attenuated EIA: the mean (± SE) maximal decrease 5 min after exercise was 9 ± 5% after pretreatment with heparin, as compared with 22 ± 5% after pretreatment with cromolyn, and 35 ± 2% after pretreatment with placebo. Because inhaled heparin prevented EIA without influencing histamine-induced bronchoconstriction, the authors felt that the action of heparin was more likely to be due to modulation of mediator release than to a direct effect on smooth muscle.

X. SUMMARY

Although β-agonists remain the preferred first-line therapy for EIA, many other agents block EIA as well. Cromolym and nedocromil provide protection from EIA and could be considered the preferred treatment after, or along with, β-agonists. Calcium channel blockers, theophylline, antihistamines, anticholinergic agents such as ipratropium, antileukotrienes, furosemide, and even heparin can prevent EIA in a subgroup of asthmatic patients. Agents such as oral steroids or steroid aerosols are potent stabilizers of asthma and thereby mitigate the effect of EIA. Thus, with the extensive array of medications available sports enthusiasts should feel reassured that single agents or combinations of medication can significantly ameliorate EIA.

REFERENCES

1. Shaw RJ, Kay AB. Nedocromil, a mucosal and connective tissue mast cell stabilizer, inhibits exercise-induced asthma. Br J Dis Chest 1985; 79:385–389.
2. Chudry N, Correa F, Silverman M. Nedocromil sodium and exercise-induced asthma. Arch Dis Child 1987; 62:412–414.
3. Henriksen JM. Effect of nedocromil sodium on exercise-induced bronchoconstriction in children. Allergy 1988; 43:449–453.
4. Boner AL, Valline G, Bennati D. Nedocromil sodium in exercise-induced bronchoconstriction in children. Ann Allgery 1989; 62:38–41.
5. Bleecker ER, Walden SM, Britt EJ, Effect of nedocromil on exercise-induced asthma. J Allergy Clin Immunol 1985; 75(1, pt 2):173.
6. Konig P, Hordvik NL, Kreutz C. The preventive effect and duration of action of nedocromil sodium and cromolyn sodium on exercise-induced asthma in adults: J Allergy Clin Immunol 1987; 79:64–68.
7. de Benedictis FM, Tuteri G, Bertotto A, Bruni L, Vaccaro R. Comparison of the protective effects of cromolyn sodium and nedocromil sodium in the treatment of exercise-induced asthma in children. J Allergy Clin Immunol 1994; 94:684–688.
8. Morton AR, Ogle SL, Fitch KD. Effects of nedocromil sodium, cromolyn sodium, and a placebo in exercise-induced asthma. Ann Allergy 1992; 68: 143–148.
9. Vilsvik J, Schaaning J. A comparative study of the effect of three doses of nedocromil sodium and placebo given by pressurized aerosol to asthmatics with exercise-induced bronchoconstriction. Ann Allergy 1988; 61:367–370.
10. Albazzaz MK, Neale MG, Patel KR. Dose–response study of nebulized nedocromil sodium in exercise-induced asthma. Thorax 1989; 44:816–819.
11. Speelberg B, Verhoeff NPLG, van den Berg NJ, Oosthoek CHA, van Herwaarden CLA, Bruijnzeel PLB. Nedocromil sodium inhibits the early and late asthmatic response to exercise. Eur Respir J 1992; 5:430–437.
12. Roberts JA, Thomson NC. Attenuation of exercise-induced asthma by pretreatment with nedocromil sodium and minocromil. Clin Allergy 1985; 15: 377–381.
13. Novembre E, Frongia G, Lombardi E, Veneruso G, Vierucci A. The preventive effect of nedocromil or furosemide alone or in combination on exercise-induced asthma in children. J Allergy Clin Immunol 1994; 94(2, pt 1):201–206.
14. Montgomery LC, Deuster PA. Ingestion of an antihistamine does not affect exercise performance. Med Sci Sports Exerc 1992; 24:383–388.
15. Pierson WE, Bierman CW, Shapiro GG, et al. Terfenadine dose–response blockage of exercise-induced bronchospasm [abstract]. J Allergy Clin Immunol 1987; 79:96.

16. Finnerty JP, Holgate ST. The contribution of histamine release and vagal reflexes, alone and in combination, to exercise-induced asthma. Eur Respir J 1993; 6:1132–1137.
17. Badier M, Beaumont D, Orehek J. Attenuation of hyperventilation-induced bronchospasm by terfenadine: a new antihistamine. J Allergy Clin Immunol 1988; 81:437–440.
18. McClean SP, Arreaza EE, Lett-Brown MA, Grant JA. Refractory cholinergic urticaria successfully treated with ketotifen. J Allergy Clin Immunol 1989; 83:738–741.
19. Nagy L, Orosz M. Effect of Zaditen on serum neutrophil chemotactic activity in exercise-induced asthma. Respiration 1985; 47:21–23.
20. Tan WC, Lim TK. Double-blind comparison of the protective effect of sodium cromoglycate and ketotifen on exercise-induced asthma in adults. Allergy 1987; 42:315–7.
21. Dorward AJ, Patel KR. A comparison of ketotifen with clemastine, ipratropium bromide, and sodium cromoglycate in exercise-induced asthma. Clin Allergy 1982; 12:355–61.
22. Petheram IS, Moxham J, Bierman CW, McAllen M, Spiro SG. Ketotifen in atopic asthma and exercise-induced asthma. Thorax 1981; 36:308–312.
23. Moreno MV, Fernandez M, de la Cuesta CG, Oehling A. The protective effect of ketotifen in exercise-induced bronchospasm. Allergol Immunopathol (Madr) 1988; 16:91–4.
24. Dorward AJ, Patel KR. A comparison of ketotifen with clemastine, ipratropium bromide, and sodium cromglycate in exercise-induced asthma. Clin Allergy 1982; 12:355–61.
25. Magnussen H, Reuss G, Jorres R, Aurich R. The effect of azelastine on exercise-induced asthma. Chest 1988; 93:937–40.
26. Motojima S, Ohashi Y, Otsuka T, Fukuda T, Makino S. Effects of azelastine on allergen- and exercise-induced asthma. Asian Pac J Allergy Immunol 1985; 3:174–8.
27. Ghosh SK, De Vos C, McIlroy I, Patel KR. Effect of cetirizine on exercise-induced asthma. Thorax 1991; 46:242–44.
28. Harries MG, Burge PS, O'Brien I, et al. Blood histamine levels after exercise testing. Clin Allergy 1979; 9:437–41.
29. Schachter EN, Rubin M. The effect of an aerosolized antihistamine, chlorpheniramine maleate, on exercise-induced bronchospasm. Ann Allergy 1985; 54:14–8.
30. Manning PJ, Watson R, O'Byrne PM. The effects of H_2-receptor antagonists on exercise refractoriness in asthma. J Allergy Clin Immunol 1992; 90: 125–126.
31. Jackson PJ, Manning PJ, O'Byrne PM. A new role for histamine H_2-receptors in asthmatic airways. Am Rev Respir Dis 1988; 138:784–8.
32. Cerrina J, Denjean A, Alexandre G, Lockhart A, Duroux P. Inhibition of exercise-induced asthma by a calcium antagonist, nifedipine. Am Rev Respir Dis 1981; 123:156–60.

33. Barnes PJ, Wilson NM, Brown MJ. A calcium antagonist, nifedipine, modifies exercise-induced asthma. Thorax 1981; 36:726–30.
34. Patel KR. The effect of calcium antagonist, nifedipine, in exercise-induced asthma. Clin Allergy 1981; 11:429–32.
35. Gordon EH, Wong SC, Klaustermeyer WB. Comparison of nifedipine with a new calcium channel blocker, flordipine, in exercise-induced asthma. J Asthma 1987; 24:261–5.
36. Olive SR, Hansen JE, Sue DY, Ben-Dov I, Wasserman K. Comparison of PY 108-068, a new calcium antagonist, with nifedipine in exercise-induced asthma. Chest 1986; 90:208–11.
37. Ben-Dov I, Sue DY, Hansen JE, Wasserman K. Bronchodilatation and attenuation of exercise-induced bronchospasm by PY 108-068, a new calcium antagonist. Am Rev Respir Dis 1986; 133:116–9.
38. Patakas D, Vlachoianni E, Tsara V, Louridas G, Argiroulou P. Nifedipine in bronchial asthma. J Allergy Clin Immunol 1983; 72:267–73.
39. Cerrina J, Denjean A, Alexandre G, Lockhart A, Duroux P. Inhibition of exercise-induced asthma by a calcium antagonist, nifedipine. Am Rev Respir Dis 1981; 123:156–60.
40. Jaiprakash SS, Chatterjee SS, Sahay JN, MacDonald G. Efficacy of nifedipine in the treatment of angina pectoris and chronic airway obstruction. Postgrad Med J 1980; 56:624–8.
41. Patel KR. Calcium antagonists in exercise-induced asthma. Br Med J 1981; 282:932–33.
42. Boner AL, Antolini I, Andreoli A, De Stefano G, Sette L. Comparison of the effects of inhaled calcium antagonists verapamil, sodium cromoglycate and ipratropium bromide on exercise-induced bronchoconstriction in children with asthma. Eur J Pediatr 1987; 146:408–11.
43. Patel KR, Peers E. Felodipine, a new calcium antagonist, modifies exercise-induced asthma. Am Rev Respir Dis 1988; 138:54–6.
44. Massey KL, Harman E, Hendeles L. Duration of protection of calcium channel blockers against exercise-induced bronchospasm: comparison of oral diltiazem and inhaled gallopamil. Eur J Clin Pharmacol 1988; 34:555–559.
45. Ibanez MD, Laso MT, Alonso E, Munoz MC, Sastre J. Effect of theophylline on airway responsiveness to methacholine and on exercise-induced bronchoconstriction. Ann Allergy 1994; 73:357–63.
46. Bierman CW, Shapiro GG, Pierson WE, Dorsett CS. Acute and chronic theophylline therapy in exercise-induced bronchospasm. Pediatrics 1977; 60: 845.
47. Pollock J, Kiechel F, Cooper D, Weinberger M. Relationship of serum theophylline concentration to inhibition of exercise-induced bronchospasm and comparison with cromolyn. Pediatrics 1977; 60:840.
48. Ellis EF. Inhibition of exercise-induced asthma by theophylline. J Allergy Clin Immunol 1984; 73:690–2.
49. Magnussen H, Reuss G, Jorres R. Methylxanthines inhibit exercise-induced bronchoconstriction at low serum theophylline concentration and in a dose-dependent fashion. J Allergy Clin Immunol 1988; 81:531–7.

50. Laursen LC, Johannesson N, Weeke B. Effects of enprofylline and theophylline on exercise-induced asthma. Allergy 1985; 40:506–9.
51. Hendeles L, Breton AL, Beaty R, Harman E. Therapeutic equivalence of a generic slow-release theophylline tablet. Pharmacotherapy 1995; 15:26–35.
52. Kanthawatana S, Ahrens RC, McCubbin M, Bronsky E, Blake K, Hendeles L. Bioequivalence of a generic slow-release theophylline tablet in children. J Pediatr 1994; 125(6 Pt 1):987–91.
53. Iikura Y, Inui H, Obata T, Nagakura T, Sugimoto H, Lee TH, Kay AB. Drug effects on exercise-induced late asthmatic responses. N Engl Reg Allergy Proc 1988; 9:203–7.
54. Waalkens HJ, van Essen-Zandvliet EE, Gerritsen J, Duiverman EJ, Kerrebijn KF, Knol K. The effect of an inhaled corticosteroid (budesonide) on exercise-induced asthma in children. Dutch CNSLD Study Group. Eur Respir J 1993; 6:652–6.
55. Vathenen AS, Knox AJ, Wisniewski A, Tattersfield AE. Effect of inhaled budesonide on bronchial reactivity to histamine, exercise, and eucapnic dry air hyperventilation in patients with asthma. Thorax 1991; 46:811–816.
56. Henriksen JM, Dahl R. Effects of inhaled budesonide alone and in combination with low-dose terbutaline in children with exercise-induced asthma. Am Rev Respir Dis 1983; 128:993–7.
57. Pederson S, et al. Budesonide treatment of moderate and severe asthma in children: a dose–response study. JACI 1995; 95:29–33.
58. Heimlich EM, Strick L, Busser RJ. An exercise response test in childhood asthma. J Allergy 1966; 37:103.
59. Jones RS. Assessment of respiratory function in the asthmatic child. Br Med J 1966; 2:972.
60. Konig P, Jaffe P, Godfrey S. Effect of corticosteroids on exercise-induced asthma. J Allergy Clin Immuno 1974; 54:14.
61. Henriksen JM, Wenzel A. Effect of an intranasally administered corticosteroid (budesonide) on nasal obstruction, mouth breathing, and asthma. Am Rev Respir Dis 1984; 130:1014–8.
62. Welsh PW, Stricker WE, Shu CP, et al. Efficacy of beclomethasone nasal solution, Nasilide, and cromolyn, in relieving symptoms of ragweed allergy. Mayo Clin Proc 1987; 62:125–34.
63. Watson RM, et al. Treatment of allergic rhinitis with intranasal corticosteroids in patients with mild asthma: effect on lower airway responsiveness. J Allergy Clin Immunol 1993; 91:97–100.
64. Corren J, Adinoff AD, Buchmeier A, Irvin CG. Nasal beclomethasone prevents the seasonal increase in bronchial responsiveness in patients with allergic rhinitis and asthma. J Allergy Clin Immunol 1992; 90:250–56.
65. Godfrey S, Konig P. Inhibition of exercise-induced asthma by different pharmacological pathways. Thorax 1976; 31:137–43.
66. Jones RS, Wharton MJ, Buston MH. The place of physical exercise and bronchodilator drugs in the assessment of the asthmatic child. Arch Dis Child 1963; 38:539.

67. Sly RM, Heimlich IM, Busser RJ, Strick I. Exercise-induced bronchospasm: effect of adrenergic or cholinergic blockade. J Allergy 1967; 40:93.
68. Hartley JPR, Davis BH. Cholinergic blockade in the prevention of exercise-induced asthma. Thorax 1980; 35:680–5.
69. Boner AL, Vallone G, De Stefano G. Effect of inhaled ipratropium bromide on methacholine and exercise provocation in asthmatic children. Clin Pediatr Univ Verona 1989; 6(2):81–5.
70. Poppius H, Sovijarvi AR, Tammilehto L. Lack of protective effect of high-dose ipratropium on bronchoconstriction following exercise with cold air breathing in patients with mild asthma. Eur J Respir Dis 1986; 68:319–25.
71. Finnerty JP, Holgate ST. The contribution of histamine release and vagal reflexes, alone and in combination, to exercise-induced asthma. Eur Respir J 1993; 6:1132–7.
72. Thomson NC, Patel KR, Kerr JW. Sodium cromoglycate and ipratropium bromide in exercise-induced asthma. Thorax 1978; 33:694–9.
73. Svenonius E, Arborelius M Jr, Wiberg R, Ekberg P. Prevention of exercise-induced asthma by drugs inhaled from metered aerosols. Allergy 1988; 43: 252–7.
74. Singh JP, Singh R, Gupta RC, Bharadwaja B. A comparative study of bronchodilator actions of ipratropium bromide (Atrovent) and salbutamol (Ventolin) on exercise-induced bronchial asthma. J Assoc Phys India 1992; 40: 545–7.
75. Pierson WE, Covert DS, Koenig JQ. Air pollutants, bronchial hyperactivity and exercise. J Allergy Clin Immunol 1984; 73:717–21.
76. Boulet LP, Turcotte H, Tennina S. Comparative efficacy of salbutamol, ipratropium, and cromoglycate in the prevention of bronchospasm induced by exercise and hyperosmolar challenges. J Allergy Clin Immunol 1989; 83: 882–7.
77. Manning PJ, Watson RM, Margoiskee DJ, et al. Inhibition of exercise-induced bronchoconstriction by MK 571, a potent leukotriene D_4 receptor antagonist. N Engl J Med 1990; 323:1736–39.
78. Finnerty JP, Wood-Baker R, Thomson H, Holgate ST. Role of leukotrienes in exercise-induced asthma. Am Rev Respir Dis 1992; 145:746–49.
79. Makker HK, Lau LC, Thomson HW, Binks SM, Holgate ST. The protective effect of inhaled LTD_4 receptor antagonist ICI 204219 against exercise-induced asthma. Am Rev Respir Dis 1993; 147:1413–18.
80. Robuscki M, Riva E, Fuccella LM, et al. Prevention of exercise-induced bronchoconstriction by a new leukotriene antagonist (SKF 104353): a double-blind study versus disodium cromoglycate and placebo. Am Rev Respir Dis 1992; 145:1285–88.
81. Mann JS, Robinson C, Sheridan AQ, et al. Effect of inhaled piriprost (U60, 257) a novel leukotriene inhibitor on allergen and exercise-induced bronchoconstriction in asthma. Thorax 1986; 41:746–52.
82. Ahmed T, Garrigo J, Danta I. Preventing bronchoconstriction in exercise-induced asthma with inhaled heparin. N Engl J Med 1993; 329:90–5.

10
The Role of Exercise Training and Conditioning in Patients with Asthma

William H. Baker and John M. Weiler
University of Iowa, Iowa City, Iowa

I. INTRODUCTION

Exercise is a common trigger for asthma, even in highly competitive, elite athletes, as is documented throughout this book. Exercise-induced asthma (EIA) is a major affliction that may prevent an elite athlete from achieving full levels of performance. Treatment of exercise-induced asthma is designed to allow athletes to compete with their nonasthmatic peers on a "level playing field." Treatment may consist of drugs, given by oral and topical routes, and nonpharmacological interventions, such as pregame warm-up and even acupuncture.

In recent years some reports have suggested that training and conditioning may also help the competitive athlete with asthma have fewer symptoms after exercise and participate at a higher level of performance [1]. Similarly, recreational athletes and nonathletes have been advised to participate in training and conditioning programs to increase their well-being and to decrease their symptoms of asthma. This chapter examines the role of training and conditioning in asthma, particularly in exercise-induced asthma. We consider the hypothesis that *exercise training and conditioning may increase the threshold of exercise necessary to induce airway obstruction in persons who have exercise-induced asthma and increase general well-being while, at the same time, decrease symptoms of asthma that occur associated with exercise.*

In this chapter, we first present an overview, and then we describe the ideal study that might be constructed to affirm or refute the hypothesis that we have stated. Next, we review the studies reported in the literature that support and refute this hypothesis. Finally, we draw conclusions based on the available evidence concerning the value of training and conditioning programs in asthma.

II. OVERVIEW

Exercise-induced asthma affects all age groups and is seen with equal prevalence in male and female subjects [2]. As many as 90% of patients with chronic asthma will have bronchial obstruction or an exacerbation of symptoms after exercise [3]. Exercise may also trigger bronchial obstruction and symptoms of asthma in individuals who do not otherwise have asthma [4]. Bierman et al. [4] in 1976, reported that 41% of those children with allergic rhinitis who do not have chronic asthma may be triggered to have an asthma attack after a 6-min free run. These authors and others have also suggested that exercise may trigger bronchial obstruction in about 7% of those who have no predisposing condition.

The prevalence of exercise-induced asthma varies depending on the type of exercise that is performed, whether the person performed exercise before the challenge, the sensitivity of the measure used to record an effect, and baseline bronchial hyperresponsiveness [5–10]. Running sports are more likely to trigger asthma than is swimming, walking, or downhill skiing [7,8].

The more intense the exercise, the more likely it will provoke asthma [6,9]. An exercise challenge, described in more detail elsewhere in this book (Chapter 2) requires about 6–8 min of strenuous exertion. Less intense exercise that is interrupted is not as likely to trigger asthma as is continuous intense exercise. Some subjects may be able to "run through" their asthma, probably as a result of a refractory period of approximately 1–4 h in which the subject is relatively resistant to an additional attack of bronchospasm following exercise [10–14]. Subjects may also be refractory to exercise after modest exertion that does not itself trigger bronchospasm [11]. The mechanism for refractoriness is not clearly understood. Subjects who are refractory to exercise may still develop bronchospasm after an antigen or histamine challenge [15,16]. Some athletes take advantage of the refractory period and run a series of sprints before a game to induce refractoriness [11].

Environmental conditions, including cold temperatures, decreased humidity, and increased pollution, may increase the likelihood of asthma occurring after exercise. Air pollution, with sulfur dioxide or ozone, will enhance bronchial reactivity and cause more severe asthma after exercise [17]. In addition, hyperventilation in cold air may provoke asthma, except that the bronchospasm that is seen is not preceded by bronchodilation or any adrenergic effect [18,19].

Parents may be reluctant to allow their children who have asthma to participate in exercise programs, and teachers may fear the consequence of a severe attack. In contrast, some teachers and coaches may fail to recognize asthma and attribute lack of performance to laziness or lack of conditioning. In either event, the consequence for the child may be very negative. Children with exercise-induced asthma may tend to avoid athletic activities. Similarly, adults who developed asthma as a child may continue to limit their involvement in exercise programs. In these subjects, asthma attacks triggered by exercise may lead to a conditioned reflex in which exercise is avoided altogether.

Exercise-induced asthma can be minimized or prevented by the following: warm-up exercise (to induce a refractory period), changing the nature of the exercise (such as from running to swimming), medication or placebo, hypnosis, prewarming air, and changing the environment [reviewed in 20]. This chapter will consider whether training and conditioning may also minimize exercise-induced asthma.

III. THE IDEAL STUDY

The ideal study to examine the hypothesis stated in this chapter would be double-blind, randomized to a block design, and "placebo-controlled" (Table 1). In a single-blind study the participants would not know which group is the "treatment group" and which is the "control group," even though they would obviously know the treatment that they are receiving and that there are two groups. In a double-blind study the investigators who are capturing the data and evaluating the results of the study would not know the identities of the interventions, and the participants would not know which group is the treatment group and which is the control group. The subject population for the ideal study would be clearly defined (as having asthma) and intervention groups would be compared for severity of asthma (mild, moderate, or severe). The type of asthma would be clearly defined in the inclusion requirement section of the protocol (exercise-induced, acute, intermittent, or chronic asthma). Intervention treatment groups would be compared for medication use, symptoms, age, ethnic origin, and gender. Groups would be matched for levels of exercise performance at the onset of the study.

Table 1 The Ideal Study to Examine the Efficacy of Training and Conditioning Interventions in Patients with Asthma

Double-blind
Randomized patients to a block design
Control group
Study population: clearly defined
Compare groups and (possibly) stratify for medication use, age, ethnic origin, symptoms and severity of disease, and exercise performance at onset of trial
Type of asthma: clearly defined
Medication use: controlled during study
Intervention duration: months to years
Intervention type: clearly defined
Outcomes: determined by objective measures; determined long-term consequence(s) of intervention
Spirometry: use FEV_1, rather than peak flows whenever possible
Significance: statistical significance *and* biologically meaningful differences defined by protocol
Statistical tests: 2-tailed

During the study, medication use would be rigidly controlled. The intervention would occur over months to years, and the method of exercise training and conditioning would be strictly defined. Objective measures of outcome would be used, rather than subjective measures. Thus, predefined, measures of effectiveness might include any of the following: spirometry; exercise challenges (pre- and post-exercise spirometry); symptoms; backup medication use; days missed from school or work; quality of life assessments; work capacity; maximum oxygen consumption rate ($\dot{V}O_2max$); ventilatory requirements; and cardiovascular parameters (heart rate or blood pressure).

In the ideal study, subjects would be asked to determine pulmonary functions away from the clinic or pulmonary function laboratory, to evaluate daytime variability and response to exercise. For these determinations, 1-S forced expiratory volume (FEV_1) is the most reproducible objective measure that can be followed to quantify airway obstruction. Other tests, such as the peak expiratory flow rate, may be more effort-dependent and less reliable in detecting airway obstruction.

The data would be analyzed using two-tailed statistical tests to determine if the intervention had a positive or negative effect on asthma. Before the study, there would also be some statement in the protocol to define a biologically significant difference. This would allow the investigators to ascertain at the end of the study whether a statistically significant change imparts a biological advantage.

A. Materials and Methods

We searched English language reports contained in the *Medline* database for all manuscripts that contained the key words "asthma" or "exercise-induced asthma" and also contained "exercise" or "exercise therapy" or "physical education and training" or "physical conditioning." Then, we reviewed abstracts of the manuscripts to determine those that may have contained reports of studies to examine the effect of a physical intervention on asthmatic subjects, although a few of the studies also included nonasthmatic subjects. Additionally, we reviewed the introduction and discussion sections of the manuscripts that were found for reference to other studies that were performed to examine the effect of a physical intervention on asthma. We quantified the length of the intervention and excluded reports in which the subjects received fewer than 5 days of training and conditioning and studies that examined the refractory period after exercise, unless there was also some physical intervention that was at least 5 days in length. Studies that met these requirements were reviewed independently by us. When we did not agree on whether the paper supported or refuted the hypothesis stated in this paper, these results were discussed and a joint conclusion was formed. Studies in which the subjects received transcendental meditation, yoga training, breathing exercises, drug therapy, or hypnosis were not included unless there was also some physical intervention that was at least 5 days in length. Forty-five studies met these criteria and were included in this analysis.

B. Study Characteristics

Table 2 lists alphabetically the 45 studies reported here [21–66]. These studies used a wide variety of training and conditioning procedures. No study fulfilled all four of the criteria that we used to evaluate study quality (double-blind, randomized, medication-controlled, and control group included). Other aspects of the studies that varied considerably were use of medication before exercise, number of sessions per week, number of weeks of training and type of training, assessment of compliance with training, location of training programs, and motivation of the subjects. In many cases important details were not included in the report. In those cases it was assumed that the investigators did not control or capture that variable.

Two studies were single-blind; none were double-blind. Six reports indicated that subjects were randomized to treatment groups. In only one

Table 2 Summary of Findings from 46 Studies

Author [Ref.] (yr)	Blinded	Randomized	Medication controlled	Control group	Overall result[a]
Afzelius-Frisk [21] (1977)	No	No	No	Yes	+
Arborelius [22] (1984)	No	No	No	No	+
Bungaard [23,24] (1982,1983)	Single	Yes	Yes	Yes	+
Cochrane [25] (1990)	No	Yes	No	Yes	+
Dean [26] (1988)	No	No	No	Yes	+
Edenbrandt [27] (1990)	No	Yes	No	Yes	−
Engström [28] (1991)	No	No	No	No	+
Fein [29] (1953)	No	No	No	Yes	Un
Fitch [30] (1976)	No	No	No	Yes	−
Fitch [31] (1986)	No	No	No	Yes	−
Freeman [32] (1989)	No	No	No	Yes	+
Geubelle [33] (1971)	No	No	No	No	−
Giordo [34] (1992)	Single	Yes	No	Yes	−
Graff-Lonnevig [35] (1980)	No	No	No	Yes	−
Hass [36] (1987)	No	Yes	No	Yes	+
Henriksen [37] (1981)	No	No	No	No	Un
Henriksen [38] (1983)	No	No	No	Yes	+
Hirt [39] (1964)	No	Yes	No	Yes	−
Holzer [40] (1984)	No	No	No	No	−
Huang [41] (1989)	No	No	No	Yes	+
Hyde [42] (1968)	No	No	No	No	−
Itkin [43] (1966)	No	No	No	No	−
Karper [44] (1988)	No	No	No	No	+
Leisti [45] (1979)	No	No	No	No	Un
Ludwick [46] (1986)	No	No	No	No	+
McElhenney [47] (1963)	No	No	No	No	+
Millman [48] (1965)	No	No	No	No	+
Nickerson [49] (1983)	No	No	No	No	−
Olivia [50] (1990)	No	No	No	No	−
Orenstein [51] (1985)	No	No	No	Yes	−
Peterson [52] (1965)	No	No	No	No	+
Ramazanoglu [53] (1985)	No	No	No	No	+
Robinson [54] (1992)	No	No	No	Yes	−
Schnall [55] (1982)	No	No	No	No	−
Schneider [56] (1980)	No	No	No	Yes	+
Schultz [57] (1955)	No	No	No	No	+
Seligman [58] (1970)	No	No	No	Un	Un
Sly [59] (1972)	No	No	No	Yes	−
Svenonius [60] (1983)	No	No	No	No	+
Szentagothai [61] (1987)	No	No	No	No	+
Tanizaki [62] (1986)	No	No	No	No	+

Table 2 Continued

Author [Ref.] (yr)	Blinded	Randomized	Medication controlled	Control group	Overall result[a]
Taylor [63] (1968)	No	No	No	No	−
Varray [64] (1991)	No	No	No	Yes	−
Varva [65] (1971)	No	No	No	No	−
Wolf [66] (1988)	No	No	No	No	+
Total = 45					
Yes or +	2	6	1	20	22
No or −	43	39	44	24	19
Un (undetermined)	0	0	0	1	4

[a] Overall supports or refutes hypothesis stated in this paper.

report was there a description that medication use was controlled during the study. This is very important because medication use may alter bronchial reactivity and symptoms, as well as many of the other endpoints that were studied by these authors, even more than the training and conditioning programs. Twenty studies included a control group, although, in many cases, the two (or more) groups were not comparable in composition.

One study met three of the criteria; it was a single-blind study. Another study met two criteria; medication use was not controlled and it was single blind. Four additional studies met two criteria; subjects were randomized to control or treatment groups. Consequently, 14 studies met only one of the four criteria and 25 failed to meet any of the criteria. Under normal circumstances these 39 studies would not be included in any analysis of a pharmacological intervention in asthma.

C. Results

Twenty-two of the reports indicated a positive outcome, or we were able to infer this overall outcome. In contrast, 19 studies failed to show a positive outcome, or we were unable to infer a positive outcome. In four reports it was not possible to categorize the outcome as either positive or negative.

Of the six studies that met two or more criteria, 3 reported positive results, and 3 reported negative results. Of the studies that met only one of the criteria, 6 reported positive results, 7 reported negative results, and 1 had results that could not be characterized as positive or negative. Of the studies that did not meet any of the criteria, 13 reported positive results, 9 reported negative results, and 3 could not be characterized as positive or negative.

The studies with the fewest controls were more likely to report a positive result than the studies that had more controls. This raises a concern that the interpretation of some of the results of the studies may have been biased. Perhaps the motivating force to perform a few of these studies was to validate, rather than to evaluate, the value of training and conditioning in subjects with asthma.

It is very important to consider publication bias in evaluating these reports. In 1991, Easterbrook et al. [67] reported that studies with statistically significant results were more likely to be published than were studies that found no differences between the treatment groups. Their report also strongly suggests that positive studies lead to a greater number of publications in journals with a high citation impact factor than do negative studies. They argue that conclusions based on literature reviews or metanalyses may be misleading if they are based only on published studies. They suggest that reviewers should be cautious in evaluating clinical trials that are small and nonrandomized. Unfortunately, the overwhelming majority of the studies we reviewed that examined the role of training and conditioning in asthma lacked these essential controls and were relatively small. In the reports reviewed by Easterbrook et al. [67] the tendency toward publication bias was particularly high with observational studies. Taken together, their findings suggest that great caution should be exercised in basing conclusions only on published data.

We also evaluated whether objective or subjective criteria were used to determine whether training and conditioning had an effect on asthma. Three studies used subjective criteria only (such as asthma symptoms or psychological factors), two reported a positive result, and one reported a negative result. Twenty-three studies used objective criteria only (such as pulmonary function tests); 11 reported a positive result, 9 reported a negative result, and 3 reports failed to allow a characterization of the outcome. Nineteen studies used a combination of subjective and objective criteria; nine reported a positive result, nine reported a negative result, and one report could not be characterized as to outcome.

Next, we examined whether the intervention (type and length) had any effect on whether the outcome was positive or negative. Unfortunately, many studies used a wide variety of training and conditioning techniques so that it was impossible to examine whether the type of physical training and conditioning had any influence on whether the results were positive or negative. Then we examined the length of intervention. One study used an intervention of 1 month or less and it was reported as positive. Twenty-one studies had interventions of more than 1 month, but not more than 3 months; 8 were reported as positive, 11 as negative, and 2 could not be characterized as to outcome. Seventeen studies had interventions lasting longer than 3 months, but not longer than 1 year; 9 were reported as positive, 6 as negative, and 2 could not be interpreted as to outcome. Five studies had interventions longer than 1 year; 3 were reported as positive and 2 as negative. One study had interventions that varied so widely that it was not included in this analysis.

IV. REPRESENTATIVE STUDIES

In this section we have highlighted some representative studies that have been reported. We have selected the six reports in which at least two criteria were met (blinded, randomized, control group, controlled medication use). These reports describe a wide range of interventions as well as a variety of endpoints to evaluate success of each intervention. These representative studies also indicate the difficulty in characterizing some studies as clearly showing an effect, or clearly not showing any capacity of the intervention(s) to have an effect on asthma.

Bungaard et al. [23,24] reported a study comparing 16 asthmatic subjects who underwent a training program with 11 control subjects. This study met three of the foregoing criteria; it was single-blind, rather than double-blind. Training continued twice a week for 1 h each session for 2 months and included running, jumping, and calisthenics. Of the original subjects who qualified for this study, 40% dropped out before study completion. The authors found that the training group had less need to use a β_2-adrenergic agonist spray, decreasing from an average of 4.94 puffs/day to 3.41 puffs/day. In contrast, there was no significant change in β_2-agonist spray use in the control group, who performed low-intensity exercise. The patients in the training group also improved their maximal oxygen consumption, whereas no change was seen in the control patients.

The study reported by Girodo et al. [34] did not control medication use and the study was single-blind. Sixty-seven asthmatic adults were randomly assigned to one of three groups of subjects. One group, the study group of interest for these authors, received deep diaphragmatic-breathing training, which resulted in decreased use of medication and decreased symptoms of asthma. This group also had about a 300% increase in time spent in physical activity. This positive outcome was not sustained;

a 2-month follow-up after completion of the training program revealed that many patients in this group had medication requirements and sedentary habits similar to those before intervention. The second group, which is the group of interest for our report, received physical exercise training, and the third group was the control group; neither of these groups had any changes in the endpoints when compared with study initiation. Consequently, this study has been judged as failing to demonstrate efficacy for training and conditioning (see Table 2).

Cochrane et al. [25] reported 36 young adult patients with asthma who were randomized to either a training group or a control group. This study was not blinded and did not control medication use. The training group performed aerobic exercise, calisthenics, and stretching for 30 min three times a week for 3 months. The training group had significant improvements in fitness and cardiorespiratory performance when compared with controls.

Edenbrandt et al. [27] reported a study in which 20 subjects trained for 3 months with circuit training, relay races, and swimming, and were taught huffing, which is a cough technique also known as forced-expiratory technique. There was no significant change in the training patients in spirometry or working capacity when compared with the 21 control patients who did not undergo any program.

Hass et al. [36] reported a comparison of 22 asthmatic subjects who participated in aerobic training with 15 asthmatic control subjects who did not participate in a fitness program. Their report indicates that the average external work capacity increased by 30% and $\dot{V}O_2max$ increased by 15% in the group that received the intervention. Pulmonary function did not change after training except for a small increase in maximal voluntary ventilation. This was attributed to respiratory muscle training. Members of this group, after participating in the training program, also had average heart rate responses that were 20 beats per minute slower than before the intervention; heart rate was not significantly changed in the control group.

Hirt et al. [39] studied 63 hospitalized asthmatic patients who were randomized to groups. Forty were assigned to the control group, and 23 were subjected to weight-resistance training and other sport activities. The authors report no statistical improvement in FEV_1 or FEV_1/FVC. There was a significant increase in $\dot{V}O_2max$ in the exercise group, but not in the control group.

A few of the studies that had fewer than two criteria were also interesting, and we highlight the reports by Robinson et al. [54] and Varray et al. [64]. In 1992, Robinson et al. [54] reported 8 asthmatic patients who completed circuit training (14 began the training) and 7 control patients

(11 began the study as controls). The $\dot{V}O_2max$ increased for both groups as did daily peak flows, but there was no change in histamine responsiveness, medication use, or symptom score.

In 1991, Varray et al. [64] reported seven asthmatic patients who participated in a swim-training program and seven control patients. They found no change in frequency of attacks, no decreased need for medication use, and no change in spirometry in the group that underwent training. The $\dot{V}O_2max$ increased after aerobic training, but did not increase further after high-intensity training.

A. Alternative Therapies

Our review of the English language literature yielded reports that described alternative therapies for the treatment of asthma in addition to physical training and conditioning. Many of these interventions involved teaching asthmatic subjects new breathing patterns or providing them with breathing exercises without other physical training and conditioning. For example, Ershine and Schonell [68] reported a randomized study that examined 12 subjects with chronic asthma who received either mental and muscular relaxation or muscular relaxation alone with the intervention, once a week for 4 weeks. They concluded that there was no change in psychological or physical measures or in spirometry.

Other studies examined the effect of breathing exercises on asthma. Fein et al. [69] studied 13 asthmatic patients and found that pursed-lip breathing and quiet diaphragmatic breathing exercises ". . . aided in the prevention of pulmonary complications of asthma and created a sense of relaxation and psychologic relief not obtained through the use of symptomatic drugs." Bolton et al. [70] in 1956, reported on 18 patients with asthma who participated in a breathing exercise program that emphasized "abdominal" breathing compared with 25 controls who were taught the "old" technique of breathing using the accessory muscles of respiration. In this study the "new" breathing exercise program resulted in improvement in diaphragmatic efficiency and vital capacity. Similarly, Weiner et al. [71], in 1992, reported a double-blind study lasting 6 months in which 15 asthmatic subjects used a threshold inspiratory muscle trainer; the control group of 15 asthmatic subjects received sham training. The active intervention group had increased inspiratory muscle strength and muscle endurance as well as improvement in symptoms, fewer hospitalizations, fewer emergency department contacts, less absence from school or work, and less medication consumption. The authors concluded that there was a clear difference between the two study groups.

Jain et al. [72] studied 46 patients in a program of yoga over 2 years and found that there was a significant increase in pumonary function test results and in exercise capacity. Scherr et al. [73] described a study in which they compared 22 asthmatic patients, who were offered biofeedback-mediated deep muscle relaxation, with 22 untrained asthmatic control patients. In this study the authors claim that there was a statistically significant improvement in behavior rating and peak flow rates and a decrease in infirmary visits, asthma attacks, and steroid use in patients in the treatment group when compared with patients in the control group. The authors do caution that this study needs to be repeated to confirm their positive outcome.

These alternative interventions suggest that some modest improvement in asthma may be seen after these programs. However, these studies are also insufficiently well controlled to have eliminated bias, suggesting that we should be cautious in interpreting the study outcomes. Furthermore, these alternative therapies do not, in general, offer the asthmatic patient the added benefits of an increase in the cardiovascular fitness that occurs in physical-training and conditioning programs regardless of whether there is also concomitant improvement in some measure of asthma.

Recently, Lacasse et al. [74] reported a metanalysis to examine the role of rehabilitation on exercise capacity and health-related quality of life (HRQL) in patients with chronic obstructive pulmonary disease (COPD). Their methods were similar to ours in that they searched the *Medline* database using specific terms, and two reviewers abstracted the data. They included inpatient, outpatient, and home-based rehabilitation programs that lasted at least 4 weeks in which there was an exercise program, with or without education or psychological support for the patients. Fourteen trials were included in their analysis. The metanalysis showed that there were significant improvements in all outcome measures. Two measures of health-related quality of life exceeded the minimum clinically important difference (''defined as the smallest difference perceived as important by the average patient''): dyspnea and mastery.

They concluded that their analysis ''. . . strongly support(s) respiratory rehabilitation that includes at least 4 weeks' exercise training as part of management for patients with COPD.'' They also suggested that rehabilitation may lead to a greater improvement in health-related quality of life and functional exercise capacity when compared with bronchodilators or oral theophylline. Interestingly, their analysis suggested that ''. . . less sophisticated rehabilitation programmes [*sic*] may be as effective as the more comprehensive programmes [*sic*] in improving HRQL.''

V. CONCLUSION

Do these studies prove the hypothesis that exercise training and conditioning may increase the threshold of exercise necessary to induce airway obstruction in individuals who have exercise-induced asthma and increase general well-being, while at the same time, decrease symptoms of asthma that occur associated with exercise? We conclude that no study was properly designed or sufficiently well controlled to allow us to support or to refute this hypothesis. Consequently, we were unable to perform a metanalysis because no study met our requirement that studies be double-blind, placebo controlled, randomized, and controlled for medication use. Eighty-seven percent of studies met either one or none of these criteria.

The majority of the studies suggest that physical training and conditioning do have a positive influence on fitness in asthmatic subjects in general. Garfinkel et al. [75] studied aerobic fitness in 27 patients with mild to moderate asthma. They concluded that in these patients "the ability to perform aerobic work is not determined by the level of NSBHR (nonspecific bronchial hyperreactivity) but by the amount of regular physical activity performed." Thus, exercise restriction in these patients was determined by deconditioning rather than limitation associated directly with asthma. None of the studies in our review suggest that the improvement that was seen was sufficient to replace pharmacotherapy. Therefore, these training and conditioning programs must be viewed only as possible adjunctive interventions in patients in whom medical therapy has been optimized. Unfortunately, we cannot make any stronger statement than to say that programs that provide asthmatic subjects with training and conditioning may help improve their asthmatic symptoms and may allow more athletic participation.

VI. SUMMARY

None of the studies that we reviewed suggest that training or conditioning is detrimental to subjects with asthma. More of the reports suggest a positive outcome (49%) than a negative one (42%). It is intuitively obvious that good physical conditioning imparts better general health for a person with or without asthma. The studies we evaluated reveal a large number of potential benefits from training and conditioning. These benefits include increased aerobic capacity, so that more exercise can be performed before reaching one's anaerobic threshold; decreased sensitivity to CO_2; decreased receptor sensitivity; decreased vagal tone; increased muscle strength; decreased symptoms; decreased medication use; improved quality of life and global evaluations; improved athletic performance; and fewer days lost from school or work. Thus, we would agree with the majority of studies that suggest that, in general, training and conditioning programs benefit asthmatic subjects. It is likely that training and conditioning programs would benefit nonasthmatic subjects in the same way by enhancing overall fitness. However, in the end, it is often impossible to ascribe improvement to a single intervention. The best results will still be obtained in a coordinated program in which physical training and conditioning is combined with appropriate pharmacotherapy and nondrug interventions [20].

ACKNOWLEDGMENT

The authors thank Dr. Jeff Wilson for his thoughtful review of this manuscript.

REFERENCES

1. Clark CJ. The role of physical training in asthma. Chest 1992; 101:293S–298S.
2. Ernst P, Demissie K, Joseph L, et al. Socioeconomic status and indicators of asthma in children. Am J Respir Crit Care Med 1995; 152:570–575.
3. Jones RS, Buston MH, Wharton MJ. The effect of exercise on ventilatory function in the child with asthma. Br J Dis Chest 1962; 56:78–86.
4. Bierman CW, Kawabori I, Pierson WE. Incidence of exercise-induced asthma in children. Pediatrics 1975; 56(suppl):847–850.
5. Karjalainen J, Lindqvist A, Laitinen LA. Seasonal variability of exercise-induced asthma especially outdoors. Effect of birch pollen allergy. Clin Exp Allergy 1989; 19:273–278.
6. Noviski N, Bar-Yishay E, Gur I, Godfrey S. Exercise intensity determines and climatic conditions modify the severity of exercise-induced asthma. Am Rev Respir Dis 1987; 136:592–594.
7. Bar-Yishay E, Gur I, Inbar O, et al. Differences between swimming and running as stimuli for exercise-induced asthma. Eur J Appl Physiol 1982; 48: 387–397.
8. Godfrey S. Exercise-induced asthma: clinical, physiological, and therapeutic implications. J Allergy Clin Immunol 1975; 56:1–17.
9. Bundgaard A, Ingemann-Hansen T, Schmidt A, Halkjaer-Kristensen J. Exercise-induced asthma after walking, running, and cycling. Scand J Clin Lab Invest 1982; 42:15–18.
10. Belcher NG, Rees PJ, Clark TJH, Lee TH. A comparison of the refractory periods induced by hypertonic airway challenge and exercise in bronchial asthma. Am Rev Respir Dis 1987; 135:822–825.

11. Reiff DB, Choudry NB, Pride NB, Ind PW. The effect of prolonged submaximal warm-up exercise on exercise-induced asthma. Am Rev Respir Dis 1989; 139:479–484.
12. Rosenthal RR, Laube BL, Hood DB, Norman PS. Analysis of refractory period after exercise and eucapnic voluntary hyperventilation challenge. Am Rev Respir Dis 1990; 141:368–372.
13. Nowak D. Jörres R, Magnussen H. Influence of exercise-induced bronchoconstriction on refractoriness. Lung 1992; 170:75–84.
14. Ohtsuka A, Koyama S, Horie T. Refractoriness of eucapnic hyperventilation-induced bronchoconstriction in rabbits. Am J Respir Crit Care Med 1994; 149:682–686.
15. Carpentiere G, Castello F, Marino S. Airway responsiveness to histamine in patients refractory to repeated exercise. Chest 1988; 93:933–936.
16. Boulet L-P, Legris C, Turcotte H. Bronchial responsiveness to histamine after repeated exercise-induced bronchospasm. Respiration 1987; 52: 237–245.
17. Yang SC, Yang SP. Respiratory function changes from inhalation of polluted air. Arch Environ Health 1994; 49:182–187.
18. Eliasson AH, Phillips YY, Rajagopal KR, Howard RS. Sensitivity and specificity of bronchial provocation testing: an evaluation of four techniques in exercise-induced bronchospasm. Chest 1992; 102:347–355.
19. Nicolai T, Mutius EV, Reitmeir P, Wjst M. Reactivity to cold-air hyperventilation in normal and in asthmatic children in a survey of 5,697 schoolchildren in Southern Bavaria. Am Rev Respir Dis 1993; 147:565–572.
20. Weiler JM. Exercise-induced asthma: a practical guide to definitions, diagnosis, prevalence, and treatment. Allergy Asthma Proc 1996; 17:315–325.
21. Afzelius-Frisk I, Grimby G, Lindholm N. Physical training in patients with asthma. Poumon Coeur 1977; 33:33–37.
22. Arborelius M Jr, Svenonius E. Decrease of exercise-induced asthma after physical training. Eur J Respir Dis Suppl 1984; 136:25–31.
23. Bundgaard A, Ingemann-Hansen T, Schmidt A, Halkjaer-Kristensen J. Effect of physical training on peak oxygen consumption rate and exercise-induced asthma in adult asthmatics. Scand J Clin Lab Invest 1982; 42:9–13.
24. Bundgaard A, Ingemann-Hansen T, Halkjaer-Kristensen J, Schmidt A, Bloch I, Andersen PK. Short-term physical training in bronchial asthma. Br J Dis Chest 1983; 77:147–152.
25. Cochrane LM, Clark CJ. Benefits and problems of a physical training programme for asthmatic patients. Thorax 1990; 45:345–351.
26. Dean M, Bell E, Kershaw CR, Guyer BM, Hide DW. A short exercise and living course for asthmatics. Br J Dis Chest 1988; 82:155–161.
27. Edenbrandt L, Olséni L, Svenonius E, Jonson B. Effect of physiotherapy in asthmatic children—a one-year follow-up after physical training once a week. Acta Paediatr Scand 1990; 79:973–975.
28. Engström I, Fällström K, Karlberg E, Sten G, Bjure J. Psychological and respiratory physiological effects of a physical exercise programme on boys with severe asthma. Acta Paediatr Scand 1991; 80:1058–1065.

29. Fein BT, Cox EP, Green LH. Respiratory and physical exercise in the treatment of bronchial asthma. Ann Allergy 1953; 11:275–287.
30. Fitch KD, Morton AR, Blanksby BA. Effects of swimming training on children with asthma. Arch Dis Child 1976; 51:190–194.
31. Fitch KD, Blitvich JD, Morton AR. The effect of running training on exercise-induced asthma. Ann Allergy 1986; 57:90–94.
32. Freeman W, Nute MGL, Williams C. The effect of endurance running training on asthmatic adults. Br J Sports Med 1989; 23:115–122.
33. Geubelle F, Ernould C, Jovanovic M. Working capacity and physical training in asthmatic children, at 1800 m. altitude. Acta Paediatr Scand Suppl 1971; 217:93–98.
34. Girodo M, Ekstrand KA, Metivier GJ. Deep diaphragmatic breathing: rehabilitation exercises for the asthmatic patient. Arch Phys Med Rehabil 1992; 73:717–720.
35. Graff-Lonnevig V, Bevegård S, Eriksson BO, Kraepelien S, Saltin B. Two years' follow-up of asthmatic boys participating in a physical activity programme. Acta Paediatr Scand 1980; 69:347–352.
36. Haas F, Pasierski S, Levine N, Bishop M, Axen K, Pineda H, Haas A. Effect of aerobic training on forced expiratory airflow in exercising asthmatic humans. J Appl Physiol 1987; 63:1230–1235.
37. Henriksen JM, Nielsen TT, Dahl R. Effects of physical training on plasma citrate and exercise-induced asthma. Scand J Clin Lab Invest 1981; 41: 225–229.
38. Henriksen JM, Nielsen TT. Effect of physical training on exercise-induced bronchoconstriction. Acta Paediatr Scand 1983; 72:31–36.
39. Hirt M. Physical conditioning in asthma. I. Preliminary results. Ann Allergy 1964; 22:229–237.
40. Holzer FJ, Schnall R, Landau LI. The effect of a home exercise programme in children with cystic fibrosis and asthma. Aust Paediatr J 1984; 20:297–302.
41. Huang S-W, Veiga R, Sila U, Reed E, Hines S. The effect of swimming in asthmatic children—participants in a swimming program in the City of Baltimore. J Asthma 1989; 26:117–121.
42. Hyde JS, Swarts CL. Effect of an exercise program on the perennially asthmatic child. Am J Dis Child 1968; 116:383–396.
43. Itkin IH, Nacman M. The effect of exercise on the hospitalized asthmatic patient. J Allergy 1966; 37:253–263.
44. Karper WB. Effects of walking on peak expiratory flow rate in four asthmatic children. Percept Mot Skills 1988; 67:847–852.
45. Leisti S, Finnilä M-J, Kiuru E. Effects of physical training on hormonal responses to exercise in asthmatic children. Arch Dis Child 1979; 54:524–528.
46. Ludwick SK, Jones JW, Jones TK, Fukuhara JT, Strunk RC. Normalization of cardiopulmonary endurance in severely asthmatic children after bicycle ergometry therapy. J Pediatr 1986; 109:446–451.
47. McElhenney TR, Petersen KH. Physical fitness for asthmatic boys: a cooperative pilot study. JAMA 1963; 185:142–143.

48. Millman M, Grundon WG, Kasch F, Wilkerson B, Headley J. Controlled exercise in asthmatic children. Ann Allergy 1965; 23:220–225.
49. Nickerson BG, Bautista DB, Namey MA, Richards W, Keens TG. Distance running improves fitness in asthmatic children without pulmonary complications or changes in exercise-induced bronchospasm. Pediatrics 1983; 71: 147–152.
50. Olivia CKW. Physical conditioning programme for children with bronchial asthma. Acta Paediatr Jpn 1990; 32:173–175.
51. Orenstein DM, Reed ME, Grogan FT Jr, Crawford LV. Exercise conditioning in children with asthma. J Pediatr 1985; 106:556–560.
52. Petersen KH, McElhenney TR. Effects of a physical fitness program upon asthmatic boys. Pediatrics 1965; 35:295–299.
53. Ramazanoglu YM, Kraemer R. Cardiorespiratory response to physical conditioning in children with bronchial asthma. Pediatr Pulmonol 1985; 1: 272–277.
54. Robinson DM, Egglestone DM, Hill PM, Rea HH, Richards GN, Robinson SM. Effects of a physical conditioning programme on asthmatic patients. NZ Med J 1992; 105:253–256.
55. Schnall R, Ford P, Gillam I, Landau L. Swimming and dry land exercises in children with asthma. Aust Paediatr J 1982; 18:23–27.
56. Schneider MR, Melton BH, Reisch JS. Effects of a progressive exercise program on absenteeism among school children with asthma. J Sch Health 1980; 50:92–95.
57. Schutz K. Muscular exercise in the treatment of bronchial asthma. Technic and physiologic basis. NY State J Med 1955; 55:635–643.
58. Seligman T, Randel HO, Stevens JJ. Conditioning program for children with asthma. Phys Ther 1970; 50:641–648.
59. Sly RM, Harper RT, Rosselot I. The effect of physical conditioning upon asthmatic children. Ann Allergy 1972; 30:86–93.
60. Svenonius E, Kautto R, Arborelius M Jr. Improvement after training of children with exercise-induced asthma. Acta Paediatr Scand 1983; 72:23–30.
61. Szentágothai K, Gyene I, Szócska M, Osváth P. Physical exercise program for children with bronchial asthma. Pediatr Pulmonol 1987; 3:166–172.
62. Tanizaki Y. Improvement of ventilatory function by spa therapy in patients with intractable asthma. Acta Med Okayama 1986; 40:55–59.
63. Taylor WF, Brkich J, Herron J, Strick L. Swim training: its effect on asthmatic children. J Allergy 1968; 41:92.
64. Varray AL, Mercier JG, Terral CM, Prefaut CG. Individualized aerobic and high intensity training for asthmatic children in an exercise readaptation program. Is training always helpful for better adaptation to exercise? Chest 1991; 99:579–586.
65. Vavra J, Macek M, Mrzena B, Spicak V. Intensive physical training in children with bronchial asthma. Acta Paediatr Scand Suppl 1971; 217:90–92.
66. Wolf SI, Lampl KL. Pulmonary rehabilitation: the use of aerobic dance as a therapeutic exercise for asthmatic patients. Ann Allergy 1988; 61:357–360.

67. Easterbrook PJ, Berlin JA, Gopalan R, Matthews DR. Publication bias in clinical research. Lancet 1991; 337:867–872.
68. Erskine J, Schonell M. Relaxation therapy in bronchial asthma. J Psychosom Res 1979; 23:131–139.
69. Fein BT, Cox EP, Malley HE. Respiratory and physical exercise in the treatment of bronchial asthma. Arch Phys Med Rehabil 1963; 44:273–277.
70. Bolton JH, Gandevia B, Ross M. The rationale and results of breathing exercises in asthma. Med J Aust 1956; 43:675–680.
71. Weiner P, Azgad Y, Ganam R, Weiner M. Inspiratory muscle training in patients with bronchial asthma. Chest 1992; 102:1357–1361.
72. Jain SC, Rai L, Valecha A, Jha UK, Bhatnager SOD, Ram K. Effect of yoga training on exercise tolerance in adolescents with childhood asthma. J Asthma 1991; 28:437–442.
73. Scherr MS, Crawford PL, Sergent CB, Scherr CA. Effect of bio-feedback techniques on chronic asthma in a summer camp environment. Ann Allergy 1975; 35:289–295.
74. Lacasse Y, Wong E, Guyatt GH, King D, Cook DJ, Goldstein RS. Meta-analysis of respiratory rehabilitation in chronic obstructive pulmonary disease. Lancet 1996; 348:1115–1119.
75. Garfinkel SK, Kesten S, Chapman KR, Rebuck AS. Physiologic and nonphysiologic determinants of aerobic fitness in mild to moderate asthma. Am Rev Respir Dis 1992; 145:741–745.

11

Exercise and Rhinitis

William C. Howland III
Allergy Center of Austin, and HealthQuest Research, Austin, Texas

David M. Lang
*Allegheny University of the Health Sciences,
Philadelphia, Pennsylvania*

I. NASAL PHYSIOLOGY DURING EXERCISE

The nose fulfills several functions that are important to the athlete during physical activity [1–3]. The nose filters out particulate matter while adjusting the humidity and temperature of inspired air. The nose can remove virtually 100% of particles larger than 10 μm in diameter [3]. Inspired air is moistened by mucous secretions, which line the nasal vestibule, through the physical process of transudation. The daily volume of fluid transudation that occurs to promote normal saturation of inspired air is approximately 1000 ml [1]. The three functions of the nose—filtration, humidification, and warming—unfortunately, may be taken for granted until one or more aspects are insufficient to serve the needs of the athlete.

The term *rhinitis* denotes inflammation of the nasal mucous membranes. Rhinitis is characterized by nasal discharge, congestion, and frequently sneezing; patients with allergic rhinitis may also have prominent pruritus. The vasomotor nerve supply to the nose consists of sympathetic and parasympathetic divisions of the autonomic nervous system [1,3]. Parasympathetic stimulation leads to vasodilation and vascular engorgement, resulting in narrowing of the airway and greater efficiency in warming inspired air [1]. Current evidence indicates that sympathetic blockade promotes nasal congestion and parasympathetic stimulation leads to rhinorrhea. Given this understanding, patients with nonallergic "vasomotor" rhinitis are said to experience this condition because of "autonomic imbalance" [3]. The prevalence of this condition is unknown, but may exceed that of allergic rhinitis [4].

Patients with angina pectoris who underwent cervical sympathectomy frequently developed nasal stuffiness [5]. These and other data have confirmed that blood vessels to the nose normally have a sympathetic vasoconstrictor tone. Vigorous physical exercise decreases nasal airway resistance. This decrease can be prevented by stellate ganglion block and use of α-adrenergic antagonists [3].

Intranasal administration of methacholine provokes watery hypersecretion [3]. This property of methacholine can be blocked by the atropine analogue ipratropium, which can be administered intranasally [6]. Ipratropium is currently used for management of various forms of nonallergic rhinitis [7].

II. IMPROVEMENT OF RHINITIS WITH EXERCISE

Renold et al. [8], in their study of adrenal cortex reactivity in oarsmen, stated: "On several occasions the men with active hay fever described a definite subjective improvement for several hours after either a strenuous rowing period or a time trial." Patients with allergic rhinitis commonly experience relief from nasal congestion with physical exercise. Formal investigation into this phenomenon has shown that vigorous exercise reduces nasal airflow resistance for up to 30–60 min [9,10]. This effect is due to capacitance blood vessel vasoconstriction with no effect on resistance vessels [11]. Recent data suggest that, rather than an effect through circulating catecholamines, the response of nasal resistance to exercise is associated with an increase in sympathetic vasoconstriction in the nasal mucosa [12].

Vasomotor rhinitis is a common syndrome that occurs as either a primary condition or secondary to other disorders [3,4], and may be characterized predominantly by congestion or rhinorrhea. Patients with the vaso-obstructive form may benefit from a disciplined and vigorous daily exercise routine [13]. The vasosecretory form entails the potential for exaggerated parasympathetic activity, and can be triggered by nonspecific stimuli, such as exposure to irritants or fumes, weather or temperature changes, or even sexual arousal [3,14]. The profuse rhinorrhea characteristic of this form of vasomotor rhinitis can be assuaged by intranasal anticholinergic agents [7].

III. IMPROVEMENT OF ASTHMA WITH EXERCISE AND NASAL BREATHING

Exercise-induced bronchospasm (EIB) can often be demonstrated in as many as 90% of asthmatics (see Chap. 4). From the standpoint of the asthmatic athlete, the nose can be viewed as having a "guard dog" role [1], such that when moderate or severe degrees of nasal congestion occur the lungs will be exposed to more substantial levels of allergens or irritants (see following). Moreover, the finding that intranasal corticosteroid treatment is associated not only with a marked improvement in allergic rhinitis symptoms, but also a significant reduction in asthma symptoms [15] underscores the importance of controlling nasal symptoms in asthmatic athletes.

Several pharmacological agents can block or modify the bronchoconstrictive response to exercise that occurs in many asthmatics (see Chap. 10). Studies have shown that severity of EIB can be successfully attenuated if nasal breathing is continued during exercise [16], by virtue of the role of the nose in humidifying inspired air [17]; however, many who exercise have difficulty with this manuever, and despite efforts to nose breathe may continue to breathe through their mouths during exercise. This may be particularly unfortunate for individuals who participate in athletic activities (football, baseball, track, or other) that entail short bursts of sprinting that require nasal breathing for optimal performance [2]. It is conceivable that a device to encourage nasal patency, such as the Breathe Right®, described later in this chapter, could have considerable usefulness in this setting; however, studies substantiating the usefulness of these devices will be required to validate this claim.

IV. WORSENING OF RHINITIS WITH EXERCISE

Although some athletes experience improvement in rhinitis with exercise, rhinitis may worsen under certain conditions [2,3]. Rhinitis in the allergic athlete could worsen with exposure to allergens. Inhalation of irritants, such as ozone, sulfur dioxide, or particulates, during outdoor exercise may also provoke or worsen rhinitis. Athletes may also note worsening of rhinitis caused by various weather conditions, particularly cold or dry air. Structural abnormalities of the nasal septum or turbinates, or trauma to the nose during exercise could also result in rhinitis.

Allergic reactions in the nasal mucosa involve the interaction of allergen with specific IgE fixed to mast cells or basophils [3]. The cross-linking of two IgE molecules results in release of mediators, including histamine, leukotrienes, prostaglandins, platelet-activating factor, tryptase, kinins, neutrophil chemotactic factor, eosinophil chemotactic factor, and others. Release of these mediators into the nasal mucosa causes sneezing, itching, excess mucus production, and dilation of blood vessels, ultimately leading to mucosal edema and nasal obstruction. Subsequent cellular infiltration of the mucosa with neutrophils, eosinophils, and mononuclear cells has been associated with a "late-phase" reaction and recurrence of symptoms 4–8 h after exposure [17]. Allergic athletes may be sensitized to seasonal allergens (pollens of tree, grass, or weed), perennial allergens (house dust mites, animal danders, mold spores), or both.

Exercising outdoors during the spring tree, summer grass, or the fall weed pollen season will increase exposure to allergen, which may provoke rhinitis in susceptible individuals. Most plants release greater quantities of pollen in the morning between 5 and 10 AM and in the afternoon from 4:30 to 6:30 PM [18]. Consequently, the athlete exercising in the morning or late afternoon may experience greater allergen exposure and a corresponding increase in rhinitis.

The athlete with perennial allergic rhinitis may have constant exposure to house dust mites or animal dander indoors or mold spores in or outdoors. These exposures can result in acute worsening of rhinitis (e.g., after petting the cat or vacuuming the house) or chronic symptoms. Because late-phase allergic reactions may occur 4–8 h later [3], the athlete with perennial allergic rhinitis may experience symptoms during exercise owing to prior exposure to allergen in the home or work place.

Priming is a term that describes the enhancing effect of allergen exposure on subsequent exposure to the same allergen. Challenge studies have demonstrated that exposure to the same amount of pollen on consecutive days results in increasing symptoms and nasal airway resistance after each challenge [19]. Priming appears to be associated with cellular infiltration in the nasal mucosa, which has been described with late-phase reactions [20]. The inflammatory response in the nasal mucosa reduces the amount of pollen needed to produce an allergic response [21]. During the pollen season, less exposure to pollen can result in clinical symptoms. It is unknown whether this response is allergen-specific or may cross over to other exposures; however, it is conceivable that the allergic athlete will experience an increase in rhinitis with exposure to outdoor pollen or mold allergens following a reaction to indoor animal dander or house dust mite.

Athletes with allergic rhinitis or asthma may exhibit paradoxical nasal obstruction following exercise. Although patients with allergic rhinitis or asthma, as well as normal subjects, show marked decreases in nasal resistance immediately after exercise with indoor treadmill exercise challenge tests, patients with allergic rhinitis or asthma show a more rapid rebound increase in nasal airway resistance (5–10 min in patients versus 20–30 min in normal subjects) [22]. Following exercise, patients with allergic rhinitis may also show rebound increases in both total and unilateral nasal resistance that surpass baseline levels [23]. These findings indicate that the athlete with allergic rhinitis and asthma may experience increased nasal obstruction after exercise, caused by underlying physiological differences in control of dilation of the capacitance vessels in the nasal mucosa.

Indoor treadmill exercise challenge has also demonstrated increases in nasal resistance and complaints of increased nasal secretions in two asthmatic athletes [24]. These athletes experienced a two- to threefold increase in nasal resistance after exercise that persisted during a 50-min postexercise observation period.

Self-reported rhinitis during exercise was seen frequently in runners participating in a 6-km race in Manhattan. Fifty-six percent of randomly surveyed runners reported nasal congestion or rhinorrhea during or after running [27]. A significantly higher percentage of runners reporting exercise-induced rhinitis experienced similar symptoms with swimming. The proportion of runners with a past history of seasonal allergic rhinitis and asthma did not differ significantly between those with and without exercise-induced rhinitis.

Rhinitis during or following exercise may also occur with exposure to irritants, pollutants, and particulates. Exposure to outdoor pollutants (ozone, sulfur dioxide, particulates) or indoor pollutants (formaldehyde, glues, paints, cleaners, tobacco smoke) may worsen rhinitis.

Ozone is a frequently encountered urban air pollutant formed by the interaction of sunlight with vehicle exhaust fumes. Human challenge studies have shown that exposure to high levels of ozone blocks the decongestant effect of exercise in nonallergic subjects [25]. High levels of ozone exposure can promote influx of inflammatory cells and increased albumin in nasal lavage secretions [26]. Additionally, 24 h after ozone exposure nonallergic subjects show increased methacholine reactivity and a nearly 50% reduction in nasal surface fluid in the anterior nasal septum [27]. These findings suggest that ozone exposure during exercise may provoke inflammation and increased reactivity of the nasal mucosa as well as block the decongestant effect of exercise.

Sulfur dioxide, another common air pollutant, may also cause rhinitis in the athlete. Patients participating in challenge studies with increasingly higher levels of sulfur dioxide complained of dryness in the nose and pharynx after 6-h exposures [28]. Nasal mucous flow also was impaired, particularly at higher levels of exposure. Twenty-seven percent of participants reported upper respiratory infection during the week following the study. Because nasal mucous flow is important in humidification of air; as well as defense against infection, exposure to this pollutant during exercise may cause subjective symptoms of dryness or irritation and possibly predispose to infection.

Particulates in outdoor air may also worsen rhinitis. These particulates include carbon particles, inert dust, and even rubber fragments. Inhalation of large numbers of particulates during exercise may further increase nasal mucosal inflammation. Exposure to a combination of inert dust and sulfur dioxide may have an additive effect [29].

Indoor exposure in gymnasiums or arenas to formaldehyde, glues, paints, cleaners, and tobacco smoke may also trigger or worsen rhinitis. Formaldehyde is a well-recognized upper respiratory irritant. Volatile organic compounds found in indoor air may cause upper respiratory irritant symptoms [30]. Challenge studies with volatile organic compounds have also demonstrated an increase in nasal lavage neutrophils [31]. Tobacco smoke exposure causes congestion or rhinorrhea in up to 67% of allergic patients and 29% of nonallergic patients [32].

Some athletes report worsening of rhinitis after swimming. In one study, 49% of subjects with running-induced exercise rhinitis and 11% of subjects without exercise rhinitis reported a greater level of rhinitis symptoms during swimming [2]. Swimming-induced rhinitis may be a vasomotor response to temperature change, or an irritant effect of chlorine or other pool chemicals.

Patients with nonallergic rhinitis often report increased symptoms with changes in air temperature, humidity, or barometric pressure. Exposure to cold, dry air is a potent stimulus resulting in rhinorrhea in up to 90% of persons and nasal congestion or sneezing in one-third to one-half. Exercise, such as skiing, in cold air may augment (see Chap. 20), and intranasal anticholinergics have been shown to inhibit, this response [33].

Sneezing, with exposure to bright light or sunlight, the solar sneeze reflex [34] may affect up to one-third of the population and may occur independently of the presence of other forms of rhinitis. Although rhinorrhea and nasal congestion do not usually occur with the solar sneeze reflex, this form of rhinitis could prove troublesome for some athletes (e.g., baseball outfielders or punt return specialists).

Viral or bacterial infections of the nose and paranasal sinuses may lead to worsening of rhinitis during exercise. Excess secretions in the nose and nasopharynx may cause cough and limit airflow required with higher ventilatory rates during exercise. Exercise in air polluted with ozone or sulfur dioxide may result in decreased nasal surface fluid and mucus, which could predispose to infection [27,28].

Internal structural abnormalities or trauma to the nose could result in rhinitis during exercise. Trauma during exercise can cause bruising or hematoma of the nasal septum and nasal tissues. Nasal trauma may also cause reflex mucosal edema or rhinorrhea. Nasal septal deviation, septal spur, or turbinate hypertrophy can increase resistance to airflow, limiting the maximal ventilation attainable through the nose and resulting in airflow turbulence with reflex increase in secretion of mucus. Nasal polyps arising in the sinuses or nasal mucosa can result in partial or complete obstruction to airflow through the nose.

An external nasal dilator (Breathe Right®) has recently been developed and may be helpful for athletes with nasal obstruction caused by structural abnormalities of the nasal turbinates or septum. The Breathe Right® positioned over the external nasal alae applies traction to dilate the nostrils. This device may be most helpful in athletes who must wear a mouthpiece during exercise and has become popular with professional football players.

V. TREATMENT

The goal of treatment of rhinitis in the athlete is to decrease symptoms and improve nasal function, without affecting athletic performance or using therapies banned by athletic governing bodies (see Chap. 24).

Avoidance of exposure to allergens and pollutants can successfully reduce rhinitis in an athlete whose symptoms are triggered by these factors. There are numerous techniques to reduce exposure to dust mites indoors [35,36]. The most effective method to reduce exposure to animal dander is to remove animals from the home environment. Exercise at times of higher pollen levels should be avoided (see foregoing). Wearing a dust or pollen mask can effectively minimize inhalation of particulates, pollens, and molds, but not gaseous air pollutants such as ozone. Athletes should avoid outdoor exercise during ozone or air pollution alerts.

Antihistamines (approved for use in international competition) may be helpful for rhinitis in the allergic athlete; however, side effects (drowsiness and anticholinergic symptoms including dry nose, mouth, throat, and eyes) can impair athletic performance. Sweating may also be impaired, owing to the anticholinergic properties of conventional antihistamines, and this may be problematic with heavy exercise [37]. Newer antihistamines, such as terfenadine, loratadine, and astemizole, cause little or no sedation and lack anticholinergic properties. However, cardiac arrhythmias can occur with elevated serum levels of terfenadine and astemizole. Appropriate precautions for use of these two agents have been recommended [39].

Topical and systemic decongestants can shrink swollen nasal mucous membranes and decrease resistance to nasal airflow. These medications may cause slight elevation of blood pressure, increased heart rate, and central nervous system stimulation, and should be avoided during athletic competition because of these potential side effects. Their use is not approved by some athletic governing bodies.

Topical sprays of cromolyn sodium (or nedocromil sodium) may be efficacious for preventing rhinitis in the allergic athlete. These drugs may function by stabilizing mast cells and decreasing inflammatory cell influx.

Use of these sprays before exercise may block reaction [5] to allergens and possibly irritants. Cromolyn sodium is approved by athletic governing bodies, and generally causes no side effects.

Topical nasal steroids may be effective in athletes with allergic rhinitis, nonallergic rhinitis, and nasal polyps. Nasal steroids appear to be effective because of their anti-inflammatory action and their effect on capillary membrane permeability. The newer synthetic topical steroids (flunisolide, beclomethasone dipropionate, fluticasone propionate, and triamcinolone acetonide) have very little systemic absorption or potential for systemic corticosteroid side effects [40,41]. These medications are presently approved by most athletic governing bodies for use during competition.

Allergen immunotherapy can effectively reduce sensitivity to pollens, mold, dust mites, and animal dander in the allergic athlete who is not well-controlled with pharmacological therapy. High-dose allergen immunotherapy has reduced both early- and late-phase responses to allergen challenge, and can achieve a significant decrease in symptoms and medication requirements [42].

Recognition and treatment of sinusitis is important in the athlete as described in Chapter 12. Because the presentation of sinusitis may be subtle, the clinician treating the athlete should maintain a high index of suspicion for sinusitis in the athlete with nasal congestion, purulent secretions, and cough. Two- to four-week courses of broad-spectrum antibiotics may be required to completely eradicate a sinus infection.

Nasal obstruction caused by polyps may improve with medical therapy, such as topical corticosteroid sprays or short courses of oral steroids. Impairment of nasal airflow caused by structural abnormalities of the nasal septum or nasal turbinates may improve with use of an external nasal dilator, such as the Breathe Right®. Patients with refractory sinusitis, nasal polyposis, or significant internal nasal structural abnormalities may require surgical intervention for long-term improvement.

REFERENCES

1. Geurkink N. Nasal anatomy, physiology, and function. J Allergy Clin Immunol 1983; 72:123.
2. Katz RM. Rhinitis in the athlete. J Allergy Clin Immunol 1984; 73:708.
3. Mygind N, Weeke B. Allergic and nonallergic rhinitis. In: Middleton E, Reed CE, and Ellis EF, eds. Allergy: principles and practice. St Louis: CV Mosby, 1983; 1107.
4. Slavin RG. Upper respiratory disorders. Immunol Allergy Clin North Am 1987; 7:9.

5. Millonig AF, Harris HE, Gardner WJ. Effect of autonomic denervation on nasal mucosa. Arch Otolaryngol 1949; 86:359.
6. Borum P. Intranasal ipratropium: inhibition of methacholine induced hypersecretion. Rhinology 1978; 16:225.
7. Druce HM, Spector SL, Fireman P, et al. Double-blind study of intranasal ipratropium bromide in nonallergic perennial rhinitis. Ann Allergy 1992; 69: 53.
8. Renold AE, Quigley TB, Dennard HE, Thorn GW. Reactions of the adrenal cortex to physical and emotional stress in college oarsmen. N Engl J Med 1951; 244:754.
9. Richerson HB, Seebohm DM. Nasal airway response to exercise. J Allergy 1968; 41:269.
10. Togawa K, Konno A, Hoshino T, et al. Respiratory function during physical exercise in normal and obstructed noses. Arch Otorhinolaryngol 1981; 232:1.
11. Paullson B, Bende M, Ohlin P. Nasal mucosal blood flow at rest and during exercise. Acta Otolaryngol (Stockh) 1984; 9:140.
12. Olson LG, Strohl KP. The response of the nasal airway to exercise. Am Rev Respir Dis 1987; 135:356.
13. Schatz M, Zeiger RS. Chronic rhinitis: a therapeutic challenge. Consultant 1980; 4:63.
14. Wald JA. An allergy to sex? JAMA 1988; 260:401.
15. Welsh PW, Stricker WE, Chu-Pin C, et al. Efficacy of beclomethasone nasal solution, flunisolide, and cromolyn in relieving symptoms of ragweed allergy. Mayo Clin Proc 1987; 62:125.
16. Shturman-Ellstein R, Zeballos RJ, Buckley JM, Souhrada JF. The beneficial effect of nasal breathing on exercise-induced bronchoconstriction. Am Rev Respir Dis 1978; 118:65.
17. Griffin MP, McFadden ER, Ingram RH. Airway cooling in asthmatic and nonasthmatic subjects during nasal and oral breathing. J Allergy Clin Immunol 1982; 69:354.
18. Platts-Mills T, Solomon W. Aerobiology and inhalent allergens. In: Middleton E, Reed CE, Ellis EF, eds. Allergy: principles and practice. St Louis: CV Mosby, 1993; 485.
19. Naclerio RM, Proud D, Adkinson NF, et al. Inflammatory mediators in late antigen-induced rhinitis. N Engl J Med 1985; 313:65.
20. Connell JT. Quantitative intranasal pollen challenge. II. Effect of daily pollen challenge, environmental pollen exposure, and placebo challenge on the nasal membrane. J Allergy Clin Immunol 1968; 41:123.
21. Wachs M, Proud D, Lichtenstein LM, et al. Observations on the pathogenesis of nasal priming. J Allergy Clin Immunol 1989; 84:492.
22. Iliopoulos O, Proud D, Adkinson NF, et al. Relationship between the early, late, and rechallenge reaction to nasal challenge with antigen: observations on the role of inflammatory mediators and cells. J Allergy Clin Immunol 1990; 86:851.
23. Syballo NC, Bundgaard A, Widdicomb JG. Effects of exercise on nasal airflow and resistance in healthy subjects and in patients with asthma and rhinitis. Bull Eur Physiopathol Respir 1985; 21:507.

24. Ohki M, Hasagawa M, Sakuma A. Exercise induced nasal obstruction in patients with allergic rhinitis. Am J Rhinol 1989; 3:1.
25. Sabinsky R, Silverman B, Dobozin B, et al. Exercise induced rhinitis (EIR) : a common entity [abstract]. J Allerg Clin Immunol 1987; 79:149.
26. Willes S, Raford P, Baroody F, Fitzgerald TK, Bascom R. Differential responses to ozone in allergic and non-allergic subjects. Am Rev Respir Dis 1991; 143:A91.
27. Bascom R, Naclerio RM, Fitzgerald TK, Kagey-Sobotka A, Proud D. Effect of ozone inhalation on the response to nasal challenge with antigen of allergic subjects. Am Rev Respir Dis 1990; 141:594.
28. Baroody F, Fitzgerald T, Raford P, Willes S, Naclerio R, Bascom R. Effect of ozone on nasal methacholine challenge of allergic and non-allergic subjects. Am Rev Respir Dis 1991; 143:A93.
29. Andersen I, Lundqvist GR, Gensen PL, Proctor F. Human response to controlled levels of sulfur dioxide. Arch Environ Health 1974; 28:31.
30. Andersen I, Molhave L, Proctor DF. Human response to control levels of combination of sulfur dioxide and inert dust. Scand J Work Environ Health 1981; 7:1.
31. Kjaergaard SK, Molhave L, Pedersen OF. Human reactions to a mixture of indoor air volatile organic compounds. Atmos Environ 1991; A:1417.
32. Karen H, Graham DE, Devlin RV. Exposure of humans to a volatile organic mixture III. Inflammatory response. Arch Environ Health 1992; 47:39.
33. Speer F. Tobacco and the non-smoker. A study of subjective symptoms. Arch Environ Health 1968; 16:443.
34. Silvers WS. The skier's nose; a model of cold induced rhinorrhea. Ann Allergy 1991; 67:32.
35. Lang DM, Howland WC. Solar sneeze reflex [letter]. JAMA 1987; 257:1330.
36. Platts-Mills T. Indoor allergens. In: Middleton E, Reed CE, Ellis EF, eds. Allergy: principles and practice. St Louis: CV Mosby, 1993; 523.
37. Korsgard J. Preventative measures in house dust allergy. Am Rev Respir Dis 1982; 125:80.
38. Kolski GB. The athlete with asthma and allergies. Clin Sports Med 1982; 1: 397.
39. Kemp J. Antihistamines—is there anything safe to prescribe? Ann Allergy 1992; 69:276.
40. Howland W, Field E, Harding S, et al. Fluticasone propionate aqueous nasal spray (fpans) is an anti-rhinitic with topical but not systemic activity [abstract]. J Allergy Clin Immunol 1995; 95:221.
41. Howland WC, Dockhorn R, Gillman S, et al. A comparison of the effects of triamicinolone acetonide aqueous nasal spray, oral prednisone and placebo on adrenocortical function in male allergic rhinitis patients. J Allergy Clin Immunol (in press).
42. Iliopoulos O, Proud D, Atkinson NF, et al. Effects of immunotherapy on the early, late and rechallenge nasal reaction to provocation with allergen: changes in inflammatory mediators and cells. J Allergy Clin Immunol 1991; 87:855.

12
Sinusitis in Athletes

Jeffrey R. Leipzig and Raymond G. Slavin
Saint Louis University School of Medicine, Saint Louis, Missouri

I. SINUSITIS

Often neglected as a clinical entity, sinusitis is being increasingly recognized as a common and important cause of morbidity. A recent survey of the annual physician visits for acute and chronic sinusitis reveals a steady increase from 1980 through 1992 [1]. Sinusitis is one of the most common chronic diseases, with a prevalence rate of 146:1000 population, which is higher than any other reported chronic conditions, such as hypertension or arthritis [2]. Despite its enormous prevalence, clinical pitfalls remain in its diagnosis and management [3]. To the sports practitioner, the occurrence of sinusitis in the athlete is particularly important for three reasons. First, there are particular athletic events that may predispose the athlete to develop sinusitis. Second, is the overall effect that sinusitis may have on athletic performance. A third reason, and most important, is that sinusitis is a reversible, treatable disease. As will be described in more detail, the initial signs and symptoms of sinusitis may be quite subtle. With thorough understanding of the structure, pathophysiology, and microbiology of the paranasal sinuses, the sports practitioner can witness extremely gratifying results with proper institution of appropriate therapy for sinusitis. This can also result in marked improvement in cough and asthma, two common complications of sinusitis.

II. STRUCTURE AND FUNCTION OF THE SINUSES

The paranasal sinuses are four paired structures surrounding the nasal cavities. Each sinus has an opening, or ostium, on the lateral side of the nose, through which drainage occurs. The maxillary sinus is located within the cheekbone. The floor of the sinus is part of the toothbearing area of the maxilla, and, in adults, is below the floor of the nasal cavity. The roof of the maxillary sinus is the base of the orbit. The maxillary sinus ostium opens into the middle meatus between the middle and inferior turbinates. The frontal sinus forms the middle portion of the roof of the orbit and is within the frontal bone. Its ostium opens into the anterior part of the middle meatus. The ethmoidal sinus lines the medial wall of the orbit in close proximity to the cranial cavity from which it is separated by the cribriform plate. Bony septa divide the ethmoid sinuses into anterior, middle, and posterior sections. The anterior and middle ethmoidal cells open into the middle meatus, and the posterior ethmoidal cells drain into the superior meatus. The sphenoidal sinus empties into the sphenoethmoidal recess above the superior turbinate. Its roof is the pituitary fossa, and its lateral aspect is formed by the cavernous venous sinuses (see Fig. 1).

Developmentally, the maxillary and ethmoid sinuses are present at birth and are evident by radiography in infancy. The frontal sinuses become recognizable anatomically by the 6th–12th month and appear radiographically between the third and seventh years. The sphenoid sinuses develop by the third year of life, but do not appear radiographically until the ninth year. There is great variation in shape and size of the sinuses at all ages, particularly the frontal sinuses. The paranasal sinuses form as invaginations of the mucous membrane of the nasal cavity; the mucosal

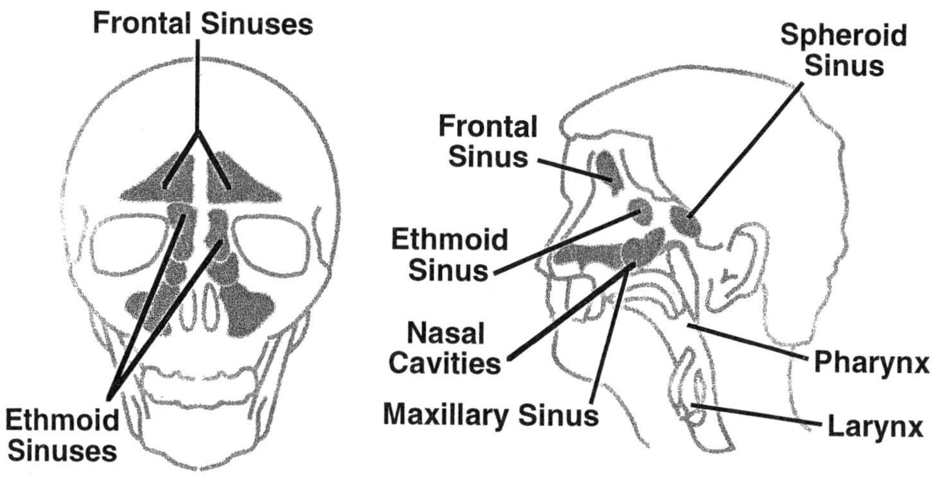

Fig. 1 Upper respiratory infections: sinusitis. Anatomy of the sinuses.

lining of the sinuses is similar to the mucosal lining of the nasal cavity, containing ciliated pseudostratified columnar epithelium and goblet cells [4].

The precise function of the paranasal sinuses is unclear: Some investigators have suggested roles in olfaction, voice response, production of protective mucus, dampening of sudden pressure changes in the nose during respiration, and lessening of skull weight.

III. PATHOPHYSIOLOGY OF SINUSITIS

The mucociliary apparatus protects against infection of the paranasal sinuses. Mucus in the sinuses traps microorganisms, pollutants, irritants, and other foreign particles that escape the filtering apparatus of the nose. Then, the mucus is removed through the draining ostia by constant movement of the mucus blanket propelled by the underlying cilia. Bacterial infection occurs when this self-cleansing mechanism is impaired. Mucus accumulates and the sinuses become infected by relatively harmless opportunistic bacteria normally found in the nose. In most instances of sinusitis, bacteria gain entrance to the sinuses through the ostia, but in some cases, such as dental abscess, bacteria can penetrate from contiguous structures. Nosocomial sinusitis can result from nasopharyngeal instrumentation in traumatized patients [5].

Several factors may result in retention of secretions in the paranasal sinuses: (a) swelling of the mucous membrane, leading to reduced patency of ostia; (b) reduced transport capacity related to abnormalities of the cilia, including quantitative reduction, retardation of movement, and insufficient coordination of movement; and (c) overproduction of secretions [6].

Patency of the ostia is the most important of these three factors in the development of sinusitis [7]. The ostia function primarily for drainage of secretions. Studies in normal persons have shown an inverse relation between the functional diameter of the maxillary ostium and the time required for emptying of contrast material [8]. The cross-sectional area of the ostium is also the primary determinant of gas exchange in the human sinuses [9].

Nasal airflow is another factor in determining gas exchange. The sinus cavity air exchanges twice as fast during nasal breathing as during oral breathing [10]. During normal nasal breathing with a patent ostium, 90% of the sinus air is exchanged in 5 min. The oxygen content of the sinus is dependent on several factors. A direct correlation between ostial size and oxygen tension has been shown in humans. The most profound changes in oxygen tension occur when infection accompanies the occlusion. Purulent maxillary sinus aspirates have a partial pressure of oxygen near zero, markedly elevated partial pressure of carbon dioxide, and decreased pH [11]. In vitro studies have demonstrated that growth of organisms, such as pneumococci, is inhibited by air exposure, compared with cultures grown with limited air access [12]. In addition to favoring increased bacterial growth and purulence, low oxygen content in the sinuses may impair local defense, including granulocyte function.

Ciliary movement is also vital in protection of sinuses against infection. The cilia beat toward the ostium in a radiating fashion to promote drainage. Even after surgical creation of a nasal antral window in the inferior meatus, which would favor gravitational drainage through the orifice, the cilia will still beat toward the natural ostium [13]. Mucociliary transport in the sinus may be compromised by a combination of low oxygen content in the sinus and in the blood. In addition to local factors, several clinical disorders have been described associated with ciliary dysfunction with loss of dynein arms, including Kartagener's syndrome [14] and immotile cilia syndrome [15].

Mucociliary activity of the sinuses is of such extreme importance in protection against sinusitis because spontaneous drainage of the maxillary sinus by gravity is nearly impossible for two reasons. First, the maxillary ostium is not simply an opening of 1–2 mm in diameter, but rather, a circuitous channel 6 mm in length that connects the maxillary antrum to the middle meatus. This is referred to as the ostiomeatal complex. Second, the maxillary ostium is located in the superior portion of the maxillary antrum. Therefore, for spontaneous drainage to occur into the nose in the upright position, the antrum must be completely filled before the contents can spill over or ciliary action must move secretions in a cephalad direction against the force of gravity.

Mucociliary activity is disturbed when purulent secretions are present owing to changes in the mucus' property, structural damage to ciliated epithelium, and slower beating of the cilia. Generally, the cilia return to normal levels after infection, but with severe empyema and scarring, portions of the cilia may be converted to squamous epithelium. Thus, if mucociliary function is congenitally deficient or damaged by scarring from previous severe infections, spontaneous drainage of the sinuses cannot occur when ostial occlusion resolves.

A third local factor important in protection of the sinuses against infection is the nature and quantity of secretions. Overproduction of sinus secretions may overwhelm the ability of the cilia to remove those secretions. In purulent secretion there is a high content of proteases that come

Table 1 Factors Predisposing to Sinusitis

Local	Systemic
Upper respiratory infection	Immune deficiency
Allergic rhinitis	Cystic fibrosis
Overuse of topical decongestants	Bronchiectasis
Hypertrophied adenoids	Immotile cilia syndrome
Deviated nasal septum	
Nasal polyps	
Tumors	
Foreign bodies	
Swimming and diving	
Cigarette smoke	
Barotrauma	
Dental extraction/injections	

principally from granulocytes. These proteases are more harmful to the mucosa than are bacteria.

Table 1 shows the most common local and systemic factors predisposing to sinusitis. Whereas, systemic factors, particularly hypogammaglobulinemia may play some role [16], the most common factors predisposing to sinusitis are local. Heading the list are viral upper respiratory infections and allergic rhinitis in which the mechanism for the development of sinusitis would appear to be similar. Acute rhinitis of either infectious or allergic etiology results in edematous obstruction of the nasal ostia, decreased paranasal sinus ciliary action, and increased production of mucus. With the subsequent accumulation of mucus in the sinus, the stage is set for secondary bacterial infection and the conversion of mucus to mucopus. Mucopus further impairs ciliary function and increases swelling around ostia when it discharges into the nose, creating a vicious cycle.

IV. MICROBIOLOGY OF SINUSITIS

Knowledge of the true microbiological picture of sinusitis has emerged from studies in which sinus aspirates are obtained by direct antral puncture or by sampling directly from the involved sinus during surgery. Nasal smears and cultures are not useful in defining the causal organism(s) of sinusitis, owing to the high rate of contamination with normal nasal flora

[17,18]. Cultures from both adults [19] and children [20] with acute sinusitis grow predominantly aerobic organisms, with the heaviest yield being *Streptococcus pneumoniae*, *Haemophilus influenzae*, and *Moraxella catarrhalis*.

Poor drainage of the chronically infected maxillary sinus reduces antral PO_2 and pH which, in turn, would be expected to encourage the growth of anaerobic bacteria by providing them with the optimal oxidation–reduction potential. In a series of 66 adult patients with chronic sinusitis reported by Brook [21], 88% of culture-positive specimens obtained during sinus surgery had anaerobes. Also, 44% of the bacteroides were β-lactamase-positive, indicating an increasing emergence of β-lactamase-producing organisms.

Chronic sinusitis in childhood has been thought to be caused by the same organisms that cause chronic sinus disease in adults, but this may not be true. Wald et al. [22] studied 40 nonallergic children with chronic sinusitis. Sinus aspirates were positive in 58%, with the predominant bacteria being *S. pneumoniae*, *H. influenzae*, and *M. catarrhalis*. No anaerobes were isolated. Goldenhersh et al. [23] also found similar results in children.

V. HISTORY AND PHYSICAL EXAMINATION

The most important clinical clue to the diagnosis of acute sinusitis is the continuation of symptoms after a typical cold has subsided. The previously clear nasal discharge becomes yellow or green. Fever persists and chills may develop. Pain that is felt in the forehead may be associated with maxillary sinusitis. The patient's discomfort is often worse when bending or straining.

On physical examination, the patient has thick, purulent, green or deep yellow secretions in the nose on the side of the diseased sinus. In the case of maxillary sinusitis, purulent secretions will be seen in the middle meatus, which is the drainage site of the maxillary sinus.

In chronic sinusitis, the general lack of pain or systemic symptoms makes chronic sinusitis difficult to diagnose from history alone. There is usually poor correlation between clinical characteristics and evidence obtained from an antral puncture. Patients with chronic sinusitis generally do not complain of headache, facial pain, fullness in the face, pain in the teeth, or discomfort when they bend over. Rather, nasal obstruction (which is sometimes unilateral), with purulent postnasal drainage, chronic cough, hyposmia, sore throat, and unpleasant breath are the most common presenting signs. Physical examination of the patient with chronic sinusitis will reveal an edematous nasal mucosa bathed in mucopus.

Complications of sinusitis are less frequent since the introduction of antibiotics, but have recently shown some increase caused by drug-resistant bacteria and by immunosuppression secondary to chemotherapy. The most commonly seen complications are in the orbit and include cellulitis, abscess, and cavernous sinus thrombosis [24]. The second most common complication is an intracranial extension of infection that may include epidural or subdural abscess, mucocele formation, and osteomyelitis. Incompletely treated acute frontal sinusitis may result in Pott's puffy tumor, which is localized edema over an area of osteomyelitis of the skull.

VI. RADIOGRAPHY AND OTHER DIAGNOSTIC TECHNIQUES

Evidence from sinus roentgenograms is the most common means of establishing a clinical diagnosis of sinusitis. The occipital mental or Waters view best demonstrates the maxillary sinuses. The head is tilted back so the dense petrous bone does not occlude the lower part of the maxillary antra. The occipital frontal or Caldwell view demonstrates both the ethmoid and frontal sinuses. The sphenoid sinus is seen on a lateral view. Correlation between antral puncture and radiographic appearance reveals that true sinusitis in the adult is associated with either mucosal thickening of 6–8 mm or greater, an air–fluid level, or opacification.

Transillumination is of very limited usefulness in the diagnosis of sinusitis, particularly with maxillary involvement [25]. Ultrasonography consists of transmitting low-power pulsed ultrasound into the selected sinus cavity by direct contact of the transducer on the patients face. At the frequency used, ultrasound does not propagate through air. When the sinus is healthy and filled with air, no echo appears from the back wall. If fluid is present, a strong echo will be reflected by the back wall of the sinus. Advantages of ultrasonography are that it is noninvasive, nonionizing, and painless. However, no consensus has yet been reached for the diagnostic accuracy and validity of ultrasonography. More studies and improvements in technology will be necessary before this technique can be recommended for general use.

A major development in the diagnosis of sinusitis is the application of computed tomography (CT) scans. There is no question that disease of the sinuses, particularly of the ethmoids, may be missed on ordinary roentgenography. CT scans will demonstrate the ostiomeatal complex, and will detect subtle disease not demonstrated on sinus x-ray films. A major problem in the past has been the rather prohibitive cost of CT scans. Through improvement in technology and the utilization of limited scans, the price of the technique has diminished to a much more reasonable level and, in some centers, is quite close to that of ordinary sinus x-ray examinations.

VII. MEDICAL MANAGEMENT

For the sports physician several important issues must be addressed concerning treatment of sinusitis in the athlete. The first concern is to relieve the infection without affecting athletic performance. Second, and especially important in the elite athlete, is to prescribe medication that will not enhance athletic performance.

The goal of medical management of sinusitis is to eradicate the infection and return the infected sinus to its normal state. Sinusitis must be

Table 2 Medical Management of Sinusitis: Sample Regimens

Therapy	Purpose	Regimen
Steam and saline	Prevent nasal crusting; liquefy secretions; mild decongestant effect	Steam inhalation several times daily. Saline nasal spray qid
Decongestants		
Phenylpropanolamine	Increases ostial diameter	25 mg q 4 h or 50 mg q 8 h, not to exceed 150 mg/day
Topical oxymetazoline	Increases ostial diameter	2–3 sprays each nostril bid for 3–5 days at start of therapy
Topical corticosteroids		
Beclomethasone	Reduces mucosal inflammation	2 sprays each nostril bid
Triamcinolone	Reduces mucosal inflammation	2 sprays each nostril bid
Budesonide	Reduces mucosal inflammation	4 sprays each nostril qd
Fluticasone	Reduces mucosal inflammation	2 sprays each nostril qd
Mucoevacuants		
Guaifenesin	Thins mucous secretions	600–1200 mg bid
Iodinated glycerol	Thins mucous secretions	60 mg qid
Potassium iodide	Thins mucous secretions	300–1000 mg after meals 2–3 times daily
Antibiotics	Eradicate bacterial infection	See Table 3

Table 3 Sample Antibiotic Regimens for Sinusitis

Drug	Dosage
Amoxicillin	500 mg tid
Amoxicillin–clavulanate	500 mg tid
Azithromycin	500 mg once, then 250 mg OD for 5 days
Clarithromycin	500 mg bid
Cefuroxime axetil	500 mg bid
Trimethoprim–sulfamethoxazole	160 mg trimethoprim and 800 mg of sulfamethoxazole bid

considered as an infection within an enclosed space; if it is approached aggressively in this fashion, a higher likelihood of achieving success in management will be realized. To achieve this, an appropriate antimicrobial agent must be delivered, and the infected contents of the sinus must, in essence, be removed (Tables 2 and 3).

Analgesics may be beneficial in relieving discomfort for the patient with sinusitis. However, it should be remembered that aspirin and nonsteroidal anti-inflammatory drug sensitivity is exceedingly common in patients with sinusitis, particularly with associated nasal polyps and asthma. Saline nasal spray is useful to liquify secretions and decrease nasal blood flow with a resultant decongestant effect [26]. Patients should be encouraged to use them liberally.

Also, sinus drainage needs to be facilitated by attempting to increase the diameter of the sinus ostia. To achieve this, oral decongestants are commonly administered. Melen et al. [27] have demonstrated that the use of oral phenylpropanolamine increases the functional diameter of the maxillary sinus. In their studies of adults with "healed and diseased" sinuses, maxillary sinus ostial diameters increased 50% in healed sinuses and 30% in diseased sinuses after use of phenylpropanolamine. Total nasal resistance decreased 33% in both groups. Aust et al. [28], however, completed a 1-week course of phenylpropanolamine (100 mg twice daily) with placebo as adjuncts to antibiotic treatment in 20 adults with acute sinusitis. There were no differences in symptoms or side effects over the 7 treatment days. There are no published controlled studies evaluating the long-term use of oral decongestants in the treatment of chronic sinusitis, and further studies are needed to prove the efficacy of the adjunctive use of decongestants for treatment or prevention of sinusitis. It is also important that the sports physician supervising elite athletes be aware that some topical and oral decongestants are considered performance-enhancing medications and may disqualify the participant.

Many clinicians prescribe a limited course of topical decongestants (3- to 5-day course) to achieve aggressive decongestion early in the treatment course. Patients must be clearly advised that the use of these agents must remain time-limited to avoid rebound effects or the possible development of rhinitis medicamentosa or atrophic rhinitis. Similarly, patients should be reassured that frequent use of topical saline sprays will not place them at risk for such complications.

Additionally, it is recommended that there be an attempt to reduce mucosal inflammation, with the goal of lessening functional anatomical barriers to drainage and to improve mucociliary clearance [29]. To this end, topical nasal corticosteroids are prescribed. Flunisolide nasal spray (100 μg to each nostril three times daily) was compared with placebo in a 7-week trial as an adjunct to a 3-week course of amoxicillin–clavulanic acid (Augmentin) in the management of sinusitis in 116 patients [30]. Reduction in turbinate swelling and patients' global assessment of effectiveness statistically favored the flunisolide group, who, in turn, demonstrated a reduced rate of recurrence after completion of antibiotic treatment. There are currently no published controlled studies evaluating the use of systemic steroids as an adjunct for the treatment of sinusitis.

Although a controlled clinical trial implementing the use of mucoevacuants as an adjunct in the comprehensive treatment of sinusitis has not been performed, we recommend the use of these agents to attempt to thin secretions and, thereby, promote improved mucociliary clearance. It is generally considered advisable to avoid the use of antihistamines in patients with sinusitis because of the theoretic concern that the anticholinergic properties of these agents may reduce nasal secretions and lead to drying and inspissation of sinus contents. If an antihistamine is necessary, the nonsedating agents are preferred, owing to their relative lack of anticholinergic properties. There are no published controlled trials investigating the use of antihistamines in the treatment of sinusitis.

Most importantly, patients must be given an appropriate antibiotic for an appropriate length of time. The first-line antibiotic for acute or chronic sinusitis remains amoxicillin. For penicillin-allergic patients, trimethoprim–sulfamethoxazole (Bactrim, Septra) may be used. Erythromycin is generally not recommended, owing to poor coverage of *H. influenzae, M. catarrhalis*, and anaerobes.

Increasingly sinusitis isolates have become β-lactamase producers and have thus become increasingly resistant to amoxicillin. This may be especially true for patients with recurrent bouts of acute sinusitis or with chronic sinusitis. Clavulanic acid, when administered in combination with amoxicillin (Augmentin), has been useful in this situation. Other antibiotics useful in this scenario include cephalosporins, such as cefuroxime axetil (Ceftin) and the newer macrolide antibiotics, clarithromycin (Blaxin) and azithromycin (Zithromax).

An extremely important consideration is the duration of therapy required to treat sinusitis successfully. A recent report by Williams et al. [31] proposes that acute maxillary sinusitis patients respond equally well to 3 or 10 days of antibiotic therapy. However, until further studies are done, 10 to 14 days of therapy for acute sinusitis is recommended. Chronic sinusitis must be treated for a minimum course of 3 weeks and frequently requires even a more prolonged course. Herein lies one of the most common errors in the treatment of chronic sinusitis. The traditional 10-day antibiotic courses may prove inadequate for the patient with chronic sinusitis, whose symptoms may transiently improve, but whose infection may smolder and lurk, only to recrudesce at a later time.

Follow-up sinus imaging may be necessary to rule out persistence of disease. If there is no significant clinical and radiographic improvement after aggressive medical management, the patient should be considered for surgical management and referred to an otolaryngologist.

After successful treatment of sinusitis, underlying causes need to be addressed. If allergic rhinitis is suspected, appropriate allergy evaluation is indicated. Environmental control should be implemented, and symptomatic therapy should be used. This may involve the use of antihistamines, decongestants, intranasal cromolyn, or intranasal corticosteroids. Immunotherapy may be necessary in selected patients. Signs and symptoms of allergic rhinitis may be obscured in the face of florid sinusitis, only to become more evident with the successful treatment of the underlying sinus infection. Nonallergic rhinitis should be treated by avoidance of irritants and by regular use of oral decongestants or intranasal corticosteroids. Also, an underlying immune disorder should be considered if history warrants. Patients with immunoglobulin deficiencies may present for evaluation of repeated attacks of sinusitis that respond only poorly to treatment.

VIII. SURGICAL MANAGEMENT

If there is no significant improvement after an appropriate period of medical therapy or if the sinusitis recurs on a regular basis, then the advice of an otolaryngologist should be sought. The task of the otolaryngologist consists of removing diseased tissue, relieving obstruction, and providing a nasal airway with drainage for all nasal and sinus compartments. The technique of functional endoscopic sinus surgery (FESS) is gaining increasing acceptance for treatment of medically resistant sinus disease and has largely supplanted other more radical procedures [32].

IX. ATHLETIC EVENTS PREDISPOSING TO SINUSITIS

Numerous athletic events may predispose the athlete to the development of sinusitis (Table 4). Events associated with an exposure to allergens can make certain athletes susceptible to sinusitis; allergic rhinitis with its corresponding inflammation can lead to sinusitis. Full contact sports, most notably wrestling, have been linked to the development of sinusitis based on mechanical obstruction of sinus ostia secondary to facial trauma [33]. Sinusitis in water skiers is thought to be related to injury of the mucosa by the forceful entry of water under high pressure into the sinus cavity [34]. Scuba diving involving sudden shifts in atmospheric pressure and resultant mucosal trauma has also been linked to sinusitis [35]. It appears that in similar sports during which barotrauma occurs, such as skydiving, the athlete may also be predisposed to sinusitis. Lastly, water sports, such as swimming and diving, have long been associated with the development of sinusitis; however the exact mechanism for this remains elusive [36–38]. Initial theories dealt primarily with chemical irritants in pool water, particulate matter, and bacterial contamination invading the sinus cavities, all of which could initiate an inflammatory process [36,37]. A recent report proposes that the pathogenesis is related to cooling of the

Table 4 Athletic Events Predisposing to Sinusitis

Seasonal exposure to allergens (allergic rhinitis)
Baseball
Football
Golf
Soccer
Track
Mechanical obstruction (trauma)
Boxing
Football
Wrestling
Barotrauma
Scuba and sky diving
Unknown (irritant vs. reflex)
Swimming and diving

skin, which could trigger a reflexive swelling of nasal mucosa and increased blood flow [38]. The exact etiology of swimmers sinusitis appears related to occlusion of the sinus ostium, but has yet to be fully defined. The sports medicine practitioner must keep a diagnostic suspicion of sinusitis high and must be aware of those conditions that predispose the athlete to its development.

X. RELATION BETWEEN SINUSITIS AND ASTHMA

The frequent association of nasal and paranasal sinus disease with bronchial asthma was first appreciated many years ago, but seemingly forgotten for some time. In recent years, attention to the clinical association of sinusitis and asthma has been revived [39,40]. Studies strongly suggest that appropriate medical or surgical management of underlying sinusitis will frequently result in an improvement of the associated asthmatic state. In our own series [41] of medically resistant adults with nasal polyps, sinusitis, and asthma, definitive nasosinus surgery resulted in significant subjective improvement in the asthmatic state in 66% of patients. Two-thirds were able to decrease their corticosteroid dose significantly, and one-third eliminated steroids entirely. In a 5-year follow-up of patients with chronic sinusitis and asthma who underwent bilateral intranasal sphenoethmoidectomy, the improvement noted within 2 years continued for 5 years [42]. Of 15 patients using frequent bursts or continuous steroids before surgery, four eliminated steroids entirely, five required only one to three bursts of steroids per year, and the other six had significantly reduced their steroid requirements from an average of 18.25 mg/day of prednisone to 7.5 mg/day. Nishioka et al. [43] also have reported dramatic results when endoscopic sinus surgery is used to treat chronic sinusitis. Thus, there does appear to be a causal relation between sinusitis and asthma.

XI. CONCLUSION

Sinusitis is an extremely common, underdiagnosed condition. The subtle clinical presentation of chronic sinusitis requires a high index of diagnostic suspicion on the part of the clinician to search for underlying sinusitis. The sports practitioner can witness dramatic results if proper therapy is given for sinusitis. The diagnosis of sinusitis is markedly enhanced by the use of CT scans, and the promise of more available scans at a reduced price is encouraging. We will no doubt see more β-lactamase-producing organisms accounting for sinusitis in the future and, one hopes, we will see the introduction of less toxic, less expensive antibiotics for these resistant organisms.

REFERENCES

1. Hughes JM, McCaig LF. Trends in antimicrobial drug prescribing among office-based physicians in the United States. JAMA 1995; 273:214–219.
2. Current estimates from the National Health Interview Survey. Vital Health Stat 10. 1994; no. 189.
3. Stafford CT. The clinician's view of sinusitis. Otolaryngol Head Neck Surg 1990; 103:870–875.
4. Rohr AS, Spector SL. Paranasal sinus anatomy and pathophysiology. Clin Rev Allergy 1984; 2:387.
5. Caplan ES. Nosocomial sinusitis. JAMA 1982; 247:639.
6. Reiner A, von Mecklenburg G, Toremalam NG. The mucociliary activity of the upper respiratory tract. III. A functional and morphologic study on human and animal material with special reference to maxillary sinus disease. Acta Otolaryngol (Suppl) 1978; 355.
7. Drettner B. The permeability of the maxillary ostium. Acta Otolaryngol 1965; 60:304.
8. Aust R, Drettner B, Hemmingson A. Elimination of contrast medium from the maxillary sinus. Acta Otolaryngol 1976; 81:468.
9. Aust R. Oxygen exchange through the maxillary ostium in man. Rhinology 1974; 12:25.
10. Aust R. Measurements of the ostial size and O_2 tension in the maxillary sinus. Rhinology 1976; 14:43.
11. Carenfelt C, Lundberg C. Purulent and nonpurulent maxillary sinus secretions with respect to pO_2, pCO_2 and pH. Acta Otolaryngol 1977; 84:138.
12. Carenfelt C, Lundberg C. The role of local gas composition in the pathogenesis of maxillary sinus empyema. Acta Otolaryngol 1978; 85:116.
13. Drettner B. Pathophysiology of paranasal sinuses with clinical implications. Clin Otolaryngol 1980; 5:277.
14. Cleveland HH. Kartagener's syndrome: a reappraisal. Acta Otolaryngol (Suppl) 1979; 368.
15. Afzelius BA. A human syndrome caused by immotile cilia. Science 1976; 193:317.
16. Stiehm ER. Immunodeficiency disorders: general considerations. In: Stiehm ER, Fulginiti VA, eds. Immunologic disorders in infants and children. Philadelphia: WB Saunders, 1980; 183–219.
17. Gill FF, Neiburger JB. The role of nasal cytology in the diagnosis of chronic sinusitis. Am J Rhinol 1989; 3:13–15.
18. Wilson NW, Jalowayski AA, Hamberger RN. A comparison of nasal cytol-

ogy with sinus x-rays for the diagnosis of sinusitis. Am J Rhinol 1988; 2: 55–59.
19. Evans FO Jr, Syndnor JB, Moore WE, et al. Sinusitis of the maxillary antrum. N Engl J Med 1975; 293:735.
20. Wald ER, Milmoe GJ, Bowen A, et al. Acute maxillary sinusitis in children. N Engl J Med 1981; 304:749.
21. Brook I. Bacteriology of chronic maxillary sinusitis in adults. Ann Otol Rhinol Laryngol 1989; 98:426.
22. Wald ER, Byers C, Guerra N, et al. Subacute sinusitis in children. J Pediatr 1989; 115:28.
23. Goldenhersh MJ, Rachelsfsky GS, Dudley J, et al. The microbiology of chronic sinus disease in children with respiratory allergy. J Allergy Clin Immunol 1990; 85:1030.
24. Sheffield RW, Cassisi, NJ, Karlan MS. Complications of sinusitis: what to watch for. Postgrad Med 1978; 63:93.
25. Spector SL, Loton A, English G, Philpotj L. Comparison between transillumination and the roentgenogram in diagnosing paranasal sinus disease. J Allergy Clin Immunol 1981; 67:22.
26. Bang BG, Mukherjee AL, Bang FB. Human nasal mucus flow rates. Johns Hopkins Med J 1967; 121:138–148.
27. Melen I, Friberg B, Andereasson L, et al. Effects of phenylpropanolamine on ostial and nasal patency in patients treated for chronic maxillary sinusitis. Acta Otolaryngol 1986; 101:494–500.
28. Aust R, Drettner B, Faluk B. Studies of the effect of peroral fenylpropanolamine on the functional size of the human maxillary ostium. Acta Otolaryngol 1979; 88:455–458.
29. Slavin RG. Sinusitis in adults. J Allergy Clin Immunol 1988; 81:1028–1032.
30. Meltzer EO, Busse WW, Druce HM, et al. Assessment of flunisolide nasal spray vs. placebo as an adjunct to antibiotic treatment of sinusitis [abstract]. J Allergy Clin Immunol 1992; 89:301.
31. Williams JW, Holleman DR, Samsa GP, Simel DL. Randomized controlled trial of 3 vs. 10 days of trimethoprim/sulfamethoxazole for acute maxillary sinusitis. JAMA 1995; 273:1015–1021.
32. Kennedy DW. Functional endoscopic sinus surgery technique. Arch Otolaryngol 1985; 3:643.
33. Tudor RB, Carson JP, Pulliam MW, Hill A. Pott's puffy tumor, frontal sinusitis, frontal bone osteomyelitis, and epidural abscess secondary to a wrestling injury. Am J Sports Med 1981; 9:390–391.
34. Kizer KW, Point B. Medical hazards of the water skiing douche. Ann Emerg Med 1980; 9:268–269.
35. Becker GD, Parell GJ. Otolaryngologic aspects of scuba diving. Otolaryngol Head Neck Surg 1979; 87:569–572.
36. Sarnaik AP, Vohra MP, Sturman SW, Belenky WM. Medical problems of the swimmer. Clin Sports Med 1986; 5:47–64.
37. Slavin RG. Sinusitis. J Allergy Clin Immunol 1984; 73:712–716.

38. Deitmer T, Scheffler R. Nasal physiology in swimmers and swimmers' sinusitis. Acta Otolaryngol (Stockh) 1990; 110:286–291.
39. Phipatanakul CS, Slavin RG. Bronchial asthma produced by paranasal sinusitis. Arch Otolaryngol 1974; 100:109.
40. Slavin RG. Relationship of nasal disease and sinusitis to bronchial asthma. Ann Allergy 1982; 49:76.
41. Slavin RG, Linford PA, Friedman WH. Bilateral intranasal sphenoethmoidectomy (BSE) in the treatment of nasal polyps, sinusitis and bronchial asthma [abstract]. J Allergy Clin Immunol 1983; 71:156.
42. Mings R, Friedman WH, Linford PA, Slavin RG. Five year follow-up of the effects of bilateral intranasal sphenoethmoidectomy in patients with sinusitis and asthma. Am J Rhinol 1987; 79:247.
43. Nishioka GJ, Cook PR, Davis WE, McKinsey JP. Functional endoscopic sinus surgery in patients with chronic sinusitis and asthma. Otolaryngol Head Neck Surg 1994; 110:494.

13

Upper Airway Disease Masquerading as Exercise-Induced Asthma

Mark T. O'Hollaren
Oregon Health Sciences University, Portland, Oregon

I. INTRODUCTION

As others have thoroughly documented throughout this book, there are many allergic and respiratory entities that may adversely affect a patient's ability to participate in sports and other strenuous physical activities. The topic of exercise-induced asthma (EIA) has already been thoroughly discussed. There are some patients, however, who appear to have exercise-induced asthma after an initial evaluation, but fail to respond to appropriate therapy. A certain proportion of these patients actually have their dyspnea originating from the larynx and upper airway. We have discussed sinusitis and rhinitis in other chapters of this book (see Chaps. 11 and 12); this chapter will mainly concentrate on dyspnea originating from the larynx and upper trachea.

Laryngeal disorders are commonly misdiagnosed, because a high index of suspicion is needed to accurately diagnose and eventually treat laryngeal pathology. To complicate diagnosis, these patients may complain of dyspnea which may be accompanied by "wheezing," and they may carry a diagnosis of "refractory asthma."

The diagnostic study with the highest yield in evaluating laryngeal causes of dyspnea is direct visualization of the larynx at the time the patient is symptomatic. Obviously, it is not always possible to do direct or indirect laryngoscopy at the time a patient is experiencing exercise-

Table 1 Symptoms That May Be Experienced by Patients with Laryngeal Pathology

Dyspnea on exertion
Shortness of breath
"Wheezing"
Hoarseness
Sense of laryngeal tightness

induced respiratory symptoms. However, pathology may also be evident on laryngeal examination at times when the patient is not symptomatic. If results of initial examinations are negative, sometimes it may be helpful to have the patient exercise outside of the physician's office and return for visualization of the larynx when they become symptomatic. If one fails to correctly establish the diagnosis of "laryngeal dyspnea," patients may experience potentially harmful iatrogenic side effects from treatment, especially when long-term oral glucocorticoids are given for what is thought to be "resistant or refractory asthma." Symptoms that a patient may experience with laryngeal abnormalities are outlined in Table 1.

II. ANATOMY AND IMPORTANCE OF NORMAL LARYNGEAL FUNCTION

The larynx is a critical and fairly complex anatomical region that extends from the superior tip of the epiglottis to the cricoid cartilage. The cricoid cartilage is actually the only complete cartilagineous ring in the tracheobronchial tree, and it forms the foundation of the larynx [1]. During the period of embryonic maturation, all major cartilages are present by 8 weeks of gestation, and both the true and false vocal cords appear at 10 weeks, with the definitive anatomical configuration of the larynx present by 28 weeks [1].

The larynx joins the airway and the superior portion of the gastrointestinal tract. It serves the critical function of providing sphincteric protection of the airway, while preventing aspiration of both fluids and food particles during swallowing. It also protects the airway from inhalation of foreign material during respiration. The act of swallowing or pharyngeal stimulation causes an automatic closing of the airway. This automatic reflex is beyond voluntary control and is a protective reflex [2].

The true vocal cords also resonate in a very complex pattern to allow the production of vocal sounds for communication. This sophisticated laryngeal function has required the development of very complex neural controls that allow precision vocal cord movements necessary to produce vocal sounds. Movement of laryngeal structures is constantly monitored through neural input of the auditory, visual, and proprioceptive systems in which the entire process is modified on an ongoing basis. Usually, this process is not done at the conscious level, and becomes apparent to both the patient and the treating physician only when something goes wrong. Some of the ways in which laryngeal and upper tracheal abnormalities may contribute to respiratory symptoms during exercise are outlined in the following sections. Before discussing what can go wrong with the movement of laryngeal structures, it is important to understand the normal anatomical relations and movements of these structures.

The average opening of the glottis is fairly constant in most patients, although it tends to be slightly wider on inspiration than with expiration [2]. The medullary respiratory center, through the vagus nerve, controls the glottic aperture. This results from contraction of the posterior cricoarytenoid (PCA) muscle [2]. Contraction of this muscle leads to abduction, which reduces resistance to airflow by opening the glottis. A PCA contraction is carefully coordinated with contraction of the diaphragmatic musculature; it may also be influenced by alterations in arterial concentrations of both oxygen and carbon dioxide, as well as intrapulmonary pressure [3]. In addition, airway obstruction and hypercapnia appear to affect posterior cricoarytenoid muscle tone, for further expiratory narrowing of the glottis may occur during experimentally induced, histamine-mediated bronchospasm [3,4]. The mechanism of this narrowing during experimentally induced bronchospasm is unclear, although some have proposed that it functions as "physiological PEEP" (positive end-expiratory pressure) to limit airway collapse [4,5]. Because of these findings, some investigators believe the glottis is capable of reflex adjustments in parallel with changes in airway caliber. For an elegant description of the principles of laryngeal movement and voice production, the reader is referred to a comprehensive summary [6].

Laryngeal pathology that may lead to dyspnea falls into two main categories. The first of these is dyspnea caused by *abnormal motion of the vocal cords* or other laryngeal structures, and the second is dyspnea caused by *structural interference with airflow*.

III. ABNORMAL MOVEMENT OF LARYNGEAL STRUCTURES PRODUCING AIRWAY OBSTRUCTION

Abnormal motion of laryngeal structures may occur in a variety of clinical situations (Table 2). These problems may occur in patients of any age,

Table 2 Abnormal Movement of Laryngeal Structures Producing Airway Obstruction

Vocal cord paralysis (unilateral or bilateral)
Laryngospasm
Paradoxical vocal cord motion (vocal cord dysfunction)
Meige syndrome (neurological condition accompanied by episodic spastic closure of the true vocal cords)
Spastic dysphonia (may rarely produce sensation of dyspnea)

and some appear to have at least a partial functional component. Most of them do not appear to be under direct voluntary control of the patient, although some disorders may have a more voluntary component than others. As previously discussed, the vocal cords are normally open wider during inspiration than expiration. "Paradoxical vocal cord motion," also known as "vocal cord dysfunction" is a condition in which the two vocal cords approximate (adduct) during inspiration. Although this syndrome may occur in men, it usually occurs in women, a striking number of which are affiliated in some way with the medical profession [7]. Their presentation may be quite dramatic and may resemble acute asthma or, alternatively, acute laryngeal edema. In many instances, emergency room personnel may move quickly to intubate the patient to secure an airway. The characteristics of this syndrome are outlined in Table 3.

Table 3 Characteristics of Vocal Cord Dysfunction (Paradoxical Vocal Cord Motion)

Most patients are female (approximately 90%)

Preponderance of patients affiliated with medical profession (e.g., nurses, medical technologists, medical records specialists)

May have strong component of inspiratory dyspnea

Clinical evaluation may disclose:

1. Arterial blood gases and arterial–alveolar oxygen gradient are usually normal, although exceptions to this have been reported.
2. The diagnosis is made by direct visualization when the patient is symptomatic.
3. Methacholine challenge test results are usually negative, although vocal cord dysfunction has been reported to accompany asthma as well.
4. Patients may have excessive airway noise ("wheezing" or stridor—often loudest over the trachea or anterior chest).

Most reports describing paradoxical vocal cord motion in the literature show that arterial blood gas determinations are normal, and the arterial–alveolar oxygen gradient remains unchanged from times when the person is asymptomatic [8].

Most of the literature also shows that patients with paradoxical vocal cord motion or laryngeal dysfunction have negative methacholine challenges; therefore, this syndrome is not a complication of asthma. However, some patients with asthma may have accompanying vocal cord dysfunction that contributes to their symptom complex [2,9]. Because various psychological factors, including emotional stress, may play a role in the pathogenesis of this condition, a multifactorial approach, including appropriate psychological or psychiatric intervention, combined with speech therapy, may be most helpful. The diagnosis is established by direct visualization of the vocal cords when the patient is symptomatic, with documentation that vocal cord movement returns to normal during times when patients are not symptomatic. The reader is referred to detailed articles on vocal cord dysfunction for further information [2,9].

It is not clear from the literature what percentage of patients with vocal cord dysfunction have symptoms when participating in strenuous exercise or vigorous physical activity. It would be reasonable to assume, however, that especially in a stressful athletic event, a patient could have dyspnea as a result of paradoxical movement of the vocal cords. The degree to which exercise would be limited in patients with ongoing symptoms from this disorder is unclear.

Another laryngeal cause of dyspnea secondary to abnormal vocal cord movement is vocal cord paralysis. Paralysis may be unilateral or bilateral, and may be the result of recurrent laryngeal nerve damage during past thyroid or parathyroid surgery, or due to other causes. Because of its relation to structures in the mediastinum, resulting in its longer anatomical path, the left recurrent laryngeal nerve is more commonly affected than the right; therefore, left vocal cord paralysis is more commonly seen than right-sided paralysis [10]. Unilateral vocal cord paralysis may also be caused by diabetic neuropathy, multiple sclerosis, sarcoidosis, alcoholic polyneuropathy, and syringomyelia [11].

In patients with vocal cord paralysis, surprisingly, some may have a voice (or a cry, in infants) that may be near normal. Some patients, however, will obviously have hoarseness. Other complications of vocal cord paralysis may include aspiration while drinking liquids or eating solid foods, with the resultant problems that may ensue from aspiration. The diagnosis is made by direct visualization of the vocal cords, especially with inadequate movement during maneuvers known to abduct the vocal cords (including coughing) or adduct the vocal cords (such as phonation).

A neurological condition known as "Meige syndrome" may also lead to inappropriate vocal cord motion [2]. This is a condition that results in episodic contractions of musculature, including facial musculature, as well as other muscle groups, including those of the larynx. Some of these patients may have true vocal cord approximation that significantly interferes with breathing. This may obstruct the airway to the point of loss of consciousness, at which point the vocal cords may relax and allow a patient airway once again [2]. This condition requires careful coordinated care with a neurologist, otolaryngologist, and a speech pathologist. Some of these patients may require tracheostomy.

Laryngeal spasm may also lead to sudden closure of the airway and may be precipitated by stressful stimuli as well as other physical stimuli, including gastroesophageal reflux [2]. Treatment is based on comprehensive medical and psychological evaluation, stress reduction, and speech therapy.

Several other conditions may lead to bilateral vocal cord paralysis, including multiple sclerosis, amyotrophic lateral sclerosis, polio, cerebral vascular accidents, trauma, malignancies of the esophagus and thyroid gland, and Parkinson's disease [11]. In addition, the cricoarytenoid joint may be affected by rheumatological conditions, such as rheumatoid arthritis [12]. Severe rheumatoid arthritis may result in fixation of the arytenoid joints and require surgical intervention [12].

Once patients with abnormal vocal cord motion have been identified, they usually require subspecialty treatment in conjunction with an otolaryngologist and speech pathologist who specialize in these disorders. Many metropolitan areas have a voice disorder center that functions as a regional referral location for these types of patients. They may document the anatomy and physiology using advanced diagnostic techniques, including both video laryngoscopy and stroboscopic examination of the larynx. After the diagnosis is established, specific treatment may be prescribed, usually using a team approach, including the primary treating physician, an otolaryngologist, and a speech pathologist.

IV. LARYNGEAL AIRFLOW OBSTRUCTION CAUSED BY STRUCTURAL INTERFERENCE

A variety of different structural abnormalities in the larynx may interfere with the laryngeal airflow. Both infectious and noninfectious processes may compromise airflow through the upper trachea or larynx (Table 4).

Table 4 Laryngeal or Tracheal Airflow Obstruction from Noninfectious Causes

Subglottic stenosis
Vocal cord polyps
Laryngocele
Saccular cysts
Foreign body aspiration
Thermal or chemical inhalation
Lye or acid ingestion
Extrinsic laryngeal compression (e.g., substernal goiter)
Anatomical disruption secondary to trauma (e.g., motor vehicle accident, prolonged intubation)
Inflammatory or vasculitic conditions (e.g., Wegener's granulomatosis)
Amyloidosis, sarcoidosis
Systemic lupus erythematosus
Relapsing polychondritis
Laryngeal vascular lesions
Laryngomalacia
Tumor
Redundant laryngeal tissue

A. Laryngeal or Tracheal Airflow Obstruction from Noninfectious Causes

Various noninfectious conditions may cause airflow obstruction as inspired air passes through the upper trachea and larynx (see Table 4). In children, the most common cause of stridor is congenital laryngomalacia. This is a condition that produces intermittent stridor and is usually precipitated by increased physical activity, including crying in infants and exercise in older children. This results from a flaccidity of the larynx, and because of a lack of rigidity of the framework supporting the larynx there is a "drawing in" of the superglottic tissues of the larynx with inspiration. These symptoms usually occur in infants and young children, and may have their onset a few weeks after birth and last up to 12–18 months. Direct visualization of the larynx, which is necessary to confirm the diagnosis, reveals a convergence of the laryngeal structures during inspiration. This disorder is usually self-limited and resolves spontaneously with observation only. In severe cases, however, tracheostomy may occasionally be indicated [13].

A number of conditions may result in subglottic stenosis. These may include laryngeal trauma from a motor vehicle accident, blunt laryngeal trauma from other causes, or prolonged endotracheal intubation. In addition, certain inflammatory or vasculitic conditions may lead to subglottic stenosis. Wegener's granulomatosis may cause dyspnea owing to laryngeal and tracheal involvement. It is rare for systemic lupus erythematosus to lead to a narrowing of the subglottic airway; however, it may be seen in relapsing polychondritis [11]. Other causes of subglottic stenosis may include infection (see Sec. IV. B), tumor, trauma, thermal or chemical inhalation, lye or acid ingestion, and tracheal malacia [14]. Redundant tissue in the larynx may also lead to symptoms of exercise-induced dyspnea. We have recently seen a patient at the Oregon Health Sciences University who complained of dyspnea on exertion, but did not have demonstrable evidence for reactive airway disease. This patient developed inspiratory stridor with exertion that was done as a part of the evaluation here, and redundant superglottic tissue collapsed in on the glottic opening with higher volume respiratory efforts during inspiration.

Inflammatory masses may also be caused by diseases such as amyloidosis and sarcoidosis. Anaphylaxis may lead to laryngeal edema, as can episodic idiopathic angioedema. Angioedema may occur in the hereditary form, characterized by C-1 esterase inhibitor deficiency, or as an acquired idiopathic condition. Acute laryngeal edema is treated with the prompt administration of subcutaneous epinephrine, maintenance of an adequate airway, other supportive measures, as well as systemic corticosteroids in most cases.

Dyspnea on exertion may also be caused in young children or toddlers by foreign body aspiration. This most commonly occurs in children or toddlers between the ages of 12 and 36 months [15]. To further complicate diagnostic accuracy, foreign bodies lodged within the esophagus of young children may also lead to respiratory compromise and stridor because of the pliability of the young larynx and its proximity to the esophagus. Young children are not the only group of patients who may suffer from foreign body aspiration; elderly patients may also present with dyspnea, wheezing, or fever as a result of foreign body aspiration. This may occur especially in elderly, debilitated patients or those who have an impaired swallowing mechanism resulting from musculoskeletal disorders, cerebral vascular accident, or other causes [16]. Dyspnea on exertion may also be caused by both benign and malignant neoplasms of the larynx. Direct visualization is mandatory for accurate diagnosis of these disorders. Laryngeal airflow may also be obstructed by various other noninfectious disorders, including saccular cysts, laryngoceles, laryngeal vascular lesions, and vocal cord polyps. Vocal cord polyps may occur either unilaterally or bilaterally, and they may need to be surgically removed if they are interfering with glottic airflow. Both substernal and cervical goiters may also cause dyspnea on exertion by interfering with tracheal or laryngeal airflow [17].

The flow–volume curve may sometimes provide hints on the location of airway obstruction, and whether it may be fixed or variable. It must be emphasized, however, that significant airway lesions may exist in the presence of a normal flow–volume curve contour.

B. Laryngeal Airflow Obstruction Caused by Infection

Several bacterial and viral infections may lead to dyspnea originating from the upper airway (Table 5). Epiglottitis is one of the most frightening and rapidly developing infectious causes of dyspnea originating in the upper airway. It is almost always due a bacterial pathogen, which causes life-threatening inflammation and edema in the supraglottic larynx. *Haemophilus influenzae* type b, pneumococci, and hemolytic streptococci are the most common causative organisms [16].

Symptoms and signs that may characterize this condition include inspiratory stridor, high-fever, drooling, and airway distress. These symptoms may be extremely rapid in onset and relentless in their progression.

Table 5 Laryngeal Airflow Obstruction from Infectious Causes

Epiglottitis
Laryngeal abscess
Bacterial tracheitis
Diphtheria
Syphilis
Trichinosis
Tuberculosis
Leprosy
Viral: croup (influenza and parainfluenza), human papilloma virus (producing laryngeal papillomatosis), cytomegalovirus (congenital infection and HIV-related disease)
Fungal: histoplasma, aspergillus, blastomyces, actinomyces, coccidioides, candida, cryptococcus, and nocardia

Although epiglottitis may occur in adults, it most commonly occurs in children between the ages of 2 and 8 years. A recent review of adults with epiglottitis disclosed that 15% required airway intervention by either endotracheal intubation or tracheostomy [18]. In that particular manuscript, risk factors associated with the need for airway intervention included the presence of stridor or sitting erect at the time of presentation. They found that major complications occurred in 5% of patients, but they had no deaths in their series of 129 cases of adult epiglottitis [18].

In patients in whom epiglottitis is suspected, visualization of the epiglottis is never done with a tongue blade because of risk of precipitation of acute airway closure [2]. The size of the epiglottis is quantified either with a lateral neck x-ray films or with the flexible fiber-optic rhinolaryngoscope. Treatment of acute epiglottitis includes appropriate antibiotic therapy, and in some patients, simultaneous use of systemic corticosteroids. If a patient with epiglottitis appears in respiratory distress, it is imperative that medical personnel capable of securing an airway are immediately available. These personnel should also be available if the patient has the potential to decompensate based on the pace at which symptoms are progressing.

In contrast to epiglottitis, which is usually caused by a bacterial pathogen, croup is generally viral in origin. The subglottic tissues and trachea are affected in croup, and although it is not a laryngeal cause of dyspnea per se, it is an important cause of stridor in children. The most common pathogens are influenza or parainfluenza viruses. Treatment of croup consists of hydration, humidification, corticosteroids, and in some patients, racemic epinephrine or a combination of these treatment options [10]. Occasionally, securing an airway is necessary by intubation or tracheostomy.

Bacterial tracheitis is a life-threatening infection of the trachea which may present with high fever, stridor, a barking cough, thick mucopurulent discharge from the trachea, and extreme leukocytosis. *Staphylococcus* is the most common causative organism producing bacterial tracheitis, although *H. influenzae* type b and group A streptococci have also been reported to cause this condition [10]. These patients may occasionally need tracheostomy or intubation, and therapeutic intervention with the appropriate antibiotics must be done expeditiously to minimize the need to artificially secure an airway. Other bacterial infections of the upper airway include laryngeal abscesses in the supraglottic, glottic, or subglottic areas, and these require surgical incision and drainage. These abscesses may be slow to increase in severity, and they may follow previous episodes of tonsilar infections.

A host of less common infections may also involve the laryngeal structures. These may include diphtheria, histoplasmosis, trichinosis, tuberculosis, syphilis, and leprosy [11]. Fungal infections have also been reported in the upper airway, including those caused by *Aspergillus*, *Coccidioides*, *Blastomyces*, *Histoplasma*, *Candida*, *Actinomyces*, *Nocardia*, and *Cryptococcus* species [11]. Viral pathogens that have been reported to cause laryngeal involvement include cytomegalovirus (CMV), although this is usually seen in patients with the acquired immune deficiency syndrome (AIDS), as well as children who acquire a congenital CMV infection.

Children who are delivered vaginally from mothers who are infected with venereal warts may acquire a laryngeal infection with the human papilloma virus. This may produce the common benign laryngeal tumor, referred to as squamous papilloma, which may occur in either a juvenile or an adult form. Patients with squamous papilloma may suffer from hoarseness, stridor, or respiratory airway compromise. This condition has lead to fatal asphyxiation in children [19]. Unfortunately, despite aggressive treatment, this condition frequently recurs. At the time of this printing endoscopic removal of the papilloma tissue with a carbon dioxide laser is the preferred form of treatment [19]. Other modalities have also been tried, including systemic interferon, although management of individual patients is dictated by the severity and frequency of recurrences of this disorder.

V. SUMMARY

Pathology involving the larynx and upper trachea may take many forms. These include infectious and noninfectious causes of laryngeal airflow obstruction, as well as abnormal movements of laryngeal structures. The cornerstone of accurate diagnosis and treatment is the combination of a high index of suspicion for these diagnostic possibilities, combined with direct visualization of the laryngeal structures. Flexible fiber-optic rhinolaryngoscopy has been a tremendous help in the complete evaluation of patients with suspected laryngeal disease. Suspicion of a laryngeal cause of dyspnea should be aroused when treatment for conditions such as exercise-induced asthma proves ineffective in controlling a patient's symptoms. An understanding of the wide diversity of problems that may lead to dyspnea on exertion will allow us to provide optimal care for our patients.

REFERENCES

1. Baxter MRN. Congenital laryngomalacia. Can J Anaesth 1994; 41:332–339.
2. O'Hollaren MT. Masqueraders in clinical allergy: laryngeal dysfunction causing dyspnea. Ann Allergy 1990; 65:351–356.
3. Wood RP, Jafek BW, Cherniak RM. Laryngeal dysfunction and pulmonary disorders. Otolaryngol Head Neck Surg 1986; 94:374.
4. Higgenbottam T. Narrowing of glottis opening in humans associated with experimentally induced bronchoconstriction. J Appl Physiol 1980; 49:403.
5. Higgenbottam T, Payne J. Glottis narrowing in lung disease. Am Rev Respir Dis 1982; 125:746.
6. Cohn JR, Spiegel JR, Sataloff RT. Vocal disorders and the professional voice user: the allergist's role. Ann Allergy 1995; 74:363–376.
7. Downing ET, Braman SS, Fox MJ, et al. Factitious asthma—physiologic approach to diagnosis. JAMA 1982; 248:2878–81.
8. Christopher KL, Wood RP, Eckert RC, et al. Vocal cord dysfunction presenting as asthma. N Engl J Med 1983; 308:1566–70.
9. Patterson DL, O'Connel EJ. Vocal cord dysfunction: what have we learned in 150 years? Insights Allergy 1994; 9(6):1–12.
10. O'Hollaren, MT, Everts EC. Evaluating the patient with stridor. Ann Allergy 1991; 67:301–306.
11. Teitel AD, MacKenzie CR, Stern R, et al. Laryngeal involvement in systemic lupus erythematosus. Semin Arthritis Rheum 1992; 22:203–214.
12. Dockery KM, Sismania A, Abedi E. Rheumatoid arthritis of the larynx: the importance of early diagnosis and corticosteroid therapy. S Med J 1991; 84: 95–95.
13. Baxter MRN. Congenital laryngomalacia. Can J Anaesth 1994; 41:332–9.
14. Spector GJ. Respiratory insufficiency, tracheal stenosis and airway control. In: Diseases of the nose, throat, ear, head, and neck. Philadelphia: Lea & Febiger, 1991:553.
15. O'Hollaren, MT, Tank JE. Shortness of breath, cough, and wheezing in a 67-year old man (review of foreign body aspiration). Ann Allergy 1991; 66: 289–293.
16. O'Hollaren MT. When dyspnea comes from the larynx. J Respir Dis 1991; 12:845–860.
17. O'Hollaren MT, Marcoux JP. Tracheal compression from substernal goiter presenting with respiratory symptoms. Ann Allergy 1986; 54:351.
18. Frantz TD, Rasgone BM, Quesenberry CP. Acute epiglottitis in adults: analysis of 129 cases. JAMA 1994; 272:1358–1360.
19. Sperry K. Lethal asphyxiating juvenile laryngeal papillomatosis. Am J Foren Med Pathol 1995; 15:146–150.

14
Exercise-Induced Urticaria and Angioedema

Christodoulos S. Christodoulou and Joseph D. Diaz
University of Texas Health Science Center at San Antonio, San Antonio, Texas

Ernest N. Charlesworth
Brenham Clinic, Brenham, Texas

I. INTRODUCTION

Since the first description by Duke in 1924 [1], the syndrome of exercise-induced urticaria (EIU), with or without associated angioedema, has become increasingly recognized as a common malady. Because of the increasing knowledge of the health benefits of exercise, there has been a growing commitment to physical fitness by the general population. This growing commitment has led to an increase in the occurrence of activity-related conditions such as EIU.

Several studies and case reports have identified patients who develop urticaria during exercise. The difficulty has been in categorizing these patients into either EIU, cholinergic urticaria (CU), or exercise-induced anaphylaxis (EIAna). The term *exercise-induced urticaria* is often discussed in the context of *cholinergic urticaria*, a form of physical urticaria triggered not only by exercise, but also by anxiety, sweating, and passive warming [2]. Most often patients who develop urticaria during exercise are categorized as either having EIU, CU, or EIAna based on the precipitating factors, such as exercise, elevation of body core temperature, or anxiety. Other clues helpful in the differentiation include the size of the wheals, presence of other systemic allergic symptoms, and provocative challenge results with either exercise or passive warming. Finally, methacholine skin test may be helpful in differentiating EIU and EIAna from CU. The signs and symptoms of EIU, as well as the results of provocative testing, such as exercise, are often indistinguishable from those of CU. Hence, the term exercise-induced urticaria is often used interchangeably with cholinergic urticaria. Cholinergic urticaria, however, is the term often used to identify the patient with exercise-induced urticarial eruptions who also develops symptoms with anxiety, activities which result in passive increase of body core temperature, and who has a positive methacholine skin test. Exercise-induced urticaria and CU, however, must be distinguished from exercise-induced anaphylaxis, in which life-threatening systemic allergic symptoms are often present (Table 1).

Interestingly, there have also been case reports defining patients with confirmed CU (positive provocative challenge to passive warming and positive methacholine skin test) in association with systemic anaphylactic symptoms, such as lightheadedness, hypotension, or laryngeal obstruction [3]. Despite the presence of anaphylactic symptoms, the diagnosis was consistent with CU because of the positive provocative challenge to passive warming and the presence of a positive methacholine skin test.

There are no biological markers that can be definitively used to differentiate patients with EIU from CU or EIAna. In fact, patients with CU and EIU have significantly elevated histamine levels during provocative testing, as is seen in exercise-induced anaphylasis [4].

Table 1 Characteristics of Cholinergic Urticaria (CU) and Exercise-Induced Anaphylaxis (EIAna)

Characteristic	Cholinergic urticaria	Exercise-induced anaphylaxis
Symptoms with exercise	Yes	Yes
Symptoms with passive elevation of body temperature	Yes	No
Symptoms with anxiety	Yes	No
Size of wheal	2–4 mm	> 5 mm
PFT[a] abnormalities and wheezing	Rarely [4]	No [39]
Hypotension	Occasionally [3,20]	Usually
Exercise challenge test	Positive	Positive
Passive-warming challenge test	Usually positive	Negative
Methacholine skin test	Positive (in 30% of patients) [11]	Negative
Elevated serum histamine level	Yes	Yes

[a] PFT, pulmonary function tests.

II. PATHOGENESIS

Although CU has been described for more than 70 years, the pathophysiology is poorly understood. Several theories have suggested the presence of a neurogenic reflex involving acetylcholine. Increased sensitivity to acetylcholine, increased numbers of cholinergic receptors, and decreased acetylcholine esterase levels have been described in patients with CU [5,6].

One theory suggests that exercise, emotional stimuli, or other stresses that induce sweating or increase body core temperature may initiate a neurogenic reflex causing the release of acetylcholine, resulting in urticaria [7]. Herxheimer et al. [8] provided strong evidence that the wheal in CU is mediated by fibers of the sympathetic nervous system innervating sweat glands that are dependent on acetylcholine. They observed that unilateral cervical sympathetic block with procaine prevented the appearance of CU on the ipsilateral side, and that generalized sympathetic block with hexamethonium nearly completely prevented the appearance of urticaria altogether following 12 min of exercise on a stationary bicycle. Because there is a relatively long interval (7 min) between the release of acetylcholine at nerve endings and the appearance of urticaria, they suggested the presence of an intermediate link, possibly sweat. The direct association between sweat and urticaria was later questioned by Kay et al., who reported a patient with both CU and anhidrosis [9].

The suggestion that acetylcholine is directly involved in the pathogenesis of CU was supported by Shelley et al. [5], who reported on a patient with CU with an unusually large number of cholinergic receptors at the urticarial sites, presumably accounting for the heightened sensitivity to acetylcholine production following exercise, heat or emotional stress. This observation, however, was contradicted by Haustein et al. [6], who reported decreased numbers of cholinergic receptors at urticarial sites. Other evidence for the role of acetylcholine in CU is obtained from studies in which decreased acetylcholine esterase levels were present in the skin of patients with CU, suggesting that increased "local" levels of acetylcholine are responsible for the symptoms of CU [10].

A possible reflex involving afferent humoral and efferent neurogenic components as the cause of CU has also been suggested [11]. A tourniquet tied proximal to a hand emersed in warm water in a patient with CU obliterates the urticarial response. When the tourniquet is released a generalized urticarial eruption may occur. It has been suggested that either a humoral component released during the warming or the central perception of a temperature change transmitted by the circulation results in an efferent reflex responsible for the urticaria [11].

Other investigators have suggested that the urticaria occurring during exercise is secondary to the production of a protease capable of causing mast cell degranulation [12]. Acetylcholine may cause the production or release of a protease that induces mast cell degranulation and that, possibly, an inhibitor of that protease is decreased in CU, resulting in increased release of histamine from mast cells. Support of this theory comes from the discovery that the plasma level of α_1-antichymotrypsin may be decreased in patients with CU [12]. This "consumption theory" was supported by clinical studies using danazol therapy, which resulted in increased levels of α_1-antichymotrypsin and resolution of the CU lesions [13,14].

Passive transfer experiments have also been carried out successfully. Investigators were able to induce local skin lesions, consistent with CU, when transferring serum locally from human to animal [15], or animal to animal [16]. In these reports the authors did not investigate the "transferred factor" responsible for the urticarial eruption. Although reports have been conflicting, there has been at least one successful report of human-to-human passive transfer of CU [17]. Because of the potential health hazards of passive transfer experiments, further documentation of passive transfer in CU is unlikely.

Since the initial report by Kaplan et al. in 1975 [18], several patients with EIU have been noted to have elevated plasma histamine levels during exercise [4,19–22]. In most patients, increased serum histamine levels parallel the onset of pruritus and urticaria. Exercise-induced urticaria, elicited experimentally in seven patients with EIU after running on a treadmill in a plastic occlusive suit, resulted in elevations of serum histamine as early as 6 min, peaking at 20 min, and returning to baseline by 40 min [4]. This does not appear to be a nonspecific finding in atopic patients. Harries et al. measured plasma histamine in 17 asthmatic patients and 6 normal controls during exercise testing and found elevated histamine levels in only 1 patient, who also developed urticaria following exercise [23]. Other mediators that are elevated in the serum of patients with EIU or CU include eosinophil and neutrophil chemotactic factors [4]. One case of elevated serotonin levels in a patient with CU during exercise has been reported [18]. Increased tryptase levels in suction blister fluid have also been observed in one patient with CU [24]. This does not appear to be specific for CU, for elevated levels of tryptase in blister fluid have been noted in other types of urticaria [24]. Also, tryptase may be insensitive as a diagnostic tool; patients have been described who have CU with systemic allergic symptoms, elevated histamine levels, but no elevation of serum tryptase [25].

Description of the histological findings in CU has been limited. Hirschmann et al. reported that seven patients who underwent biopsy had perivascular inflammatory infiltrates and interstitial edema. Six of those patients had perivascular neutrophils, four had a perifollicular inflammatory infiltrate, and eosinophils were demonstrated in three cases [26]. Winkelmann obtained biopsies from three patients with urticaria produced by exercise and noted that two patients had a "neutrophilic urticarial infiltrate," consisting of a polymorphonuclear cell infiltration in and about the walls of vessels. The third patient had only lymphocytes present in the surrounding vessels of the dermis [27]. James et al. took biopsy specimens from 21 patients with urticaria, two of whom had CU. They found no histological difference between patients with CU and those with chronic urticaria [28].

III. CUTANEOUS MANIFESTATIONS

In general, individuals with EIU or CU develop small punctate pruritic skin lesions, usually measuring 2–4 mm in diameter [29], surrounded by areas of erythema that may coalesce, making them difficult to distinguish from ordinary urticaria [3]. The rash may occur within 30 min following the onset of exercise, usually beginning on the thorax and neck, and frequently spreading to the entire body [2]. In the vast majority of cases the hives last for 30 min, distinguishing them from the hives seen in idiopathic urticaria, which may persist for several hours. Angioedema [19,30,31] and dermatographism [32] have also been described in association with the urticaria of EIU–CU. It is not uncommon to elicit a history of pruritus during exercise, without the appearance of true urticaria [33]. *Cholinergic erythema* has been described as a variant of CU in which exercise or hot bathing provokes erythema with pruritus in which no papular eruptions occur [34].

IV. SYSTEMIC MANIFESTATIONS

Although most patients with CU do not complain of systemic allergic symptoms, several case reports have described patients with CU and systemic allergic symptoms. These reports note the presence of pulmonary, gastrointestinal, or other generalized allergic symptoms occurring in conjunction with CU (see later discussion). Czarnetzki et al. compared pulmonary function testing in 21 patients with CU before and after bronchial provocation with acetylcholine [35]. Patients with "severe" CU demonstrated increased reactivity. These patients, however, did not complain of pulmonary symptoms, such as dyspnea, cough, or wheezing, during exercise. On the other hand, Soter et al. [4] reported that experimental exercise produced wheezing and shortness of breath in six of seven patients with CU or EIU. These symptoms were accompanied by a statistically significant drop in 1-s forced expiratory volume (FEV_1), maximal midexpiratory flow rates (MMEF), and specific conductance (sGaw), along with a rise in residual volume (RV). Simultaneous occurrence of exercise-induced asthma, abdominal pain, nausea, diarrhea, and dizziness with CU have also been reported [30,36,37].

Although exercise-induced anaphylaxis will be discussed elsewhere in this book (see Chap. 15), it is important to differentiate it from CU, because both can occur with exercise and have similar manifestations. The wheals of exercise-induced anaphylaxis are usually larger (5–15 mm) compared with the smaller urticarial eruptions of CU (2–4 mm). Cholinergic urticaria may be associated with pulmonary symptoms, as noted; however, hypotension and vascular collapse are more often seen in exercise-induced anaphylaxis, but are rarely seen in association with CU [29,38,39] (see Table 1).

Several reports have challenged the distinction between exercise-linked anaphylaxis and CU by performing exercise challenges on patients with a history of exercise-induced urticaria and hypotension [3,20,40]. These patients had both punctate hives usually characteristic of CU and hypotension characteristic of EIAna. A subset of these patients were eventually felt to have CU and not EIAna, based on clinical investigation. Casale et al. [3] reported two patients with anaphylactic symptoms noted after vigorous exercise. Both had a positive exercise challenge test, but only one patient had a positive provocative challenge to passive heating and a positive methacholine skin test, differentiating him from the other patient with EIAna. The term "variant CU," has been suggested by some investigators referring to exercise-induced punctate urticaria and angioedema, which may involve systemic symptoms or progress to vascular collapse [19,41].

V. EPIDEMIOLOGY AND NATURAL HISTORY

The true incidence of EIU–CU is unknown and has been reviewed in few reports. A large prospective study of 493 high school and university students suggested a prevalence of 11.2%, of which only 22% sought medical attention [42]. The authors suggested that the discrepancy between the high prevalence of disease and the surprisingly low number of patients seeking medical advice was because only a small percentage suffered sufficiently enough to seek medical advice.

Most studies suggest that CU is responsible for the urticaria in 4–7% of patients with a diagnosis with chronic idiopathic urticaria [43,44]. Although in adults, the cause of chronic idiopathic urticaria may be secondary to CU in as many as 11% of the patients [45,46], lower rates may be found in children. In one report only 6 (2.7%) of 226 children with chronic urticaria had CU [47]. Similarly low rates have also been described by Quaranta et al. [48].

The age of onset of CU is usually the second or third decade of life [26,43]. In most patients, the symptoms are regular and predictable. Cholinergic urticaria is a chronic condition that persists for more than 5 years in 60% of patients and for more than 10 years in 31% [26]. The duration of CU has been documented in one study to be from 9 months to 27 years [26]. In this study, 89% of patients developed CU after exercise, whereas hot baths or showers provoked eruptions in 80% and stress in 60%. This underscores the importance of questioning patients presenting with EIU about whether or not exposure to hot temperatures, such as hot showers or baths, or stress provoke symptoms, thereby, suggesting a diagnosis of CU. Also, patients with EIU–CU have a much higher incidence of atopy present, up to 45% in one study [42].

VI. FOOD-ASSOCIATED, EXERCISE-INDUCED URTICARIA AND ANGIOEDEMA

Although there are several reports describing postprandial exercise-induced anaphylaxis, postprandial EIU or angioedema, have been less frequently described. Kushimoto et al. reported six patients with a history of type I hypersensitivity to wheat, presenting with urticaria, angioedema, or anaphylaxis during exercise after eating wheat [49]. Elimination of wheat from diet completely eradicated symptoms during exercises. The authors suggested that this phenomenon was due to increased cardiovascular activity during exercise, resulting in larger amounts of allergen deposition, leading to increased allergic symptoms. Another group of investigators evaluated five patients with EIU or angioedema after food ingestion to which they were skin-test positive [60]. The implicated food alone, or exercise alone, did not induce symptoms. The authors suggested that the urticaria or angioedema appearing after the introduction of both food and exercise was the result of the combined effects on mast cells. Further support of this entity comes from a recent case report of a woman with angioedema provoked by the combined ingestion of food plus exercise. Daily exercise before breakfast has resulted in no symptoms [51].

VII. COMBINATION OF CHOLINERGIC URTICARIA WITH OTHER PHYSICAL URTICARIAS

Cholinergic urticaria has been described in association with cold and aquagenic urticaria. Coexistence of EIU and cold urticaria is significant because patients may exercise under cold conditions such as jogging in cold weather or swimming in cold water. Two different syndromes have been described and include combined cold urticaria with CU and cold-induced CU. In combined cold urticaria and CU, symptoms appear after exposure to either cold or exercise [7,52,53]. Evaluation of these patients has revealed both a positive ice cube test and independently performed exercise challenge test. In cold-induced CU the development of urticaria is dependent on exposure to cold and appears while exercising in cold weather. The urticaria does not occur with elevation of body temperature, as exercising in a warm environment sufficient to cause sweating does not precipitate urticaria; furthermore, the ice cube test is negative [54]. This entity was first described in 1981 [54]. Neittaanmäki reported that of 220 patients with cold urticaria, 21 patients (8%) also had coexistent CU, and 2 patients (1%) had cold-induced CU [55]. The frequent association of these two forms of urticaria suggests a common etiological factor. A circulating factor, possibly IgE, which recognizes epitopes revealed during both cold and hot stimuli, has been suggested. Cold-induced CU may be a consequence of neuronal involvement, as in true CU. In the cold-induced CU reactions, autonomic pathways that recognize and respond to cold stimuli may be involved [53].

Aquagenic urticaria coexisting with CU was first described by Shelley et al. in 1964 [56]. They reported three patients with CU who developed urticaria when exposed to water of any temperature or following strenuous exercise. They postulated that water reacts with a component in the sebum, or sebaceous glands, to produce a histamine "liberator" that is absorbed and leads to release of histamine from mast cells. They demonstrated that inert oil coating prevented the occurrence of symptoms. Similar associations of CU with aquagenic urticaria have been described by other investigators [57,58].

VIII. DIAGNOSIS

As with almost all medical conditions, the diagnosis of EIU–CU is often suggested by the initial history. A feeling of cutaneous warmth occurring shortly after beginning exercise with associated pruritus and urticaria are highly suggestive of EIU–CU. Although provocative diagnostic testing is seldom necessary, exercise challenge is often helpful in establishing the presumed diagnosis, and allows the clinician to observe the specific urticarial eruptions. Other provocative diagnostic tests may be helpful in establishing the diagnosis of EIU and differentiate it from CU or exercise-induced anaphylaxis.

A. Exercise Challenge Test

Exercise provocation is often a reliable test and will reproduce symptoms and objective findings in most patients. Although there is no universally accepted standardized exercise procedure, this tool, which is sensitive and efficient, is the most frequently used provocation procedure in EIU, angioedema, and CU [3,4,11,20,21,26,30,37,40,59,60]. Patients may perform any type of exercise until sweating is induced. The urticarial eruptions may occur during, or shortly following, the exercise maneuver. A standardized and more quantitative and reproducible evaluation may be performed using a bicycle ergometer exercise [20]. A treadmill programmed at 6.44 km/h (4 miles/h) and 12° grade has also been used [21]. In one report all nine patients (100%) with a clinical history of EIU or CU had positive exercise challenges [60]. In contrast, another report revealed that exercise provoked urticaria in only 14 of 22 patients (64%) with a history consistent with EIU [26]. Other studies have reported positive exercise challenge tests in patients with CU. Soter et al. reported on seven patients (100%) with a clinical diagnosis of CU who developed urticaria while running on a treadmill wearing plastic occlusive suits [4]. Exercise without the plastic occlusive suit did not consistently reproduce the urticarial lesions in two subjects tested. Although exercise is a reliable test, it may not always result in the production of urticaria. This may be explained either by "refractoriness," especially if the patient had recent symptoms, or because the provocation test was suboptimal [2]. Finally, exercise challenge while wearing an occlusive plastic suit may provide the most reproducibility, although this approach may be impractical.

B. Passive Warming Challenge

Passive warming may be another useful and practical provocative challenge procedure in patients with EIU or CU. Under investigational conditions the passive heat challenge test can be performed by raising the subject's body core temperature by 1–1.5°C. This may be accomplished by immersion of half the body in a bath with a temperature of 43°C [60,61], or by using a hyperthermic blanket [29]. The patient can be observed for the development of the characteristic wheals after sweating has been induced. In one study [60], all but one of nine patients with EIU or CU developed symptoms following passive warming. Most patients developed symptoms within 20 min of immersion and, interestingly, nonimmersed skin developed more lesions than immersed skin.

C. Methacholine Skin Challenge Test

The methacholine skin challenge test requires the intradermal injection of 100 μg of methacholine in 0.1 mL of saline solution [11]. It is considered positive if a characteristic wheal-and-flare reaction occurs often surrounded by satellite lesions. This test is felt to be diagnostic when such satellite lesions are present [22]. Unfortunately, only 30% of patients with CU have a positive skin test to methacholine [11,29]. Consequently, the skin test can be used to confirm the diagnosis, but not as the sole diagnostic test, because a negative test does not rule out the presence of CU. Usually, individuals who test positive to methacholine tend to have a more severe form of CU [60]. Singler et al. examined the ability of atropine to inhibit the formation of satellite lesions following methacholine intradermal injection in patients with CU. One-hundred micrograms of atropine was mixed with 100 μg of methacholine. Although prominent satellite lesions were noted when methacholine–saline control was used, the combination of atropine with methacholine inhibited satellite lesion formation, suggesting the presence of a "true" cholinergic receptor in the pathogenesis of CU [7].

Other substances used as skin-testing material have also been investigated. Czarnetzki et al. studied cutaneous reactions to histamine, compound 48/80, kallikrein, ATP, and acetylcholine [35]. Compared with controls and patients with "moderate disease," patients with severe CU developed larger urticarial eruptions following histamine skin testing, but not following skin testing with any of the other substances [35]. Skin testing using the neuromuscular blocking agent D-tubocurarine, which is analogous in structure to acetylcholine, has also been investigated [62]. Patients with CU were at least ten times more sensitive to D-tubocurarine than the controls. The authors suggested that caution should be used during general anesthesia with compounds such as tubocurarine in patients with CU because of the theoretical risk of precipitating anaphylactic or anaphylactoid reactions.

IX. TREATMENT

Depending on the severity of symptoms and the patients' willingness to alter their exercise lifestyle, many patients with EIU or CU may obtain relief by avoiding the precipitating stimuli, such as exercise, stressful situations, or other activities that may result in increased body core temperature. Unfortunately, avoiding such activities may not be acceptable. Many patients are willing to tolerate the symptoms of EIU or CU without seeking medical attention. Zuberbier et al. [42] reported that 78% of patients with CU were "not troubled" by their symptoms, and 80% had never sought medical advice. If exercise restriction is not acceptable by the patient, modification of exercise should be considered. Patients should be advised to avoid exercising in warm environments or reduce the intensity of exercise to minimize sweating. Also, patients should discontinue exercise immediately with the onset of symptoms [29]. These measures may reduce the severity, duration, and frequency of symptoms in patients with EIU or CU.

Successful desensitization to EIU–CU has been reported by Kaplan et al. [20]. They reported a patient subjected to a 4-day exercise protocol in which the patient ran at full speed for at least 15 min/day. The severity of symptoms dramatically decreased, and by the fourth day total resolution of symptoms occurred. This improvement in symptoms was associated with a progressive decrease of histamine levels from 26 ng/mL on the first day to 0.8 ng/mL on the fourth day. This patient remained symptom-free with a daily exercise program. However, after discontinuing exercise for a 3-week period, a severe reaction occurred during subsequent exercise. Other desensitization attempts have been unsuccessful [53].

Exacerbations of CU may occasionally be aborted or decreased by applying cold water to the skin after activities that may provoke sweating [61]. Also, purposely inducing an attack has been suggested as a way to prevent symptoms during a specific time, such as an anticipated social event. This "prevention" may be secondary to the refractory period, which may last for several hours, during which exercise will not provoke symptoms [43,61]. Because the aforementioned measures are often not felt to be practical by the patient or clinician, or may be ineffective in preventing exacerbations of CU–EIU, pharmacological therapy must often be used. Antihistamines remain the mainstay of this therapy [63].

Although any antihistamine may be useful in controlling the symptoms of EIU–CU, hydroxyzine is the most widely used H_1-antagonist because of its potent antipruritic effects [2,63]. In a double-blind, placebo-controlled crossover trial of 14 patients with CU–EIU, hydroxyzine was compared with brompheniramine and placebo [43]. All patients were treated with hydroxyzine, brompheniramine, and placebo. Eight patients improved while receiving hydroxyzine and four with brompheniramine. Two patients did not respond to either antihistamine, and no patients responded to placebo. In another double-blind, placebo-controlled crossover trial, ten patients were treated prophylactically with hydroxyzine compared with acrivastine and placebo. Both hydroxyzine and acrivastine were more efficient than placebo in controlling the symptoms provoked by exercise challenge. There was no statistical difference between hydroxyzine and acrivastine in preventing symptoms [63]. Many other reports have supported the beneficial effects of hydroxyzine therapy in patients with CU [2,29,53]. Regular use of hydroxyzine and other conventional antihistamines may be limited by their sedative effects. Patients must be warned of the potential sedation associated with conventional antihistamine therapy. Furthermore, patients should be educated about the fact that, despite the absence of obvious clinical sedation, the use of conventional antihistamines may be associated with decreased cognitive function [64]. A combination of hydroxyzine and cyproheptadine (8–16 mg/day) may be the most effective treatment of CU when associated with cold urticaria [2,11].

Cetirizine, a hydroxyzine metabolite with H_1-antagonistic properties, recently approved for use in the United State, has been successful in treating patients with CU [65]. A double-blind, placebo-controlled crossover trial involving 24 patients treated with 10 or 20 mg/day of cetirizine versus placebo, revealed significant improvement in the cetirizine-treated group [65]. All patients had a history of moderate to severe symptoms and had failed therapy with multiple other conventional antihistamines.

Doxepin, a tricyclic antidepressant with potent antihistaminic properties, dosed at 75 mg twice a day, was effective in a patient who failed hydroxyzine therapy [52]. Adding cimetidine, an H_2-antagonist (300 mg qid) virtually obliterated all symptoms.

Although one would suspect that any antihistamine with H_1- and possibly H_2-antagonistic properties will result in improvement in patients with EIU–CU, most of the newer antihistamines have not been specifically investigated in patients with CU. In one report, four of seven patients with CU reported significant improvement following the use of terfenadine. In a double-blind, placebo-controlled study in one patient with CU–EIU, no statistical difference was observed in symptom scores between terfenadine and placebo therapy [66].

Ketotifen, which possesses both H_1-receptor–blocking and mast cell-stabilizing properties, was effective in controlling symptoms in four patients with CU, who had associated cardiac and respiratory symptoms refractory to conventional antihistamine therapy [25]. Treatment with ketotifen, 3–8 mg/day, resulted in overall dramatic clinical improvement, suppression of exercise challenge provocation test, and decreased histamine release following exercise. Huston et al. reported a patient with EIU, treated with 4 mg/day of ketotifen, noting complete resolution of symptoms [67]. Different results were reported by Czarnetzki et al. [68], who observed that only 61–70% of 13 patients participating in a double-blind cross-over study noted significant reduction in symptoms following therapy with ketotifen [68]. In this study ketotifen therapy did not exceed 2 mg/day, as opposed to higher doses used in the previous studies.

Inhaled cromoglycate has been reported to be effective in preventing the symptoms of EIU–angioedema [69]. Interestingly, oral cromoglycate was ineffective. Danazol has also been successful in alleviating the symptoms of EIU–CU in two prior studies [13,14].

Anticholinergics, such as atropine, applied locally decrease the symptoms of EIU on treated skin. These drugs are not recommended for routine use because of the possible absorption of the drug through the skin [8].

The assessment of the effectiveness of these medications may be difficult because of the variable course of the disease and the extent of daily activity. Symptom scores on a daily basis are the most reliable indicator and should be used when evaluating medication efficacy. Frequently, the relief provided by medications and avoidance measures is incomplete, often requiring the use of increased doses of conventional medications or instituting combination therapy. More controlled studies are needed to better evaluate the effectiveness of the newer antihistamines or other infrequently used medications in the treatment of EIU–CU.

X. CONCLUSION

Because of the high prevalence and potential morbidity of exercise-induced allergic symptoms, the clinician must be knowledgeable in the correct diagnosis and therapy of patients with EIU, CU, and EIAna. The changing lifestyle of many patients and the desire to increase exercise activities should prompt physicians to be aware of the possible diagnostic tests available to confirm the correct diagnosis.

Patients with exercise-induced cutaneous symptoms may also have associated systemic allergic symptoms. The differentiation of EIU–CU from exercise-induced anaphylaxis is critical, for the latter can often be life-threatening.

Although avoidance of the precipitating activity is often the ideal therapy, it is impractical in many circumstances, and pharmacological therapy remains the mainstay of treatment. Only a few antihistamines have been scientifically investigated; nevertheless, it is presumed that all antihistamines may be useful in the therapy of patients with EIU–CU. The sedative and other possible adverse effects of conventional antihistamine therapy must be considered and discussed with each individual patient. Finally, other therapeutic modalities may include the use of tricyclic antidepressants, cromolyn and other mast cell-stabilizing agents, danazol and other anabolic steroids, or topically applied parasympatholytic agents. None of these alternatives have been well investigated, even though individual case reports do suggest their effectiveness in treating patients with EIU–CU.

ACKNOWLEDGMENT

The authors would like to thank Kelly Littlejohn for her excellent secretarial assistance.

REFERENCES

1. Duke WW. Urticaria caused specifically by the action of physical agents. JAMA 1924; 83:3–8.
2. Horan RF, Sheffer AL, Briner WW Jr. Physical allergies. Med Sci Sports Exerc 1992; 24:845–848.
3. Casale TB, Keahey TM, Kaliner M. Exercise-induced anaphylactic syndromes; insights into diagnostic and pathophysiologic features. JAMA 1986; 255:2049–53.
4. Soter NA, Wasserman SI, Austen KF, McFadden ER. Release of mast-cell mediators and alterations in lung function in patients with cholinergic urticaria. N Engl J Med 1980; 302:604–8.
5. Shelley WB, Shelley ED, Ho AKS. Cholinergic urticaria: acetylcholine–receptor-dependent immediate-type hypersensitivity reaction to copper. Lancet 1983; I:843.
6. Haustein UF, Schliebs R, Schaller J. Changes in muscarinic acetylcholine receptor binding in skin slices of cholinergic urticaria. Acta Derm Venereol 1990; 70:208–11.
7. Sigler RW, Levinson AI, Evans R III, Horakova Z, Kaplan AP. Evaluation of a patient with cold and cholinergic urticaria. J Allergy Clin Immunol 1979; 63:35–8.
8. Herxheimer A. The nervous pathway mediating cholinergic urticaria. Clin Sci 1956; 15:195–205.

9. Kay DM, Maibach HI. Pruritus and acquired anhidrosis, two unusual cases. Arch Dermatol 1969; 100:291–3.
10. Magnus IA, Thompson RHS. Cholinesterase activity of human skin. Br J Dermatol 1954; 66:163–73.
11. Kaplan AP. Exercise-induced hives. J Allergy Clin Immunol 1984; 73:704–7.
12. Eftekhari N, Ward AM, Allen R, Greaves MW. Protease inhibitor profiles in urticaria and angioedema. Br J Dermatol 1980; 103:33–9.
13. Wong E, Eftekhari N, Greaves MW, Ward AM. Beneficial effects of danazol on symptoms and laboratory changes in cholinergic urticaria. Br J Dermatol 1987; 116:553–6.
14. Berth-Jones J, Graham-Brown RAC. Cholinergic pruritus, erythema and urticaria: a disease spectrum responding to danazol. Br J Dermatol 1989; 121: 235–7.
15. Murphy GM, Greaves MW, Zollman PE, Winkelmann RK. Cholinergic urticaria, passive transfer experiments from human to monkey. Dermatologica 1988; 177:338–40.
16. Logas D, Kunkle G, Galderwood-Mays M, Frank L. Cholinergic pruritus in a horse. J Am Vet Med Assoc 1992; 201:90–1.
17. Illig L, Heinicke A. Zur Pathogenese der cholinergischen Urticaria. IV. Zur frage einer echten Antigen-Antikorperreaktion. Arch Klin Exp Dermatol 1967; 229:360–71.
18. Kaplan AP, Gray L, Shaff RE, Horakova Z, Beaven MA. In vivo studies of mediator release in cold urticaria and cholinergic urticaria. J Allergy Clin Immunol 1975; 55:394–402.
19. Stephansson E, Koskimies S, Lokki ML. Exercise-induced urticaria and anaphylaxis. Acta Derm Venereol 1991; 71:138–42.
20. Kaplan AP, Natbony SF, Tawil AP, Fruchter L, Foster M. Exercise-induced anaphylaxis as a manifestation of cholinergic urticaria. J Allergy Clin Immunol 1981; 68:319–24.
21. Tse KS, Yeung M, Ferreira P. A study of exercise-induced urticaria and angioedema. J Allergy Clin Immunol 1980; 65:227.
22. Kaplan AP, Beaven MA. In vivo studies of the pathogenesis of cold urticaria, cholinergic urticaria and vibration-induced swelling. J Invest Dermatol 1976; 67:327–32.
23. Harries MG, Burge PS, O'Brien I, Cromwell O, Pepys J. Blood histamine levels after exercise testing. Clin Allergy 1979; 9:437–41.
24. Deleuran B, Kristensen M, Larsen CG, Matsson P, Enander I, Andersson AS, Thestrup-Pedersen K. Increased tryptase levels in suction-blister fluid from patients with urticaria. Br J Dermatol 1991; 125:14–7.
25. McClean SP, Arreaza EE, Lett-Brown MA, Grant JA. Refractory cholinergic urticaria successfully treated with ketotifen. J Allergy Clin Immunol 1989; 83:738–41.
26. Hirschmann JV, Lawlor F, English JSC, Louback JB, Winkelmann RK, Greaves MW. Cholinergic urticaria. Arch Dermatol 1987; 123:462–7.
27. Winkelman RK. Cholinergic urticaria shows neutrophilic inflammation. Acta Derm Venereol 1985; 65:432–4.

28. James MP, Eady RAJ, Kobza-Black A, Hawk JLM, Greaves MW. Physical urticaria: a microscopal and pharmacological study of mast cell involvement. J Invest Dermatol 1980; 74:451.
29. Nichols AW. Exercised-induced anaphylaxis and urticaria. Clin Sports Med 1992; 11:303–12.
30. Lawrence CM, Jorizzo JL, Kobza-Black A, Coutts A, Greaves MW. Cholinergic urticaria with associated angioedema. Br J Dermatol 1981; 105:543–50.
31. Hopkins JG, Kesten BM, Hazel OG. Urticaria provoked by heat or by psychic stimuli. Arch Dermatol Syphilol 1938; 38:679–91.
32. Mayou SC, Kobza-Black A, Eady RAJ, Greaves MW. Cholinergic dermographism. Br J Dermatol 1986; 115–371–7.
33. Silvers WS. Exercise-induced allergies: the role of histamine release. Ann Allergy 1992; 68:58–63.
34. Murphy GM, Kobza-Black A, Greaves MW. Persisting cholinergic erythema: a variant of cholinergic urticaria. Br J Dermatol 1983; 109:343–8.
35. Czarnetzki BM, Galinski C, Meister R. Cutaneous and pulmonary reactivity in cholinergic urticaria. Br J Dermatol 1984; 110:587–91.
36. Blumberg MZ. Cholinergic urticaria and asthma. Ann Allergy 1978; 41: 99–100.
37. Kounis NG, MacMahon RG. Cholinergic urticaria with systemic manifestations. Ann Allergy 1975; 35:243–5.
38. Tiles S, Schocket A, Milgrom H. Exercise-induced anaphylaxis related to specific foods. J Pediatr 1995; 127:587–9.
39. Sheffer AL, Soter NA, McFadden ER Jr, Austen F. Exercise-induced anaphylaxis: a distinct form of physical allergy. J Allergy Clin Immunol 1983; 71:311–6.
40. Lewis J, Lieberman P, Treadwell G, Erffmeyer J. Exercise-induced urticaria angioedema and anaphylactoid episodes. J Allergy Clin Immunol 1981; 68: 432–7.
41. Sheffer AL, Austen KF. Exercise-induced anaphylaxis. J Allergy Clin Immunol 1980; 66:106–11.
42. Zuberbier T, Althaus C, Chantraine-Hess S, Czarnetzki BM. Prevalence of cholinergic urticaria in young adults. J Am Acad Dermatol 1994; 31:978–81.
43. Moore-Robinson M, Warin RP. Some clinical aspects of cholinergic urticaria. Br J Dermatol 1968; 80:794–9.
44. Champion RH, Roberts SOB, Carpenter RG, Roger JH. Urticaria and angioedema. A review of 554 patients. Br J Dermatol 1969; 81:588–97.
45. Barlow RJ, Warburton F, Watson K, Kobza-Black A, Greaves MW. Diagnosis and incidence of delayed pressure urticaria in patients with chronic urticaria. J Am Acad Dermatol 1993; 29:954–8.
46. Juhlin L. Recurrent urticaria: clinical investigation of 330 patients. Br J Dermatol 1981; 104:369–81.
47. Volonakis M, Katsarou-Katsari A, Stratigos J. Etiologic factors in childhood cholinergic urticaria. Ann Allergy 1992; 69:61–5.

48. Quaranta JH, Rohr AS, Rachelefsky GS, Siegel SC, Katz RM, Spector SL, Mickey MR. The natural history and response to therapy of chronic urticaria and angioedema. Ann Allergy 1989; 62:421–4.
49. Kushimoto H, Aoki T. Masked type I wheat allergy. Arch Dermatol 1985; 121:355–60.
50. Kivity S, Sneh E, Greif J, Topilsky M, Mekori YA. The effect of food and exercise on the skin response to compound 48/40 in patients with food associated exercise-induced urticaria–angioedema. J Allergy Clin Immunol 1988; 81:1155–8.
51. Zuberbier T, Bohm M, Czarnetzki BM. Food intake in combination with a rise in body temperature: a newly identified cause of angioedema. J Allergy Clin Immunol 1993; 91:1226–7.
52. Farnam J, Grant JA, Lett-Brown MA, Lord RA, Russel WL, Henry DP. Combined cold-and-heat-induced cholinergic urticaria. J Allergy Clin Immunol 1986; 78:353–7.
53. Ormerod AD, Kobza-Black A, Milford-Ward A, Greaves MW. Combined cold urticaria and cholinergic urticaria. Clinical characterization and laboratory findings. Br J Dermatol 1988; 118:621–7.
54. Kaplan AP, Garofalo J. Identification of a new physically induced urticaria: Cold induced cholinergic urticaria. J Allergy Clin Immunol 1981; 68:438–41.
55. Neittaanmäki H. Cold urticaria. J Am Acad Dermatol 1985; 13:636–44.
56. Shelley WB, Rawnsley HM. Aquagenic urticaria. Contact sensitivity to water. JAMA 1964; 189:895–8.
57. Parker RK, Crowe MJ, Guin JD. Aquagenic urticaria. Cutis 1992; 50:283–4.
58. Davis RS, Remigio LK, Schocket AL, Bock SA. Evaluation of a patient with both aquagenic and cholinergic urticaria. J Allergy Clin Immunol 1981; 68:479–83.
59. Jorizzo JL. Cholinergic urticaria. Arch Dermatol 1987; 123:455–7.
60. Commens CA, Greaves MW. Tests to establish the diagnosis in cholinergic urticaria. Br J Dermatol 1978; 98:47–51.
61. Jorizzo JL, Smith EB. The physical urticarias. Arch Dermatol 1982; 118: 194–201.
62. Wolf R, Wolf D, Sanbank M. Positive Intradermal tests to D-tubocurarine in patients with cholinergic urticaria. Ann Allergy 1984; 53:355–7.
63. Kobza-Black A, Aboobaker J, Gibson JR, Harvey SG, Marks P. Acrivastine versus hydroxyzine in the treatment of cholinergic urticaria. Acta Derm Venereol 1988; 68:541–4.
64. Tharion WJ, McMenemy DJ, Rauch TM. Antihistamine effects on the central nervous system, congnitive performance and subjective states. Neuropsychobiology 1994; 29:97–104.
65. Zuberbier T, Aberer W, Burtin B, Rihoux J-P, Czarnetzki BM. Efficacy of cetirizine in cholinergic urticaria. Acta Derm Venereol 1995; 75:147–9.
66. Duffull SB, Begg EJ. Terfenadine ineffective in the prophylaxis of exercise-induced pruritus. J Allergy Clin Immunol 1992; 89:916–7.
67. Huston DP, Bressler RB, Kaliner M, Sowell LK, Baylor MW. Prevention

of mast cell degranulation by ketotifen in patients with physical urticarias. Ann Intern Med 1986; 104:507–10.
68. Czarnetzki BM. Ketotifen in cholinergic urticaria. J Allergy Clin Immunol 1990; 86:138–9.
69. Hatty S, Mufti GJ, Hamblin TJ. Exercise-induced urticaria and angioedema with relief from cromoglycate insufflation. Postgrad Med J 1983; 59:586–7.

15

Exercise-Induced Allergy Syndromes

Lawrence M. Du Buske, Richard F. Horan, and Albert L. Sheffer
Brigham and Women's Hospital, Boston, Massachusetts

I. INTRODUCTION

A variety of allergic and respiratory diseases may afflict athletes, including mild dermatological conditions, such as cholinergic urticaria, and annoying upper respiratory conditions, such as rhinitis, associated with exercise. The physician who tends to athletes, however, must be acutely aware of the more serious exercise-associated syndromes, including exercise-induced asthma and exercise-induced anaphylaxis; the latter is a potentially life-threatening condition [Briner, 1992].

II. EXERCISE-ASSOCIATED URTICARIA

A. Cholinergic Urticaria

Urticaria that occur consequent to physical agents represent nearly 17% of all urticaria cases, being more frequent in adolescents than in adults. Cholinergic urticaria accounts for 5% of all urticaria, and it may manifest either as locally or systemicly [del Rio Navrro, 1993]. Typically, patients with cholinergic urticaria experience punctate hives, 2 to 4 mm in diameter, occurring during exercise or after passive warming, as with a hot shower or steam bath [Briner, 1993]. The diagnosis of cholinergic urticaria may be confirmed using intradermal methacholine challenge [Briner, 1993]. Life-threatening anaphylaxis or angioedema typically do not occur with cholinergic urticaria [Briner, 1993]. However, cases have been described wherein patients with exercise-induced anaphylaxis had urticarial lesions similar to those of cholinergic urticaria, rather than the larger, coalescent lesions normally seen in exercise-induced anaphylaxis [Silvers, 1992].

Discrimination between cases of cholinergic urticaria and exercise-induced anaphylaxis can usually be made clinically based on history and presentation of the patient. Exercise testing of patients with cholinergic urticaria may raise plasma histamine levels concomitant with the development of hives, as occurs in patients with exercise-induced anaphylaxis. Passive warming of patients with cholinergic urticaria sufficient to raise core body temperature 0.7°C elicits urticaria and elevates plasma histamine levels, whereas endogenous warming, induced by infused endotoxin, fails to induce either urticaria or elevated histamine levels [Casale, 1986]. Patients with exercise-induced anaphylaxis do not become symptomatic with passive warming or endotoxin infusion [Casale, 1986]. Thus, thermoregulatory abnormalities may underlie the pathogenesis of exercise-induced cholinergic urticaria [Casale, 1986].

Tolerance may be induced in patients with cholinergic urticaria by employing slowly progressive exercise, similar to the tolerance that occurs in patients with exercise-induced asthma who gradually "warm-up" as they begin to exercise. Therapy suggested for cholinergic urticaria generally includes antihistamines, which can be used prophylactically. Hydroxyzine has been most often mentioned as the antihistamine of choice for this condition [Briner, 1993]; however, newer nonsedating antihistamines, such as astemizole, terfenadine, and loratadine, certainly could be considered as therapy to avoid the potential sedation associated with hydroxyzine use. Cetirizine, the natural biological metabolite of hydroxyzine, demonstrates minimal sedation at the 10-mg dose, a dose-dependent increase in somnolence from 10 to 18% incidence being noted as one advances from 5- to 20-mg–daily dosage [Du Buske, 1995]. Cetirizine is rapidly effective for the relief of symptoms of urticarias and can be given as a single daily dose in the evening to minimize any sedative effects.

Sedating antihistamines could adversely affect athletic performance, making the newer nonsedating or low-sedating antihistamine alternatives more attractive [Montgomery, 1993]. Among the choices available, astemizole requires daily therapy to be optimally effective, whereas terfenadine, loratadine, and cetirizine are rapidly effective within 2–4 h of dosing, allowing them to be used on an as-needed basis. Astemizole and terfenadine also pose potential risk of accidental drug interactions with macrolide antibiotics and antifungal agents. Inhibition of the metabolism of astemizole and terfenadine by these is antibiotics is associated with increased serum concentrations of the unmetabolized parent compounds, which can inhibit potassium repolarization channels in the ventricular conduction system, leading to QT prolongation and possible ventricular arrhythmia including life-threatening torsades de pointe [Honig, 1992; Hanrahan, 1992; Honig, 1993]. Hypokalemia, as can occur with vigorous exercise or consequent to diuretic use, may also induce QT prolongation in patients using terfenadine or astemizole.

Loratadine, although subject to similar inhibition of metabolism by macrolide antibiotics and antifungal agents, does not affect potassium repolarization channels in the myocardium, nor has it been associated with QT prolongation or ventricular arrhythmias [Good, 1994]. Cetirizine, which is more potent than loratadine, terfenadine, or astemizole [Simons, 1987] in suppressing histamine-induced wheals in the skin on a single-dose basis, largely depends on renal elimination, rather hepatic metabolism; consequently, it has little potential for drug interactions. Cetirizine also tends to be devoid of nonselective central nervous system receptor interactions when compared with terfenadine, which shows less selectivity for central nervous system receptors, including dopaminergic and serotonergic receptors [Spencer, 1993]. This perhaps accounts for the failure of cetirizine to affect activity performance in several studies in which it has been compared with antihistamines such chlorpheniramine and hydroxyzine [Goetz, 1989]. All antihistamines, including those of the second generation, can potentially induce resting supraventricular tachycardias that are not due to ventricular conduction abnormalities, but consequent to effects on the sinoatrial node. These resting supraventricular tachycardias tend to be mild and generally are not clinically significant [Smith, 1994].

Ultimately, further studies are needed to define the roles of first-generation sedating antihistamines versus second-generation antihistamines in the treatment of cholinergic urticaria. It is possible that some of the non—H_1-receptor antagonistic effects of the older agents could be therapeutically useful, such as their anticholinergic activity, which could be beneficial in limiting symptoms of cholinergic urticaria [Wyngaarden, 1951]. The absence of these nonselective receptor antagonistic attributes may potentially limit the efficacy of second-generation antihistamines for certain types of urticaria. Further study is needed to establish the relative efficacy of the first-versus second-generation antihistamines in the treatment of physical urticarias.

B. Other Physical Urticarias

Other physical urticarias may occur in athletes including cold-induced urticaria, localized heat-induced urticarias, dermatographism, delayed pressure urticaria and angioedema, solar urticarias, and aquagenic urticaria. Similar to exercise-induced urticaria, cold-induced urticaria may be associated with elevated plasma histamine levels at the onset of symptoms [Silvers, 1992]. Development of an area of wheal-and-flare after application of an ice cube to the forearm of patients with cold-induced urticaria is a simple diagnostic test. Similar testing can be done for localized heat-induced urticaria using a warm stimulus. Delayed pressure urticaria can be diagnosed historically; deep pressure, induced by running or recurrent trauma to the hands, induces angioedema and urticaria usually hours after the initiating event. Solar urticaria typically is manifested as hives in sun-exposed areas, and can require sophisticated testing, using exposure to selected ultraviolet light frequencies, to discriminate among at least six variants of this condition that have been described. Dermatographism is a very common condition occurring in up to 5% of the general population in whom stroking of the skin elicits a wheal-and-flare response. This condition is not dangerous, does not lead to systemic urticaria or anaphylaxis, and is essentially an annoying affliction without significant morbidity.

Treatment of these physical urticarias essentially involves the avoidance of the physical stimulus for the urticaria. Appropriate measures to cover the body and keep warm can avert symptoms of cold urticaria. Cold urticaria commonly occurs in athletes who go from a warm to cold environment, such as rapidly going from a warm environment out of doors into the cold water of a swimming pool or lake. Occasionally, life-threatening urticaria has occurred in patients with cold urticaria, because the occurrence of diffuse hives can lead to hypotension and syncope. It is essential that the athlete with cold urticaria avoid the sudden change of body temperature that can occur when going into a cold swimming pool. It is advisable that persons with cold urticarias swim only in warm-water pools. The use of sun screens and proper covering of the body can diminish solar urticaria symptoms. Symptomatic and prophylactic therapy may also include use of antihistamines. Cyproheptadine has been used as a therapy for cold urticaria, but second-generation antihistamines can be considered for all of these conditions, with the same caveats for use as outlined for cholinergic urticaria. Delayed pressure urticaria and angioedema tends to respond poorly to antihistamines and may require corticosteroids if symptoms are sufficiently intense.

II. RHINITIS ASSOCIATED WITH EXERCISE

Rhinitis associated with exercise may be an annoying condition that potentially affects ultimate athletic performance. Athletes who exercise outdoors may suffer from seasonal allergic rhinitis, the occurrence of pollen-induced symptoms in the months of March through May suggesting tree allergy, June through July suggesting grass allergy, and mid-August through October typical of weed allergy.

Exercise-induced rhinitis has been recognized in athletes who develop rhinorrhea, congestion, and sneezing during vigorous activity, such as running, cycling, and skiing [Silvers, 1992]. Laboratory challenges employing cold air may show mediator release similar to that which occurs during allergen challenge [Silvers, 1992].

Vasomotor rhinitis, a nonallergic form of rhinitis associated with changes in temperature, irritant fumes, and noxious stimuli, is believed to be induced by a relative excess of parasympathetic nasal nervous stimulation in the nose; it may also occur in athletes. Treatment of these forms of rhinitis in athletes generally includes use of either antihistamines or topical anti-inflammatory therapies, including cromolyn sodium or corticosteroids, such as beclomethasone, triamcinolone, budesonide, flunisolide, or fluticasone. Topical anticholinergic therapy using 0.03% ipratropium bromide spray giving one to two sprays in each nostril three times a day is also helpful in decreasing rhinorrhea in nonallergic perennial rhinitis patients. Most studies of allergic rhinitis patients have demonstrated that topical corticosteroids are more efficacious than antihistamines in relieving rhinitis symptoms: approximately 80% symptomatic relief occurring in corticosteroid-treated cohorts, whereas antihistamine responses approach 50–60% symptomatic relief. Studies specifically of patients with exercise-induced rhinitis are needed to adequately assess the responses to various potential therapies.

III. EXERCISE-INDUCED ANAPHYLAXIS

Exercise-induced anaphylaxis is the most serious of the conditions that can affect athletes; the adverse consequences of this syndrome include not only morbidity, such as impaired performance, but also the potential for mortality [Kobayashi, 1991]. Indeed, recognition of this condition mandates that physicians' "game day" medical kits now include epinephrine for the treatment of exercise-induced anaphylaxis [Kyle, 1994].

The exact incidence of exercise-induced anaphylaxis is unknown. In a survey of 179 patients who presented to the Mayo Clinic for evaluation of anaphylaxis over a 3-year period, 7% were identified as having exercise-induced anaphylaxis. [Yocum, 1994]. A survey of Japanese teachers inquiring about food-associated exercise-induced anaphylaxis revealed that only 31% of the teachers were aware of this entity. Including 11,647 pupils in 11 kindergartens, 11 elementary schools, and 5 junior high schools. The incidence of food-dependent exercise-induced anaphylaxis was 0% in the kindergarten children, 0.06% in the elementary school children, and 0.21% in the junior high school pupils [Tanaka, 1994].

Anaphylaxis is a systemic condition that occurs consequent to mast cell and basophil activation. The signs and symptoms of anaphylaxis are induced by diffuse affects of mast cell mediators, including histamine, leukotriene C_4, and prostaglandin D_2, all of which induce vasodilation, vascular leakage, and bronchospasm. Symptoms of anaphylaxis are seen in the skin, including flushing, pruritus, urticaria, and angioedema. Respiratory tract symptoms include rhinitis, laryngeal edema, and bronchospasm. Gastrointestinal symptoms are nausea, colicky pain, diarrhea, and intestinal bleeding. Cardiovascular symptoms include hypotension, tachycardia, and vascular collapse caused by diffuse movement of fluid from the vascular system into the surrounding tissues consequent to microvascular leakage. Mortality may be related to respiratory events, including severe bronchospasm or laryngeal edema, or maybe due to shock with end-organ damage related to hypotension, consequent to vascular collapse.

Exercise-induced anaphylaxis typically is heralded by the development of generalized pruritus and flushing sensations, a feeling of warmth, and the development of urticarias in association with vigorous exercise. The urticaria includes lesions of 10–15 mm, which coalesce, in contrast to the punctate 2- to 4-mm lesions of cholinergic urticaria [Briner, 1992]. Cutaneous mast cell degranulation and increased serum histamine levels occur concomitant with these symptoms [Gerth van Wijk, 1991; Sheffer, 1980]. These symptoms of exercise-induced anaphylaxis appear variably with exercise, vigorous exercise being often required to elicit anaphylaxis [Briner, 1992]. This syndrome has now been recognized as frequently occurring consequent to exercise after ingestion of food, suggesting that, usually, exercise-induced anaphylaxis is related to a food allergy, whereas in other patients, exercise alone without food ingestion may be sufficient to induce anaphylaxis [Gerth van Wijk, 1991]. The initial reports of exercise-induced anaphylaxis by Mathews and Pan [1970] included a description of postexercise-induced wheezing, dermatographism, and elevated plasma histamine [Mathews, 1970].

The first systematized and rigorous description of exercise-induced anaphylaxis was that of Sheffer and Austen [1980], wherein 16 patients, all of whom were regularly involved in athletic activity, including 11 men and 5 women from 12 to 54 years of age, were reported as having anaphylaxis associated with their exercise [Sheffer, 1980]. Typically, symptoms occurred over several years and varied from isolated to recurrent attacks among athletes involved in jogging, running, tennis, and soccer. Although all 16 patients exercised frequently, the exercise-induced anaphylaxis occurred sporadically, in contrast with other physical urticarias for which a known provocative stimulus almost invariably produces symptoms. Apparently consistent levels of exercise did not always result in reproducible symptoms of anaphylaxis [Sheffer, 1980]. A variety of factors were suggested as contributing to the development of exercise-induced anaphylaxis, including prior ingestion of food noted in 3 patients, aspirin noted in 5 patients, prior drinking of coffee, exercise in the rain, or exercise in high ambient temperatures.

Clinical evaluation of this initial cohort of patients with exercise-induced anaphylaxis revealed a consistent progression of symptoms in most of them. The onset of anaphylaxis was heralded by the development of fatigue, warmth, and cutaneous erythema associated with pruritus. Urticarial lesions, which develop rapidly and coalesce, are often associated with angioedema of the palms, soles, and face. The urticaria and angioedema will persist throughout the duration of the exercise-induced anaphylactic episode, which typically lasts 30 min to 4 h. Symptoms of gastrointestinal colic, nausea, and vomiting are common, as are respiratory symptoms, including stridor and choking. Loss of consciousness with vascular collapse occurred in 12 of the 16 patients. Severe headache, which persisted for up to 3 days, was often noted to follow episodes of exercise-induced anaphylaxis [Sheffer, 1980; Sheffer, 1984].

This clinical evaluation of exercise-induced anaphylaxis was reaffirmed in an epidemiological study of 199 persons believed to have exercise-induced anaphylaxis, of whom 134 were female and 65 were male, the mean age being 24.7 years. The most common activity producing symptoms was jogging, followed by bicycling, tennis, racquetball, skiing, and aerobic exercise. While isolated attacks of anaphylaxis were reported, typically symptoms occurred two to three times a week [Wade, 1989]. The dermatological symptom of pruritus was the most common early expression of anaphylaxis, with urticaria, angioedema, and flushing also being frequently encountered. Upper respiratory symptoms developed in 59% of patients, and gastrointestinal symptoms, including colic, occurred in 30%. Loss of consciousness occurred in 32%. Headache was a usual late sequelae in these patients. Most episodes of exercise-induced anaphylaxis resolved in 2 h with only a few episodes lasting as long as 12 h.

This study suggested that certain environments promoted the occurrence of exercise-induced anaphylaxis; 64% felt that exercise in a warm environment precipitated an attack, 23% felt that cold environments triggered attacks, and 32% identified high humidity as an associated factor. Among the females surveyed, 18% felt that a phase of the menstrual cycle was critical. Prior ingestion of medication was identified by several respondents, including aspirin ingestion in 6% and alcohol ingestion in 5% [Wade, 1989].

A. Food-Associated Exercise-Induced Anaphylaxis

Many reports have suggested a strong linkage between food ingestion and the development of exercise-induced anaphylaxis. Most of these reports implicate one or several foods identified by clinical history and suggested by either prick test or radioallergosorbent test (RAST) as being potential allergens. Specific food ingestion is requisite before exercise for anaphylaxis to occur in some patients. However, other patients have been described as having exercise-induced anaphylaxis postprandially, irrespective of the food ingested, the postprandial state alone being sufficient to precipitate an attack when eating is followed by vigorous exercise. Ingestion of aspirin has been reported to be an exacerbating factor in some cases of food-dependent exercise-induced anaphylaxis [Dohi, 1990]. Nonsteroidal anti-inflammatory agents and aspirin can increase gut permeability, thereby allowing relatively intact food antigens to be more readily absorbed [Bjarnason, 1989]. Three cases of food-dependent exercise-induced anaphylaxis have been reported to have enhanced symptoms of anaphylaxis when taking aspirin in addition to the offending food before exercise. Although aspirin ingestion alone failed to induce exercise-induced anaphylaxis symptoms with exercise challenge, ingestion of aspirin, in conjunction with the food to which the person was allergic, before the attack of exercise-induced anaphylaxis resulted in more severe attacks, with less strenuous exercise required to induce them [Dohi, 1990].

The identification of a specific food that could cause exercise-induced anaphylaxis was first noted by Maulitz [1979], who reported the case of a 31-year-old atopic long-distance runner who experienced anaphylaxis when running after eating either shrimp or oysters. Skin-prick test revealed positive reactions to oysters, shrimp, clams, crabs, peanuts, and aeroallergens. Neither indigestion of shrimp nor oysters without running, nor running without shellfish ingestion provoked anaphylaxis in this man. This case exemplified the exquisite relation between selected food ingestion and the development of exercise-induced anaphylaxis completely dependent on the association of the exercise with proximate ingestion of a specific food [Maulitz, 1979].

Subsequently, many cases of food-associated exercise-induced anaphylaxis have been reported. Further reports of shellfish-induced anaphylaxis were noted by several investigators [Dohi, 1990; McNeil, 1988; Watanabe, 1990]. The occurrence of anaphylaxis in an otherwise healthy male athlete 3½ h after ingestion of shrimp, was noted in a case wherein anaphylaxis occurred shortly after onset of exercise [Novey, 1983]. A 15-year-old male runner had anaphylaxis 4 h after a lunch containing fried shrimp. Skin test and RAST to shrimp were positive, and exercise challenge after ingestion of boiled shrimp resulted in a marked elevation of plasma histamine [Watanabe, 1990]. A 17-year-old girl in Japan experienced anaphylaxis while riding a bicycle 55 min after eating *sulculas* shellfish and while running 30 min after eating *Turbo cornutus* shellfish. Exercise challenge was positive with an elevation of plasma histamine, and RASTs to both of these shellfish were positive. RAST inhibition revealed poor cross-inhibition by either shellfish; however, good inhibition of RAST by both shellfish occurred when antigens from keyhole limpit hemocyanin were employed. This result suggested some cross-allergenicity between these two shellfish [Juji, 1990]. In a survey of 25 exercise-induced anaphylaxis cases in Japan, 10 of 25 were related to shrimp allergy and 13 of 25 were related to prior ingestion of wheat [Watanabe, 1990].

Wheat and other grain flours have been reported as the likely causes of exercise-induced anaphylaxis, often without other signs of grain allergy being present before the exercise-related event [Kushimoto, 1985; Armentia, 1990; Sabbah, 1989]. A patient was described who had a positive skin test and RAST to grain flours, but who tolerated ingestion of these grains without symptoms, and developed anaphylaxis only with grain ingestion followed by exercise [Armentia, 1990]. A case of wheat-induced anaphylaxis has also been reported in a person who reacted only when eating toasted wheat [Akutsu, 1989]. A farmer in Japan, who experienced 12 episodes of anaphylaxis while doing strenuous farm work, was reported to be skin-test positive to wheat and to have 9 anaphylactic episodes occurring typically in the afternoon, 2 h after ingestion of wheat cake [Okazahi, 1992]. A positive food exercise challenge to wheat in the form of ingestion of a sandwich was noted in a 25-year-old woman with a history of three episodes of exercise-induced anaphylaxis after eating a meal including wheat flour. Her exercise challenge resulted not only in symptoms of anaphylaxis, but also in an elevation of plasma histamine to three times normal concentrations [Tashiro, 1993]. In a comprehensive study of six persons with exercise-induced anaphylaxis related to wheat ingestion, wheat or gluten allergens obtained by simple extraction were less related to the symptoms of anaphylaxis than were gliadin, glutenin, or gluten that had been digested with pepsin. Trypsin digestion abolished reactivity to gluten, gliadin, and glutenin. This suggested that certain wheat allergens may have enhanced allergenicity after pepsin exposure in the stomach, but reduced allergenicity after trypsin exposure in the jejunum [Kushimoto, 1985]. This sequence of events, may partly explain the timing of the onset of exercise-induced anaphylaxis symptoms after wheat ingestion as being related to the timing of the digestive process [Kushimoto, 1985].

Other foods reported to cause exercise-induced anaphylaxis include peaches, grapes, celery, apples, a variety of grains, fruits, and vegetables [Buchbinder, 1983; El-Dieb, 1984; Kidd, 1983; Kivity, 1998; Lin, 1993; Silverstein, 1986; Dohi, 1991; Anaut, 1994]. Several cases of celery-induced exercise-induced anaphylaxis have been documented by observation of symptoms in persons who exercise shortly after ingestion of celery [Silverstein, 1986]. Three cases noted by Kidd [1983] had documentation of celery-dependent exercise-induced anaphylaxis by skin testing with a fresh celery extract with further prevention of the episodes by avoidance of ingestion of celery before exercise [Kidd, 1983]. Nuts as the cause of exercise-induced anaphylaxis has been reported in a person reacting to hazelnut on both skin test and RAST, who had a positive exercise challenge only after hazelnut ingestion [Martin, 1994]. Chicken was noted to be a possible cause of food-associated exercise-induced anaphylaxis in another report, the quantity of chicken ingestion before exercise being related to the tendency to develop anaphylaxis [Laufer, 1987]. A survey of persons experiencing exercise-induced anaphylaxis implicated shellfish in 8%, celery in 6%, and cabbage in 6%, as foods ingested before exercise that are likely related to the occurrence of anaphylaxis [Wade, 1989].

Sometimes the food that induces exercise-induced anaphylaxis escapes exact identification, as in the case of a 33-year-old Chinese woman who reacted with anaphylaxis on exercise after ingestion of Chinese seafood noodle soup. This woman was skin-prick test negative for all the putative ingredients of the soup, but was skin-prick test positive to the actual soup broth [Lin, 1993].

It is uncertain if there is a requirement for a specific food allergy for exercise-induced anaphylaxis to occur. Several investigators have reported postprandial exercise-induced anaphylaxis in the absence of a detectable food allergy, the postprandial state apparently being sufficient to induce the symptoms of exercise-induced anaphylaxis [Dohi, 1991; Novey, 1983]. The report of 16 cases of exercise-induced anaphylaxis by Sheffer and Austen identified only 3 persons who had anaphylaxis associated with the postprandial state [Sheffer, 1980]. The subsequent numerous reports of exercise-induced anaphylaxis associated with foods, some of them quite subtle, including spices and foods contaminated with latex or dust mites, suggest that the occurrence of food-associated exercise-induced anaphylaxis may be more common than initially believed [Beuers, 1993]. Cross-reacting allergens present in some foods and in natural rubber latex, can lead to systemic reactions following latex exposure or food ingestion [Ownby, 1995]. Cases of anaphylaxis in persons previously tolerant to avocado and banana have occurred after these individuals have become sensitized to natural rubber latex. A case of an individual previously tolerant to bananas, who developed exercise-induced anaphylaxis after eating them subsequent to developing latex allergy, has been reported in a health care worker. This patient had latex allergy documented by whole blood leukocyte histamine release testing and RAST and was also noted to be RAST-positive to bananas and avocados, precluding further ingestion of these fruits before exercise [Anderson, 1996]. The cross-reactivity between latex and a variety of fruits, including kiwi, pears, apples, strawberries, grapes, and tomatoes, suggests that latex-allergic persons be wary of eating within 3–4 h of exercise [Bush, 1995].

The timing of a meal relative to exercise may be critical, for most respondents, in one survey of exercise-induced anaphylactic patients, indicated that they had eaten 3–4 h before exercise [Wade, 1989]. The survey of 11,647 Japanese school children revealed that the longest interval between beginning exercise and the onset of anaphylaxis was 50 min and the longest time between eating and the onset of anaphylaxis was 3½ h, suggesting that close attention should be paid to children with a history of anaphylaxis who exercise within 4 h of eating [Tanaka, 1994].

A familial tendency to develop exercise-induced anaphylaxis in addition to a familial tendency towards atopy has been noted by several authors, with early age of onset of exercise-induced anaphylaxis associated with increased incidence of atopy [Grant, 1985; Longley, 1987]. Patients who develop exercise-induced anaphylaxis before 20 years of age, have been noted to have elevated serum IgE levels, frequent presence of food-specific IgE, and atopic personal and family histories, frequently being skin-test-positive for a variety of allergens. Persons who develop exercise-induced anaphylaxis after 30 years of age, however, are less atopic and often have normal serum total IgE levels, but still may have discrete food allergen association with exercise-induced anaphylactic symptoms. Wheat is a common allergen associated with exercise-induced anaphylaxis in this older cohort [Dohi, 1991].

In most patients with exercise-induced anaphylaxis, a precedent atopic history is present [Dohi, 1991]. The association of allergy with specific foods and the occurrence of exercise-induced anaphylaxis definitely mandates careful evaluation of any one who participates in sports and undergoes unexplained cardiovascular collapse or respiratory collapse during exercise, especially if there is an association with giant urticaria, angioedema, or gastrointestinal symptoms. Assessment for possible food allergy is absolutely essential in all cases of postprandial exercise-induced anaphylaxis [Romana, 1992].

B. Exercise Challenge in Exercise-Induced Anaphylaxis

Some patients with exercise-induced anaphylaxis may demonstrate symptoms with exercise challenge, including running on a treadmill while wearing a plastic occlusive suit. In a report of seven persons with exercise-induced anaphylaxis challenged in this manner by Sheffer and colleagues, clinical responses were noted in only four of the subjects, typically including pruritus, flushing, and generalized erythema, sometimes without urticaria. Symptoms typically resolved within 30 min after conclusion of the exercise challenge. Two persons were noted to develop angioedema, one of whom had upper respiratory obstruction, including angioedema-associated cough, which required administration of epinephrine for symptomatic relief. Late-occurring, severe headache also occurred after rechallenge of the this patient, in addition to the recurrence of symptoms of angioedema. No cases of loss of consciousness or vascular collapse occurred consequent to the exercise challenges in this study. Neither wheezing nor changes in pulmonary function tests were noted. Those persons having a positive challenge to exercise were noted to have elevated serum histamine levels, which normalized within 20 min often before resolution of clinical symptoms of anaphylaxis [Sheffer, 1983] (Table 1). Serum complement levels were normal in all cases studied in this manner, whereas some reports have noted a perturbation of the complement values during exercise-induced anaphylaxis [Obata, 1989].

Exercise challenge may discriminate between cholinergic urticaria and exercise-induced anaphylaxis. Passive elevation of body temperature induces symptoms of cholinergic urticaria in patients with this condition, but not in exercise-induced anaphylaxis patients; exercise is required to induce symptoms of exercise-induced anaphylaxis [Casale, 1986].

Table 1 Classification of Exercise-Induced Physical Allergy

Type	Precipitating event	Urticaria: morphology	Associated collapse	Bronchospasm: Clinical	Bronchospasm: Functional	Elevated serum histamine
Cholinergic	Heat, stress, exercise	Punctate (2–5 mm)	−	±	+	+
Variant	Exercise	Punctate	+	−	−	+
Anaphylactic	Exercise	Conventional (10–15 mm)	+	−	−	+

−, absent; +, present; ±, equivocal.
Source: Sheffer et al., 1983.

C. Pathophysiology of Exercise-Induced Anaphylaxis

The association of positive experimental challenges in persons with exercise-induced anaphylaxis with increases in mast cell and basophil mediators, including elevation of serum histamine levels, suggests the participation of mast cells or basophils in the development of this anaphylactic syndrome. Elevations of tryptase levels, implicating mast cell involvement, have also been noted during exercise-induced anaphylaxis in some persons. Mast cell degranulation occurring consequent to exercise challenge was reported in a morphological study of mast cell ultrastructure in patients with exercise-induced anaphylaxis [Sheffer, 1985]. This study, conducted by Sheffer and Austen, revealed that before exercise challenge, cutaneous mast cells demonstrated normal morphology. After exercise challenge in exercise-induced anaphylaxis patients, there were significant ultrastructural changes, including a decrease in the number of intact granules within the mast cells and a loss of internal granule substructure and density. Fusion of granule membranes with mast cell membranes was noted to be similar to that observed after challenge of dispensed pulmonary mast cells with anti-IgE or challenge of dermal mast cells with specific allergen in clinically sensitized individuals [Sheffer, 1985].

Complement abnormalities have been noted only occasionally in cases of exercise-induced anaphylaxis [Silverstein, 1986]. Abnormal complement levels, in general, have not been noted in studies in which controlled exercise challenge has been performed [Sheffer, 1980; Sheffer, 1985; Novey 1983]. In one such controlled exercise challenge study of six patients with exercise-induced anaphylaxis, five developed symptoms during running and two developed hypotension associated with elevated histamine levels to 11.2 and 23.2 ng/ml, respectively. Subjects who had solely cutaneous symptoms, without associated vascular collapse, did not demonstrate elevated blood histamine levels. Serum complement levels, including C3 and C4 levels, were normal in all subjects both before and during exercise challenge [Lewis, 1981].

However, several case reports have suggested perturbation of complement in exercise-induced anaphylactic patients. In a study of five patients having exercise-induced anaphylaxis symptoms in Finland, two patients who presented with urticaria similar to cholinergic urticaria, which then progressed to angioedema and vascular collapse, were noted to have elevated plasma histamine levels with exercise challenge. Three patients who had anaphylactic symptoms without elevation of plasma histamine levels, however, had signs of alternative complement pathway activation [Stephansson, 1991]. In another case, an 18-year-old Hispanic male, with a history of exercise-induced anaphylaxis, had a clinically negative exercise test and a clinically negative response to hot water emergence, but on both tests, plasma histamine levels rose, from undetectable to 1.0 and 3.7 ng/mL respectively. During the exercise challenge, C2 and C5 were reduced and fell further with prolonged exercise [Grant, 1985]. A 17-year-old Japanese girl, with a history of ten episodes of exercise-induced anaphylaxis, had significant elevation of plasma histamine to 13.2 ng/mL and a decrease in C_H50 to 17 U/mL and C3 to 70 mg/dL during one documented episode of exercise-induce anaphylaxis. On remission from the anaphylactic episode, C_H50 remained relatively low at 26 U/mL as did the C3 level at 83 mg/dL and the C4 level at 15 mg/dL. The patient's mother also had a relatively low C4 level of 14 mg/dL, suggesting a genetic basis for her relatively low complement. Although her exercise challenge was negative, it was associated with a decrease in C_H50 level suggesting a role for complement in the pathogenesis of her exercise-induced anaphylaxis [Obata, 1989]. Most studies using controlled exercise challenge, however, have failed to reveal significant perturbation in the complement system [Sheffer, 1985; Lewis, 1981].

The participation of the mast cell in exercise-induced anaphylaxis appears well substantiated by studies that have demonstrated that the threshold for mast cell degranulation may be affected by physiological factors, including cytokine production, histamine-releasing factors, endogenous opiates, and neurohumoral peptides [Holgate, 1989; White, 1989].

Neurological factors contributing to exercise-induced anaphylaxis include the enhanced increase in norepinephrine versus epinephrine levels during exercise-induced anaphylaxis, suggesting that heightened α-adrenergic tone could influence mast cell degranulation during exercise [Dimsdale, 1984]. The nonadrenergic, noncholinergic autonomic tone which may be affected consequent to exercise, may also affect mast cell degranulation and releasability of mast cell mediators [Dimsdale, 1984]. Other physiological factors associated with exercise can enhance mast cell degranulation, including dehydration, with a subsequent increase in osmolality of the mast cell milieu, or electrolyte fluctuation, which could enhance mast cell mediator releasability.

A study of autonomic nervous system physiological activity in four patients with exercise-induced anaphylaxis who underwent food-associated exercise challenge test, revealed a significant decrease in systolic blood pressure and an increase in heart rate after the postural test, a decrease in heart rate after the Ascher tests, and reduction in the increase in systolic blood pressure during the cold pressor test. Overall, after food-associated exercise challenge, the activity of the parasympathetic nervous system increased, whereas the response of the sympathetic nervous system was reduced [Fukutomi, 1992].

Postprandial exercise-induced anaphylaxis may also be partially related to enhanced responsiveness to autonomic efferent nervous impulses or neuropeptide generation. For instance, it has been noted that gastrin, both in vivo and in vitro, can enhance cutaneous mast cell mediator release, suggesting that enhanced production of gastrin during the postprandial state could increase the tendency toward mast cell activation [Tharp, 1984]. The association with responses from the gastrointestinal tract to the development of exercise-induced anaphylaxis is further substantiated by the development of shifts in blood flow consequent to anaphylactic events. Although vasodepressor mediators are liberated during episodes of exercise-induced anaphylaxis, part of the mechanism for postprandial exercise-associated syncope is likely attributed to a shift of blood flow to the splanchnic microvasculature [Novey, 1983].

The association between certain foods and postprandial exercise-induced anaphylaxis suggests that clinical mast cell-related food allergy becomes manifested in certain persons only when exercise-associated factors enhance mast cell responsiveness [Wade, 1989; Kivity, 1988]. In a study of mast cell reactivity in exercise-induced anaphylaxis, five patients with this syndrome related to food ingestion were evaluated by Kivity [1988]. Among these cases, four of five had positive exercise challenges after food ingestion. Enhanced cutaneous wheal response, induced by the mast cell secretogogue compound 48/80, was noted only in persons challenged with exercise after ingestion of the food to which they had clinically relevant exercise-induced anaphylactic symptoms and to which they had been demonstrated to be positive on skin-prick test. Exercise alone without concomitant prior specific food ingestion, or food ingestion alone without concomitant exercise, did not alter skin reactivity to compound 48/80. Skin response to injected histamine was unaffected by exercise, food ingestion, or exercise after food ingestion [Kivity, 1988]. This experiment suggests that subclinical responses to foods to which a person has allergen-specific IgE may become clinically evident owing to the synergistic effects of exercise and prior food ingestion, the exercise perhaps enhancing mast cell reactivity, which is likely ongoing consequent to the ingestion of a food to which the person is subclinically allergic [Kivity, 1988].

A variety of postulates have been developed for the possible etiologies of the exercise-induced anaphylaxis phenomenon related to mast cell degranulation and food ingestion. Exercise may enhance mast cell secretogogue concentrations, such as gastrin, thus relating anaphylaxis to the postprandial state in which enhanced gastrin production occurs. Aberration of autonomic neural tone, especially postprandially, may enhance the development of anaphylaxis in susceptible individuals. There may be significant differences in mast cell sensitivity in susceptible persons to secretogogues, or neural tone fluctuation leading to exercise-induced anaphylactic events. The occurrence of an ongoing food-associated subclinical mast cell response may become clinically evident only consequent to these exercise-associated neural or humeral factors influencing mast cell activation. During exercise, also, it is possible that food allergen distribution may be enhanced by changes in splanchnic blood flow; the ongoing allergic reactivity of an otherwise subclinical allergic event being manifested only by the combination of exercise and prior food ingestion. Additionally, exercise-induced anaphylactic patients tend to have heightened responses during times when their allergic reactivity is greatest, such as during the specific pollen season in those patients who have concomitant seasonal allergic rhinitis [Sheffer, 1980, 1983, 1985]. This phenomenon implicates priming of the allergic response induced by seasonal allergic rhinitis may enhance reactivity to foods such that otherwise subclinical responses become clinically evident.

The potential influence of genetic susceptibility to allergic disease may also be important in the genesis of exercise-induced anaphylaxis. A genetic tendency to exercise-induced anaphylaxis has been noted in two siblings with this syndrome who had exercise-induced anaphylaxis during running, but not swimming, cycling, or racquetball; one also had concomitant allergic rhinitis, as did the children's father. An association between the HLA haplotype A3-B8-DR3 and exercise-induced anaphylaxis in this family was noted in these two siblings [Longley, 1987].

D. Differential Diagnosis of Exercise-Induced Anaphylaxis

Exercise-induced anaphylaxis can be clinically differentiated from other exercise-related events, such as arrhythmias, asthma, and cholinergic urticaria. The syndrome of exercise-induced anaphylaxis includes pruritus, flushing, cutaneous erythema, urticaria sometimes associated with vascular collapse, upper respiratory distress, gastrointestinal colic, and subsequent headaches, making exercise-induced anaphylaxis an entity similar to IgE-mediated anaphylactic responses, such as the anaphylaxis that occurs in persons having food or drug allergy. Cardiac arrhythmias associated with syncope or collapse during exercise lacks these associated signs of anaphylaxis, including cutaneous, respiratory, or gastrointestinal symptoms.

Patients with exercise-induced asthma develop clinically significant wheeze and alteration of pulmonary function consequent to exercise, whereas pulmonary function abnormalities have been minimal in patients with exercise-induced anaphylaxis who undergo controlled exercise challenge. The prominent cutaneous symptoms of urticaria, angioedema, and flushing are likewise absent in persons with exercise-induced asthma, as are anaphylactic consequences including vascular collapse [Sheffer, 1983].

The entity that must be critically distinguished from exercise-induced anaphylaxis is cholinergic urticaria, a physical urticaria characterized by punctate hives, typically 1–3 mm in diameter that occur on elevation of core body temperature by exercise, hot baths, hot showers, or fever. The typical lesions of exercise-induced anaphylaxis are larger than those of cholinergic urticaria, although occasionally, patients with exercise-induced anaphylaxis symptoms will experience hives similar in size to those of patients with cholinergic urticaria [Sheffer, 1984, 1983; Casale, 1986]. Signs of vascular collapse are absent in cholinergic urticaria, whereas pulmonary manifestations including abnormal pulmonary function tests are common in patients with cholinergic urticaria, but are typically minimal in exercise-induced anaphylaxis [Soter, 1980]. Furthermore, easily reproducible symptoms of cholinergic urticaria occur experimentally with passive heat challenge or naturally with exposure with hot showers, or even during periods of anxiety and stress. The induction of exercise-induced anaphylaxis by exercise challenge, however, is much less predictable [Casale, 1986].

Serum histamine levels may be elevated in either exercise-induced anaphylaxis or cholinergic urticaria. Both entities are associated with mast cell degranulation. In exercise-induced anaphylaxis, ultrastructural changes occur in mast cells identical with those that occurs in IgE-dependent degranulation of dispersed pulmonary mast cells, including diffuse and widespread changes in the mast cell secretory granules [Maulitz, 1979]. In cholinergic urticaria, more focal zonal degranulation of mast cells occurs. An IgE-dependent mechanism of a mast cell degranulation has been demonstrated in some older studies of patients with cholinergic urticaria through the utilization of passive transfer of serum IgE from one individual to another. Ethical considerations now preclude passive serum transfer experiments in patients with exercise-induced anaphylaxis, although the strong association of exercise-induced anaphylaxis with food allergy suggests an IgE-dependent mechanism in many persons. Although the precise mechanisms of both cholinergic urticaria and exercise-induced anaphylaxis remain to be determined, both of these conditions clearly represent states of enhanced mast cell lability induced by a combination of endogenous and exogenous factors [Sheffer, 1983].

E. Treatment of Exercise-Induced Anaphylaxis

The initial treatment of exercise-induced anaphylaxis includes the use of subcutaneous epinephrine, intravenous volume repletion, oxygen, and protection of the upper airway patency, including intubation or tracheostomy if severe airway compromise is evident. Such therapy is identical with that for other forms of anaphylaxis. The use of antihistamines, which may diminish urticarial symptoms and pruritus, while helpful, should not preclude more valuable therapies, such as subcutaneous epinephrine and volume replenishment. Constant assessment of airway function is critical to avoid life-threatening upper airway occlusion. Inhaled bronchodilators or aminophylline may be useful if bronchospasm occurs in association with exercise-induced anaphylaxis. Empiric use of glucocorticoids early in the course of treatment of anaphylaxis has been noted to be useful in patients with idiopathic anaphylaxis, and likely should be considered in the management of exercise-induced anaphylaxis patients [Wong, 1990]. Prolonged observation of at least 6 h in the emergency ward seems prudent for assessment of the patient with exercise-induced anaphylaxis for any late-occurring or recurrent symptoms of anaphylaxis.

F. Prevention of Exercise-Induced Anaphylaxis

Identification of historical factors associated with the occurrence of exercise-induced anaphylaxis is essential to prevent further attacks. Recent meals, prior ingestion of specific foods, prior ingestion of medications, including aspirin and nonsteroidal anti-inflammatory drugs, prior ingestion of alcohol, high ambient temperature, high ambient humidity, and association with a specific allergy season in patients who have concomitant seasonal allergic rhinitis, all should be considered in patients with exercise-induced anaphylaxis. It is essential that these patients avoid those situations that may predispose to this syndrome.

Evaluation of food-dependent exercise-induced anaphylaxis can include skin-prick testing using commercial food extracts, skin-prick testing using freshly prepared food extracts, and allergen-specific IgE testing for foods, in addition to exercise challenge done either with or without prior ingestion of the suspected food [Romano, 1995]. In a study of 14 patients with food-dependent exercise-induced anaphylaxis, all patients showed evidence of possible allergic responses to at least 2 foods, and 10 patients demonstrated reactivity to 11 or more foods (Romano, 1995). Only 3 of 8 patients who agreed to undergo food-associated exercise challenge test were positive on exercise challenge in this study, 2 of whom reacted to wheat ingestion followed by exercise and 1 of whom reacted to tomato ingestion when followed by exercise [Romano, 1995]. In the 9 cases with negative exercise challenge tests, positive skin-prick tests or positive RAST using the Pharmacia CAP RAST for foods, including celery, fennel, basil, kiwi, parsley, soybeans, peach, apple, tomato, garlic, lettuce, onion, walnuts, and bananas, were noted [Romano, 1995]. In general, skin testing with freshly prepared food confirmed the positive results obtained using commercial food extracts and also allowed identification of some sensitivities not recognized using only the commercial food extract. Curiously, in this study, none of the patients were positive on any of the tests for reactivity towards cows' milk, fish, or eggs, all very common causes of classic food allergy. The in vitro detection of allergen-specific IgE with the Pharmacia CAP system gave exact concordance in 270 instances where RAST results for specific allergens were compared to skin-prick test results. There were 80 instances of discordance between RAST results and skin-prick test results, among which 54 were RAST-positive and skin-prick test-negative. When using skin-prick test results to native freshly prepared foods, 156 cases of concordance between RAST and skin-prick test results were noted, with only 26 instances of the RAST being positive when the skin-prick test result was negative. As several patients had symptoms related to the foods identified by a positive Pharmacia CAP RAST test result associated with a negative skin-prick test result, the authors felt that all of the assays were required for comprehensive identification of all those foods possibly associated with exercise-induced anaphylaxis [Romano, 1995].

It is essential that the patient with exercise-induced anaphylaxis recognize its earliest signs and symptoms, so that exercise can be stopped before progression of the anaphylactic event occurs. Among the measures that may decrease the occurrence of exercise-induced anaphylaxis is modification of the exercise regimen to decrease the duration and intensity of exercise, and limitation of exercise on warm and humid days. In addition, it is recommended that patients with this syndrome avoid exercise for 4–6 h after eating or after ingesting alcohol. Those persons who have had exercise-induced anaphylaxis after ingestion of aspirin or nonsteroidal anti-inflammatory drugs, should avoid further exercise after the use of these medications. Given the risk of anaphylaxis after administration of allergen immunotherapy being potentially enhanced by changes in blood flow consequent to exercise, patients who have exercise-induced anaphylaxis who are receiving allergy immunotherapy for inhalant allergens probably should not exercise after receiving their allergen injections [Du Buske, 1992]. The use of β-adrenergic-blocking agents or angiotensin-converting enzyme (ACE) inhibitors may compromise therapy for anaphylaxis. For instance, patients receiving β-adrenergic blocking agents may have more refractory symptoms of anaphylaxis when treatment with epinephrine is attempted [Hepner, 1990]. Angiotensin II, epinephrine, and norepinephrine are produced as a consequence of plasma volume loss during anaphylaxis [Van der Linden, 1992]. Angiotensin II also inactivates bradykinin, a potential mediator of anaphylaxis. Thus, use of ACE inhibitors could adversely affect the course of anaphylaxis. [Brunnet, 1992; Pegues, 1992; Tunon-de-Lara, 1992]. In the study of 179 cases of anaphylaxis evaluated at the Mayo Clinic, 7 were patients using β-adrenergic blocking agents and 4 were patients using ACE inhibitors, suggesting that these agents should not be used in patients at risk for anaphylaxis [Yocum, 1994].

The first signs of anaphylaxis, including flushing, hives, or enhanced skin warmth or erythema, should be a sign to the person with exercise-induced anaphylaxis that exercise must be immediately stopped. Prophylactic measures in patients with exercise-induced anaphylaxis may include the use of antihistamines. However, although antihistamines may blunt an attack of exercise-induced anaphylaxis, these drugs typically fail to fully prevent these attacks. Prior treatment of the exercise-induced anaphylactic patient with antihistamines thus cannot be relied on to prevent this syndrome [Montgomery, 1993].

Several novel prophylactic measures for persons with exercise-induced anaphylaxis have been noted in case reports from the Japanese literature. One report describes an 18-year-old girl who has documented wheat allergy by skin-prick test and RAST and who also had exercise-induced anaphylactic symptoms during exercise challenge following wheat ingestion, including a significant rise in plasma histamine level and an 18.7% decrease in 1–S forced expiratory volume (FEV_1) on pulmonary function tests. When she received oral disodium cromoglycate before ingestion of wheat, all symptoms were blocked, with no decrease in FEV_1 or increase in plasma histamine [Juji, 1994]. Another case of wheat-associated exercise-induced anaphylaxis was reported to be prevented by pretreatment of the patient with sodium bicarbonate, which inhibited exercise-induced anaphylactic symptoms and prevented a decrease in blood pH that was associated with elevation in plasma histamine levels in this person during exercise challenge [Katsunuma, 1992].

All patients with exercise-induced anaphylaxis should have one or two doses of epinephrine available when they exercise. This can be in the form of an anaphylaxis kit or by carrying one or two Epi-Pens during exercise. Patients should also be instructed in the proper use of self-administered epinephrine devices and should be ready to treat anaphylaxis promptly with these devices should signs and symptoms of exercise-induced anaphylaxis occur. In cases of food-induced anaphylaxis not associated with exercise, prompt administration of epinephrine has been associated with generally favorable outcomes, whereas delayed use of epinephrine has been associated with fatalities [Sampson, 1992; Yocum, 1994]. The relative safety of dosages of 0.3 mL of 1 : 1000 concentration of epinephrine and the high risk entailed if one fails to treat anaphylaxis, clearly mandate early use of subcutaneous epinephrine in persons having exercise-induced anaphylactic symptoms. Another prudent measure for the athlete who has exercise-induced anaphylaxis includes always exercising with a companion who is aware of the condition and is instructed in the treatment of anaphylaxis, including use of epinephrine. It is also useful for persons having exercise-induced anaphylaxis to wear an emergency identification bracelet.

Serious morbidity has occasionally been reported with exercise-induced anaphylaxis, including a case of ventricular fibrillation occurring with signs of coronary spasm in an athlete in whom subsequent coronary artery disease was excluded. In this person, ergonovine provocation was positive, suggesting an H_2-dependent histamine-induced provocation of coronary artery spasm [Attenhofer, 1994].

As other forms of anaphylaxis, including drug- and food-induced anaphylaxis have been associated with significant morbidity and mortality, it would appear always prudent to treat exercise-induced anaphylaxis as a potentially life-threatening event in which epinephrine is promptly administered, preferably by the patient early in the course of the anaphylactic episode, and the patient is then rapidly transported to an emergency facility for further observation and treatment [Sheffer, 1985; Wade, 1989; Sonsiridej, 1983]. Ultimately, prevention of attacks of exercise induced anaphylaxis is essential to minimize morbidity and mortality of this condition, including such measures as modification of the exercise regimen and avoiding postprandial exercise.

REFERENCES

Adelman DC, Spector SL. Acute respiratory emergencies in emergency treatment of the injured athlete. Clin Sports Med 1989; 8:71–79.

Akutsu I, Motojima S, Ikeda Y, et al. [Three cases of food-dependent exercise-induced anaphylaxis]. Arerugi 1989; 38:277 [in Japanese].

Anaut A, Iglesias A, Zapatero L, et al. Exercise-induced anaphylactic reaction to apple. Allergy 1994; 49:67.

Anderson G, Li T, Malki J, et al. Assessment by Hycor RAST and Pharmacia CAP of cross-sensitization to banana and avocado among latex-sensitive hospital employees. JACI 1996; 97(1 pt 3):320.

Anderson SD. Current concepts of exercise-induced asthma. Allergy 1983; 38: 289.

Anderson SD, Rodwell LT, Du Toll J, Young IH. Duration of protection by inhaled salmeterol in exercise-induced asthma. Chest. 1991; 100:1254–1260.

Armentia A, Martin-Santos JM, Blanco M, et al. Exercise-induced anaphylactic reaction to grain flours. Ann Allergy 1990; 65:149.

Attenhofer C, Speich R, Salomon F, Burkhard R, Amann FW. Ventricular fibrillation in a patient with exercise-induced anaphylaxis, normal coronary arteries, and a positive ergonovine test. Chest 1994; 105:620–622.

Beuers U, Baur X, Schraudolph M, Richter WO. Anaphylactic shock after game of squash in atopic woman with latex allergy. Lancet 1993; 335:1095.

Bjarnason I, Smethurst P, Clark P, et al. Effect of prostaglandin on indomethacin-induced increased intestinal permeability in man. Scand J Gastroenterol Suppl 1989; 164:97–102.

Bleecker ER. Exercise-induced asthma. Physiologic and clinical considerations. Clin Chest Med 1984; 5:109–119.

Briner WW Jr. Introduction: exercise and allergy. Med Sci Sports Exerc 1992; 24:843–844.

Briner WW Jr. Physical allergies and exercise. Clinical implications for those engaged in sports activities. Sports Med 1993; 15:365–373.

Briner WW Jr, Sheffer AL. Exercise-induced anaphylaxis. Med Sci Sports Exerc 1992; 24:849–850.

Brunet P, Jaber K, Berland Y, Baz M. Anaphylactoid reactions during hemodialysis and hemofiltration: role of associating AN69 membrane and angiotensin I-convertin enzyme inhibitors. Am J Kidney Dis 1992; 19:444–447.

Buchbinder EM, Bloch KJ, Moss J, et al. Food-dependent exercise-induced anaphylaxis. JAMA 1983; 250:2973.

Bush RK, Hefle SL. Lessons and myths regarding cross-reacting foods. Allergy Proc 1995; 16:245–246.

Casale TB, Keahey TM, Kaliner M. Exercise-induced anaphylactic syndromes. Insights into diagnostic and pathophysiologic features. JAMA 1986; 255: 2049–2053.

Custovic A, Arifhodzic N, Robinson A, Woodcock A. Exercise testing revisited. The response in normal and atopic children. Chest 1994; 105:1127–1132.

del Rio Navarro BE, Sol Monterrey EG, Paredes Novelo C, Siernra Monge JJ. Anaphylaxis and urticaria caused by exercise. Review of the literature and report of 2 cases. Rev Alerg Mex 1993; 40(3):63–66.

De Vos C, Maleux M-R, Baltes E, Gilbert J. Inhibition of histamine and allergen skin weal by cetirizine in four animal species. Ann Allergy 1978; 59:278–282.

Dhillon DP. Studies in exercise-induced asthma. Eur Respir Rev 1991; 1:265–267.

Dimsdale JE, Hartley LH, Guiney T, et al. Postexercise peril: plasma catecholamines and exercise. JAMA 1984; 251:630.

Dohi M, Suko M, Sugiyama H, et al. Three cases of food-dependent, exercise-induced anaphylaxis in which aspirin exacerbated anaphylactic symptoms. Arerugi 1990; 39:1598.

Dohi M, Suko M, Sugiyama H, et al. Food-dependent, exercise-induced anaphylaxis. A study on 11 Japanese cases. J Allergy Clin Immunol 1991; 87:34.

Du Buske LM. Dose-ranging comparative evaluation of cetirizine in patients with seasonal allergic rhinitis. Ann Allergy Asthma Immunol 1995; 74:345–353.

Du Buske LM, Ling CJ, Sheffer AL. Special problems regarding allergen immunotherapy. Immunol Allergy Clin North Am 1992; 12:145.

Eggleston PA, Kagey-Sobotka A, Schleimer RP, Lichtenstein LM. Interaction between hyperosmolar and IgE-mediated histamine release from basophils and mast cells. Am Rev Respir Dis 1984; 130:86.

El-Dieb MR. Food-dependent, exercise-induced anaphylaxis [letter]. JAMA 1984; 251:3224.

Fukutomi O, Kondo N, Agata H, et al. Abnormal responses of the autonomic nervous system in food-dependent, exercise-induced anaphylaxis. Ann Allergy 1992; 68:438–445.

Gerth van Wijk R, Roovers MH, Dieges PH. Exercise-dependent anaphylaxis. Ned Tijdschr Geneeskd 1991; 135:2293–2295.

Goetz DW, Jacobson JM, Murnane JE, et al. Prolongation of simple and choice reaction time in a double-blind comparison of twice-daily hydroxyzine versus terfenadine. J. Allergy Clin Immunol 1989; 84:316–322.

Good AP, Rockwood R, Schad P. Loratadine and ventricular tachycardia. Am J Cardiol 1994; 74:207–209.

Grant JA, Farnam J, Lord RA, et al. Familial exercise-induced anaphylaxis. Ann Allergy 1985; 54:35.

Hanrahan JP, Choo PW, Carlson W, et al. Antihistamine-associated sudden death, ventricular arrhythmias, syncope and QT-prolongation: a comparison of terfenadine and other antihistamines. PostMarketing Surveillance 1992; 6: 23–24.

Hepner MJ, Ownby DR, Anderson JA, et al. Risk of systemic reactions in patients taking beta-blocker drugs receiving allergen immunotherapy injections. J Allergy Clin Immunol 1990; 86:407–411.

Holgate S, Benyon RC, Lowman MA, et al. Activation of human mast cells after immunoglobin E-dependent and neuropeptide stimulation. Prog Clin Biol Res 1989; 297:103.

Honig PK, Wortham DC, Zamani K, et al. Terfenadine–ketoconazole interaction. JAMA 1993; 12:1513–1518.

Honig PK, Woosleu RL, Zamani K, et al. Changes in the pharmocokinetics and electrocardiographic pharmacodynamics of terfenadine with concomitant administration of erythromycin. Clin Pharmacol Ther 1992; 52:231–238.

Hough DO, Dec KL. Exercise-induced asthma and anaphylaxis. Sports Med 1994; 18:162–172.

Juji F, Suko M. Effectiveness of disodium cromoglycate in food-dependent, exercise-induced anaphylaxis: a case report. Ann Allergy 1994; 72:452–454.

Juji F, Takashima H, Suko M, et al. [A case of food-dependent-exercise induced anaphylaxis possibly induced by shellfish (*Sulculus* and *Turbo cornutus*)]. Arerug 1990; 39:151–22 [In Japanese].

Katsunuma T, Iikura Y, Akasawa A, et al. Wheat-dependent exercise-induced anaphylaxis: inhibition by sodium bicarbonate. Ann Allergy 1992; 68: 184–188.

Kidd JM III, Cohen SH, Sosman AJ, et al. Food-dependent, exercise-induced anaphylaxis. J Allergy Clin Immunol 1983; 71:401.

Kivity S, Sneh E, Greif J, et al. The effect of food and exercise on the skin response to compound 48/80 in patients with food-associated, exercise-induced urticaria–angioedema. J Clin Immunol 1988; 81:1155.

Kobayashi RH, Mellion MB. Exercise-induced asthma, anaphylaxis, and urticaria. Primary Care 1991; 18:809–831.

Konig P. The use of cromolyn in the management of hyperreactive airways and exercise. J Allergy Clin Immunol 1984; 73:686.

Kushimoto H, Aoki T. Masked type I wheat allergy. Relation to exercise-induced anaphylaxis. Arch Dermatol 1985; 121:355.

Kyle JM. Exercise-induced pulmonary syndromes. Med Clin North Am 1994; 78: 413–421.

Latimer KM, O'Byrne PM, Morris MM, et al. Bronchoconstriction stimulated by airway cooling: better protection with combined inhalation of terbutaline sulphate and cromolyn sodium than with either alone. Am Rev Respir Dis 1983; 128:440.

Laufer P. Exercise-induced anaphylactic reaction to chicken dependent on the quantity ingested. Immunol Allergy Pract 1987; 9:213.

Lee TH, Nagakura T, Papegorgiou N, et al. Exercise-induced late asthmatic reactions with neutrophil chemotactic activity. N Engl J Med 1983; 308:1502.

Lewis J, Lieberman P, Treadwell G, et al. Exercise-induced urticaria, angioedema, and anaphylactoid episodes. J Allergy Clin Immunol 1981; 68:432.

Lin RV, Barnard M. Skin testing with food, codeine, and histamine in exercise-induced anaphylaxis. Ann Allergy 1993; 70:475.

Longley S, Panush RS. Familial exercise-induced anaphylaxis. Ann Allergy 1987; 58:257.

Martin Munoz F, Lopez Cazana JM, Villas F, Contreras JF, Diaz JM, Ojeda JA. Exercise-induced anaphylactic reaction to hazelnut. Allergy 1994; 49: 314–316.

Mathews KP, Pan P. Post-exercise hyperhistaminemia, dermographia, and wheezing. Ann Intern Med 1970; 72:241.

Maulitz RM, Pratt DS, Schocket AL. Exercise-induced anaphylactic reaction to shellfish. J Allergy Clin Immunol 1979; 63:433.

McNeil D, Strauss RH. Exercise-induced anaphylaxis related to food intake. Ann Allergy 1988; 61:440.

Montgomery LC, Deuster PA. Effects of antihistamine medications on exercise performance. Implications for sportspeople. Sports Med 1993; 15:179–195.

Morton AR, Kitch KD, Davis T. The effect of "warm-up" on exercise-induced asthma. Ann Allergy 1979; 42:257–260.

Novey HS, Fairshter RD, Salness K, et al. Postprandial exercise-induced anaphylaxis. J Allergy Clin Immunol 1983; 71:498.

Obata T, Kishida M, Okuma M, et al. A case of exercise-induced anaphylaxis: evidence of an association with the complement system. Acta Paediatr Jpn Overseas Ed 1989; 31:340.

Okazaki M, Kitani H, Mifune T, Mitsunobu F, Saito S, Asaumi N, Tanizaki Y. Food-dependent exercise-induced anaphylaxis. Int Med 1992; 31: 1052–1055.

Ownby DR. Mechanisms in adverse reactions to food. The whole body. Allergy 1995; 50(20 suppl):26–30.

Pegues DA, Beck-Sague CM, Woollen SW, et al. Anaphylactoid reactions associated with reuse of hollow-fiber hemodialyzers and ACE inhibitors. Kidney Int 1992; 42:1232–1237.

Romana A, Di Fonso M, Venuti A, Pamieri V, Zeppilli P. Food-dependent exercise-induced anaphylaxis; report of two cases. Int J Sports Med 1992; 13: 585–587.

Romano A, Di Fonso M, Guiffreda F, et al. Diagnostic work-up for food-dependent, exercise-induced anaphylaxis. Allergy 1995; 50:817–824.

Sabbah A, Drouet M, Bonneau JC. [Anaphylaxis induced by exercise]. Allerg Immunol (Paris) 1989; 21:381–388 [In French].

Sampson HA, Mendelson L, Rosen JP. Fatal and near-fatal anaphylactic reactions to food in children and adolescents. N Engl J Med 1992; 327(6): 380–384.

Sheffer AL, Austen KF. Exercise-induced anaphylaxis. J Allergy Clin Immunol 1980; 66:106.

Sheffer AL, Austen KF. Exercise-induced anaphylaxis. J Allergy Clin Immunol 1984; 73:699.

Sheffer AL, Soter NA, McFadden ER Jr, et al. Exercise-induced anaphylaxis: a distinct form of physical allergy. J Allergy Clin Immunol 1983; 71:311.

Sheffer AL, Tong AK, Murphy GF, et al. Exercise-induced anaphylaxis: a serious form of physical allergy associated with mast cell degranulation. J Allergy Clin Immunol 1985; 75:479.

Silvers WS. Exercise-induced allergies: the role of histamine release. Ann Allergy 1992; 68:58–63.

Silverstein SR, Frommer DA, Dobozin B, et al. Celery-dependent exercise-induced anaphylaxis. J Emerg Med 1986; 4:195.

Simons FER. H_1-receptor antagonists: comparative tolerability and safety. Drug Safety 1994; 10:350–380.

Simons FR, McMillan JL, Simons KJ. A double-blind, single-dose crossover comparison of cetirizine, terfenadine, loratadine, astemizole and chlorpheniramine versus placebo, suppression effects on histamine-induced weals and flares during 24 hours in normal subjects. J Allergy Clin Immunol 1990; 86: 540–547.

Sly RM. Management of exercise-induced asthma. Drug Ther 1982; 12:956–999.

Smith CM, Anderson SD. Hyperosmolarity as the stimulus to hyperventilation asthma. J Allergy Clin Immunol 1985; 75:143.

Smith SJ. Cardiovascular toxicity of antihistamines. Otolaryngol Head Neck Surg 1994; 111:348–354.

Sonsiridej V, Busse WW. Exercise-induced anaphylaxis. Clin Allergy 1983; 13: 317.

Soter NA, Wasserman SI, Austen KF, et al. Release of mast cell mediators and alterations in lung function in patients with cholinergic urticaria. N Engl J Med 1980; 302:604.

Spencer CM, Faulds D, Peters DH. Cetirizine; a reappraisal of its pharmacological properties and therapeutic use in selected allergic disorders. Drugs 1993; 46:1055–1080.

Stephansson E, Koskimies S, Lokki ML. Exercise-induced urticaria and anaphylaxis. Acta Derm Venereol 1991; 71:138–142.

Tanaka S. An epidemiological survey on food-dependent exercise-induced anaphylaxis in kindergartners, schoolchildren and junior high school students. Asia Pac J Public Health 1994; 7:26–30.

Tashiro H, Hori S, Shinozawa Y, et al. [A case of food-dependent exercise-induced anaphylaxis associated with repeated episodes of syncope]. Kokyu To Junkan 1993; 41:587–90 [in Japanese].

Tharp MD, Thirlby R, Sullivan TJ. Gastrin induces histamine release from human cutaneous mast cells. J Allergy Clin Immunol 1984; 75:159.

Thompson NC, Patel KR, Kerr JW. Sodium cromoglycate and ipratropium bromide in exercise-induced asthma. Thorax. 1979; 33:694.

Tunon-de-Lara JM, Villanueva P, Marcos M, Taytard A. ACE inhibitors and anaphylactoid reactions during venom immunotherapy [letter]. Lancet 1992; 340:908.

Van der Linden P-WG, Hack CE, Poortman J, et al. Insect-sting challenge in 138 patients: relation between clinical severity of anaphylaxis and mast cell activation. J Allergy Clin Immunol 1992; 90:110–118.

Wade JP, Liang MH, Sheffer AL. Exercise-induced anaphylaxis: epidemiologic observations. Prog Clin Biol Res 1989; 297:175.

Watanabe T, Sakamoto Y, Tomonaga H, et al. A case of food-dependent exercise-induced anaphylaxis. Arerugi 1990; 39:1523.

Wyngaarden JB, Seevers MH. The toxic effects of antihistamine drugs. JAMA 1951; 145:277–282.

White MV, Kowalski ML, Kaliner MA. Mast cell secretagogues. Prog Clin Biol Res 1989; 297:83.

Yocum MW, Khan DA. Assessment of patients who have experienced anaphylaxis: a 3 year survey. Mayo Clin Proc 1994; 69:16–23.

Yunginger JW. Fatal food-induced anaphylaxis. JAMA 1988; 260:1450–1452.

Wong S, Dykewicz MS, Patterson R. Idiopathic anaphylaxis. A clinical summary of 175 patients. Arch Intern Med 1990; 150:1323–1328.

16

Effects of High Altitude

Robert C. Roach
Copenhagen Muscle Research Center, Copenhagen, Denmark

Pope L. Moseley
University of New Mexico, Albuquerque, New Mexico

I. INTRODUCTION

Around the world many people travel to high altitudes for work or leisure. This chapter introduces the physiological challenges faced on ascent to high altitudes, and discusses the concerns and consequences for pulmonary patients. The medical problems encountered at high altitude range from the relatively benign symptoms of acute mountain sickness (AMS) to life-threatening high-altitude pulmonary (HAPE) and cerebral edema (HACE).

II. THE HIGH-ALTITUDE ENVIRONMENT

How high is high altitude? It is useful to categorize altitudes above sea level into high altitude (1500–3000 m), very high altitude (3000–5000 m) and extreme altitude (above 5000 m). The primary physiological challenge of high altitude is a decreased partial pressure of oxygen and resulting hypoxemia (Fig. 1). The consequence for persons visiting high altitudes can be an arterial Po_2 equivalent to that seen at sea level in patients with chronic obstructive pulmonary disease. How healthy travelers adjust and thrive in such an environment is explained by the process of acclimatization.

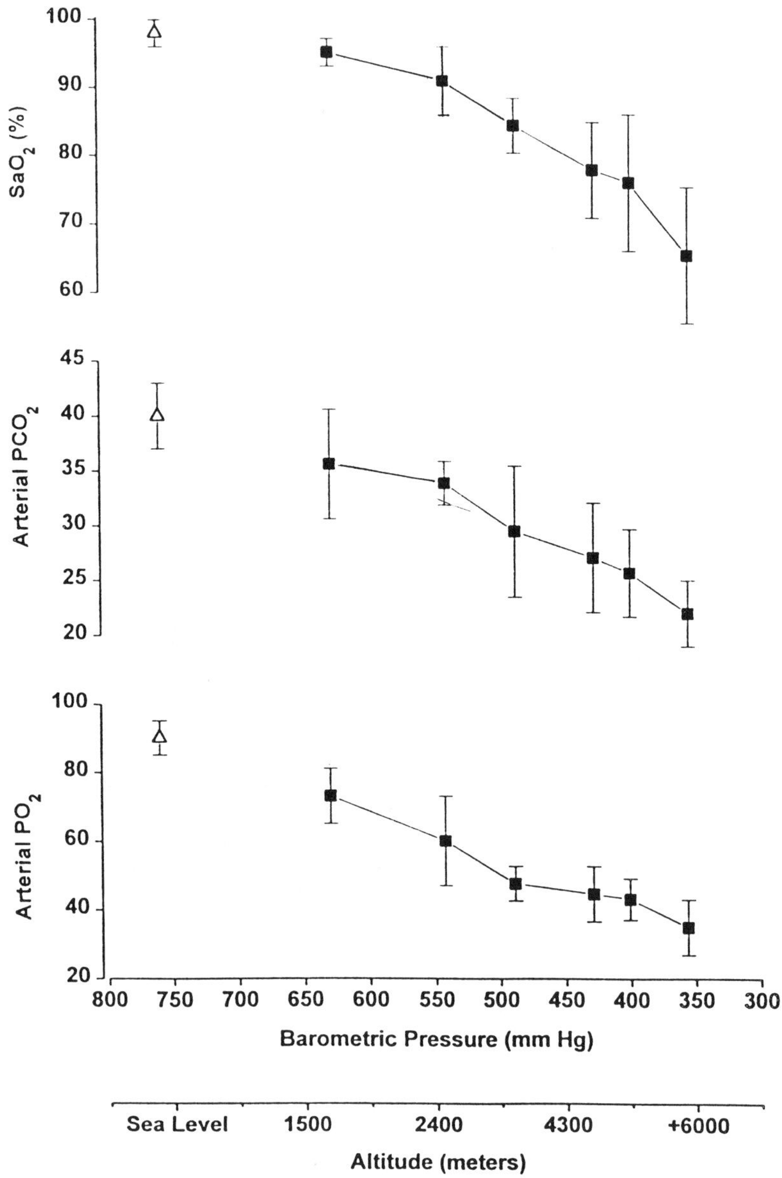

Fig. 1 Resting arterial blood gases from sea level to above 6000 m in young, healthy male subjects. (Data from Ref. 81 for 1646 m; from Refs. 82–84 for other altitude data.)

III. THE PROCESS OF ACCLIMATIZATION

Acclimatization is the process by which people gradually adjust to high altitudes [1,2]. The success of acclimatization determines survival and performance at high altitude. Acclimatization is a series of physiological changes that increase oxygen delivery and improve hypoxic tolerance. Several factors determine the degree and rate of acclimatization that an individual can attain. These factors include the severity of the high-altitude hypoxic stress, rate of onset of the hypoxia, and an individual's physiological response to hypoxia.

Some individuals acclimatize quickly, whereas others develop AMS [3,4]. A few fail to acclimatize even with gradual exposure. The best predictor of an individual's tendency to acclimatize well or to become ill is that individual's past history at altitude [5]. Prolonged exposure to high altitude over weeks to months improves submaximal exercise capacity, but if the altitude is high enough (more than 5000 m) a long-term stay may result in loss of physical capacity. These adjustments of acclimatization disappear after descent to low altitude, although the rate of loss is not well documented. Susceptibility to HAPE after return from a brief trip to sea level by high-altitude residents illustrates the important and temporary nature of high-altitude acclimatization. A few days at sea level may be sufficient to render a person susceptible to altitude illness, especially HAPE, on reascent [6,7]. Recent work suggests that ventilatory acclimatization may persist for many days or even weeks after return to sea level [8,9]. The mechanism for persistent ventilatory acclimatization after descent from high altitude is unknown.

The basic physiology of acclimatization is organized as oxygen flows from the environment to the tissues. Thus, ventilation, circulation, blood and tissue adjustments to the decreased partial pressure of oxygen encountered at high altitude are described sequentially (Fig. 2).

A. Ventilatory Acclimatization

The first step in acclimatization to high altitude involves increased ventilation. This response starts within the first few hours of exposure to altitudes as low as 1500 m (P_{IO_2} = 122 torr). The carotid bodies, sensing a decrease in arterial P_{O_2} (see Fig. 1), stimulate the central respiratory center to increase ventilation [10,11]. Numerous studies have shown that a good ventilatory response to altitude enhances acclimatization and performance, and a low ventilatory response may contribute to illness [12,13]. After several hours to days at altitude the cerebrospinal fluid (CSF) pH has adjusted to the respiratory alkalosis produced by the hyperventilation

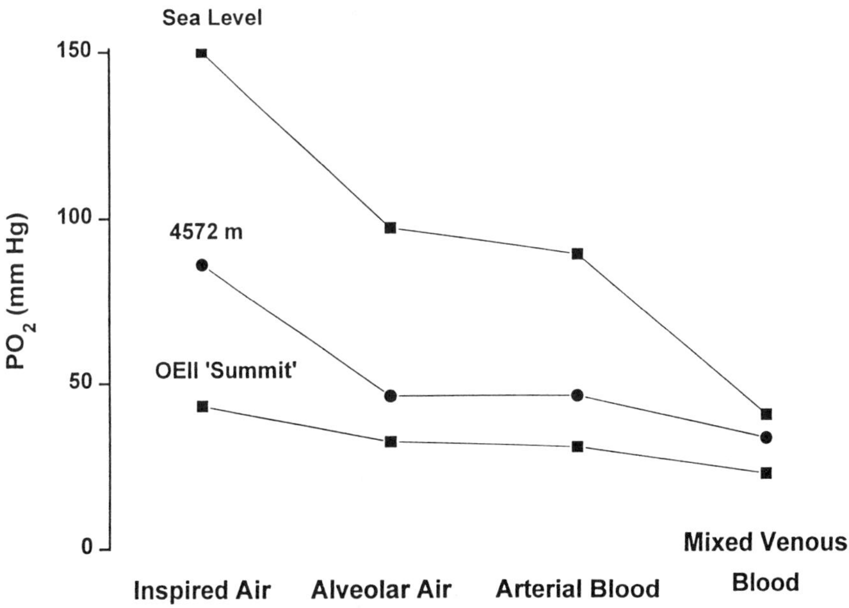

Fig. 2 The oxygen cascade, at rest, from inspired air to mixed venous oxygen tension at sea level [83], in high-altitude native residents (4572 m [84]), and in research subjects exposed to the simulated summit of Mt. Everest in a pressure chamber during Operation Everest 2 (OEII, [83]) Note that acclimatization improves oxygen extraction and utilization so that differences in mixed venous oxygen are much smaller than differences in inspired, alveolar, or arterial blood oxygen levels.

of acclimatization [14], and a new steady state is reached and maintained throughout the stay at high altitude.

B. Circulatory Acclimatization

Circulatory adjustments complete the next step in acclimatization by moving oxygenated blood from the lungs to the tissues. During the initial phase of acclimatization (hours to days), plasma volume drops, stroke volume is decreased, and resting heart rate is elevated, resulting in a slight increase or no change in resting cardiac output. These adjustments effectively counter the fall in arterial oxygen content so that oxygen transport remains adequate [15,16]. Most of the cardiovascular adjustments to altitude are regulated by increased sympathetic tone [17].

After acclimatization, the resting heart rate returns to near sea-level values except at altitudes above 5000 m [18]. Maximal heart rate during exercise follows the decline in maximal oxygen uptake with increasing altitude [19]. The maximal heart rate response to sudden altitude exposure is variable, with some studies reporting no change [20] and a recent study, at higher altitude, reporting decreased peak heart rate with sudden ascent [21]. Whether the sinoatrial node is susceptible to brief, severe hypoxemia is unknown. At higher altitudes, generally above 5000 m, the limits to hypoxic acclimatization are approached, and maximum and resting heart rates converge. During Operation Everest II, cardiac function was appropriate for the level of work performed, and cardiac output was not a limiting factor for performance [18].

C. Blood and Tissue Changes During Acclimatization

Scientists have long thought that the increased erythropoiesis is an important component of the acclimatization process [22]. As red blood cell mass is increased secondary to increased erythropoietin production, the oxygen-carrying capacity of the blood is increased [23]. Coupled with ventilatory and cardiovascular acclimatization, the increase in oxygen-carrying capacity secondary to an increased red cell mass largely accounts for the increased work capacity observed after successful acclimatization.

Transport of oxygen from the capillary to the cell is the final link in the oxygen transport chain considered here. Any factor that impedes oxygen transfer, such as hypoxia or anemia, will hinder acclimatization. Similarly, factors that enhance cellular oxygen utilization will enhance acclimatization and physical performance. In studies of humans exposed to high altitude for several weeks, months [24,25], or years [26,27] an intriguing pattern of adjustments in the skeletal muscle occurs and serves to maximize oxygen delivery to working muscles. The most important adjustments are a reduction in muscle fiber size and an increase in the capillary/fiber ratio [24,28,29]. These two changes effectively shorten the pathway for oxygen to travel from the capillary to the muscle cell, thereby enhancing oxygen delivery and physical work capacity [26].

D. Exercise

The ability to exercise drops dramatically on ascent to high altitude, and is a nearly universal experience at altitudes higher than 2500 m that was well-described over 100 years ago:

> The most important and striking symptom (of climbing at high altitude) was the disastrous result of the least muscular exertion. Twenty steps

> on the gentle slope of the glacier sufficed to produce a feverish quickening of the pulse to 160 per minute [30].

Maximal oxygen uptake (Vo_2max) decreases from sea level approximately 10% for each 1000 m of altitude gained above 1500 m. Consequently, at 4500 m a climber has only 70–75% of his or her sea level exercise capacity. Above 4500 m exercise tolerance falls rapidly, being only 60% at 5900 m, and less than 40% at 7400 m [31]. Those with the highest sea level Vo_2max values have the greatest decrement in Vo_2max [31,32] at altitude. Furthermore, the world's elite mountaineers are distinguished by their average Vo_2max values [33], in contrast with other endurance athletes [34]. With long-term acclimatization, Vo_2max remains depressed, but submaximal exercise capacity increases dramatically. In one study, submaximal endurance time was increased more than 60% from initial altitude values after less than 2 weeks at altitude [35]. Enhancement of submaximal work capacity is observed up to altitudes of approximately 5200 m; at higher altitudes physical deterioration outpaces acclimatization.

Athletes have special interests and concerns about training at high altitude. Some must prepare for athletic events held at high altitudes, whereas others are concerned with enhancement of sea level performance from altitude training. To compete in endurance activities (longer than 3- to 4-min duration) at altitudes above 1500 m, acclimatization is necessary [36]. For competition at 1500 m, 5 days acclimatization at that altitude may be sufficient, whereas up to 20 days is likely necessary for events staged at altitudes up to 4000 m. For events above 4000 m, staging, or acclimatization at an intermediate altitude, is recommended.

Athletes and coaches claim altitude training for sea level competition is very effective [37], whereas scientists are divided [38]. One clear advantage of altitude training is an increased hemoglobin concentration and, thus, enhanced oxygen-carrying capacity. If endurance, power, and strength are maintained during altitude training, then the altitude-trained athlete will be environmentally blood-boosted compared with sea-level counterparts. Recently, American [39] and Finnish [40] scientists have shown that athletes that sleep while hypoxic (in a low-oxygen room or at moderate altitude) and then train at or near sea level significantly improve their exercise performance at sea level.

IV. WHEN ACCLIMATIZATION FAILS: THE HIGH-ALTITUDE SYNDROMES

The high-altitude syndromes include acute mountain sickness (AMS), high-altitude pulmonary edema (HAPE), and high-altitude cerebral edema

(HACE). The least-threatening and most common syndrome is AMS. Occasionally, AMS progresses to life-threatening HAPE or HACE. The high-altitude syndromes have several features in common, and all respond to descent or oxygen. The ease of travel to high-altitude areas and the popularity of mountain-area recreation have increased the number of AMS, HAPE, and HACE cases worldwide.

A. Acute Mountain Sickness

The syndrome of AMS has long been recognized, but the first modern description in English comes from TH Ravenhill. Writing of his experiences as a mining camp physician in the Andes mountains, his descriptions of AMS from early in this century are as clear as any yet written:

> As a rule, towards the evening the patient begins to feel rather slack and disinclined for exertion. He goes to bed, but has a restless and troubled night, and wakes up next morning with a severe frontal headache. There may be vomiting, frequently there is a sense of oppression in the chest, but there is rarely any respiratory distress or alteration in the normal rate of breathing so long as the patient is at rest. The patient may feel slightly giddy on rising from bed, and any attempt at exertion increases the headache, which is nearly always confined to the frontal region [41].

The incidence and severity of AMS depend on the rate of ascent and the altitude attained, length of time at altitude, degree of physical exertion, and the individual's physiological susceptibility. AMS can be classified as mild, moderate, or severe on the basis of symptoms (Table 1 [42]). Age and prior physical condition have little influence on incidence. Although hemoglobin concentration increases with acclimatization, it is not related to susceptibility to altitude illness. Controlled studies have not yet determined whether men and women differ in their susceptibility to AMS. Limited epidemiological studies suggest that women have the same or slightly greater incidence of AMS, but may be less susceptible to HAPE [43]. The chief significance of AMS is that it may progress to life-threatening HAPE or HACE.

The most striking symptoms of AMS are headache, fatigue, dizziness, and anorexia. The headache is usually throbbing, bitemporal or occipital, and typically worse during the night and on awakening [44]. Anorexia and nausea are common. Afflicted persons commonly complain of a deep inner chill, unlike mere exposure to cold temperature, accompanied by facial pallor [44]. Other symptoms may include vomiting, marked dys-

Table 1 The Ten Most Frequent Symptoms of AMS in 840 Men at Altitudes Between 3350 and 5500 m

1. Headache
2. Nausea
3. Loss of appetite
4. Breathlessness
5. Insomnia
6. Muscular weakness
7. Fullness or pain in the chest
8. Giddiness
9. Vomiting
10. Disinclination to work

Source: Ref. 4.

pnea on exertion, and irritability [6,45]. A simple, easy to use scoring system has been developed to classify AMS in the field (Table 2).

Because everyone experiences dyspnea on exertion at high altitude, it may be difficult to distinguish normal from abnormal. Dyspnea at rest is definitely abnormal and often precedes HAPE. Although a dry cough is quite common in the mountains, especially after exercise in the cold, any pulmonary symptomatology calls for a careful examination for HAPE [45].

B. High-Altitude Pulmonary and Cerebral Edema

High-altitude pulmonary edema is the most common cause of death related to high altitude. Complete recovery is easily attained with early diagnosis and proper treatment. Ignoring the signs and symptoms of HAPE in the high-altitude setting can lead to rapid deterioration and death within hours. Fewer than 1:10,000 skiers in the western United States develop HAPE, but up to 1:50 climbers on McKinley succumb to HAPE [6]. An epidemiological study of visitors to moderate altitude in Colorado also found a greater incidence of HAPE during the winter, compared with summer months, even when the differences in number of visitors per season were taken into account [46]. As with AMS, individual physiology, rate of ascent to high altitude, and the final altitude reached play a role in the incidence of HAPE [6,47].

In contrast to AMS, which occurs in the first 24 h at a new altitude, HAPE usually is noticed only after 24–48 h and commonly occurs after

Table 2 The Lake Louise Acute Mountain Sickness (AMS) Score

1. Self assessment
   a. *Headache*
      0 No headache
      1 Mild headache
      2 Moderate headache
      3 Severe headache, incapacitating
   b. *Gastrointestinal symptoms*
      0 No gastrointestinal symptoms
      1 Poor appetite or nausea
      2 Moderate nausea or vomiting
      3 Severe nausea or vomiting, incapacitating
   c. *Fatigue or weakness*
      0 Not tired or weak
      1 Mild fatigue/weakness
      2 Moderate fatigue/weakness
      3 Severe fatigue/weakness, incapacitating
   d. *Dizziness or lightheadedness*
      0 Not dizzy or lightheaded
      1 Mild dizziness or lightheadedness
      2 Moderate dizziness or lightheadedness
      3 Severe dizziness or lightheadedness, incapacitating
   e. *Difficulty sleeping*
      0 Slept as well as usual
      1 Did not sleep as well as usual
      2 Woke many times, poor night's sleep
      3 Could not sleep at all
2. Clinical assessment
   a. *Change in mental status*
      0 No change in mental status
      1 Lethargy or lassitude
      2 Disoriented or confused
      3 Stupor or unconsciousness
   b. *Ataxia (heel to toe walking)*
      0 No ataxia
      1 Maneuvers to maintain balance
      2 Falls down
      3 Cannot stand
   c. *Peripheral edema*
      1 No peripheral edema
      2 Peripheral edema at one location
      3 Peripheral edema at two or more locations
3. Functional score
   Overall, if you had any symptoms, how did they affect your activity?
      0 No reduction in activity

Table 2 Continued

1 Mild reduction in activity
2 Moderate reduction in activity
3 Severe reduction in activity

This score provides a system for both self-assessment and clinical assessment of the symptoms and signs of AMS. The self-assessment score can also be administered by a health care provider or researcher. Only if a person has a headache score of at least mild severity and one additional symptom are they considered to have AMS. In this case, the total number of points on the scale (maximum 15) are summed and become that person's AMS score. [see Ref. 2 for a complete discussion].

the second night [45]. Symptoms of AMS, such as headache, anorexia, and lassitude, are often present. Dyspnea on exertion is often the first clear sign of HAPE; whereas dyspnea at rest and audible râles suggest fulminant pulmonary edema [6]. A persistent dry cough develops. Nail beds and lips become cyanotic. Misdiagnosis is common, with early HAPE often attributed to influenza or lack of physical condition. Although HAPE develops slowly, because the early signs are often missed HAPE often appears to strike suddenly. Severe hypoxemia (or cerebral edema) may produce mental changes, ataxia, depressed level of consciousness, and coma.

The early symptoms and signs of high-altitude cerebral edema suggest that HACE is a severe form of AMS. Most authors estimate that the incidence of HACE is less than 1% up to about 4000–4500 m [44], with a slightly higher incidence above 5000 m [4]. Truncal ataxia and change of mental status help differentiate early HACE from AMS [48]. The progression from mild AMS to unconsciousness may be as fast as 12 h, but usually requires 1–3 days [49].

Fulminant HACE is characterized by ataxic gait, severe lassitude, and altered consciousness, including confusion, impaired mental capacity, drowsiness, stupor, and coma [44]. Exaggerated hypoxemia is present, probably secondary to concomitant pulmonary edema [50].

C. Pathophysiology of the High-Altitude Syndromes

The pathophysiology of the high-altitude syndromes includes many common features, some well understood and others that remain obscure despite intense scientific scrutiny. Singh [4] proposed in 1969 that the high-altitude syndromes are secondary to the body's responses to hypobaric hypoxia, not simply due to hypoxemia. He based this conclusion on the observations that (a) the delay between onset of hypoxia and onset of symptoms after ascent (from hours to days), and (b) all symptoms are not immediately reversed with oxygen. In this section we present a concise review of the pathophysiology of the high-altitude syndromes. For a more in-depth discussion, several recent reviews are available on AMS [51–53], HAPE [6,47], and HACE [48,54,55].

Findings documented in moderate to severe AMS that relate to pathophysiology include relative hypoventilation [51], fluid retention and redistribution [52], increased intracranial pressure and brain swelling [50], and impaired pulmonary gas exchange [56] and mechanics [57]. One quickly recognizes both pulmonary and cerebral components in the pathophysiology of AMS. Just what factor(s) determine how AMS will progress are not yet known.

The findings documented in HAPE that relate to pathophysiology include exaggerated pulmonary symptoms seen with AMS, elevated pulmonary artery pressure and pulmonary vascular resistance [58], a low to normal pulmonary wedge pressure, and low to normal cardiac output and systemic arterial blood pressure [59]. The electrocardiogram usually reveals sinus tachycardia. Arterial blood gas levels consistently reveal respiratory alkalosis and exaggerated hypoxemia. The radiographic findings reveal fluffy and patchy infiltrates, with areas of aeration between infiltrates [60]. Infiltrates may be unilateral or bilateral, with a propensity for the right middle lung field, which corresponds to the usual area of râles. The findings documented in HACE that relate to pathophysiology include elevated CSF pressures [61,62], evidence of cerebral edema on computed tomography (CT) scans [63] and magnetic resonances imaging (MRI) [64], and gross cerebral edema on necropsy [50]. Well-documented HACE cases have often included pulmonary edema [50].

Common to AMS, HAPE, and HACE is a global increase in microvascular permeability. The signs that fluid has leaked into the alveolar spaces are present in AMS [65], and from recent MRI reports, it seems likely a similar process occurs in the brain during AMS [66]. Once a patient has developed HAPE, the alveoli are overcome with fluid, as is true in the brain with HACE. Vasoactive mediators of vascular permeability (leukotriene B_4; LTB_4) are increased in AMS [67] and HAPE [68]. Whether such mediators are central to the pathogenesis of the high-altitude syndromes remains to be determined.

D. Prevention and Treatment of the High-Altitude Syndromes

The fundamentals of prevention are similar for AMS, HAPE, and HACE, and are based on slow ascent, time for acclimatization, a low sleeping altitude, and avoidance of any factors that increase hypoxemia (e.g., sedative hypnotics, alcohol). Gradual ascent, with time spent to acclimatize at intermediate altitudes, aids acclimatization and decreases the incidence and severity of AMS [9]. The rules for how high and how fast one can safely ascend to high altitude are summarized in the simple phrase: "climb high, sleep low" [69]. The lower altitude for sleeping aids acclimatization and allows high-quality sleep. The higher the destination sleeping altitude, the longer needed for acclimatizing. Travelers to Rocky Mountain ski resorts that spent at least 38 h in Denver (1500 m) on their way to higher-destination altitudes (2500–3000 m) had significantly less AMS than counterparts who spent no time acclimatizing. At even higher sleeping altitudes, the benefits of acclimatization are even greater, and the costs of going too high, too fast are even more severe [43].

When rapid ascent is unavoidable, or known susceptibility to AMS, HAPE, or HACE exists, several drugs are helpful in the prevention of the high-altitude syndromes (Table 3). Acetazolamide and dexamethasone are useful for the prevention of AMS (and HACE) [70,71]. Acetazolamide is a respiratory stimulant and mild diuretic; both actions are of clear benefit for AMS. How dexamethasone works to prevent AMS is unknown. Dexamethasone is as effective as acetazolamide, but is generally reserved for use in cases in whom acetazolamide is contraindicated or is not well-tolerated. Nifedipine is useful for preventing HAPE in persons with a known history of HAPE [72].

Treatment of mild AMS can include additional time to acclimatize at the present altitude, or symptomatic therapy for headache and nausea. Symptoms often resolve in 1–2 days. Moderate to severe AMS, HAPE, and HACE should all be treated with immediate descent. In a patient with mild AMS, any deterioration of neurological status or signs of pulmonary edema demand immediate descent. Simulated descent in one of the recently available portable pressure chambers is a good option when actual descent is difficult, and oxygen is unavailable. Oxygen immediately relieves the symptoms of AMS, the hypoxemia and pulmonary hypertension in HAPE, and can also be an effective treatment for HACE. Depending on the severity, in more severe HAPE and HACE cases oxygen can be a life-saving, temporizing measure. Clinicians have repeatedly observed that a rapid descent of 500–1000 m brings profound relief to HAPE and HACE victims, more relief than seemed apparent from supplemental oxygen alone [49]. It appears that descent (increasing the barometric pressure) may cause a more rapid reversal of pulmonary edema, but the improvement is nearly identical after several hours of descent or a similar time breathing oxygen [73].

When descent is not possible, acetazolamide and dexamethasone successfully treat AMS and HACE (see Table 3 for dosage regimen) [65,74]. No controlled studies are yet available on the effectiveness of

Table 3 Treatment of High-Altitude Illness

Mild acute mountain sickness
Stop ascent, rest, acclimatize at same altitude
Acetazolamide 125–150 mg bid to speed acclimatization
Symptomatic treatment as necessary with analgesics and antiemetics *or* Descend 500 m or more
Moderate acute mountain sickness
Low-flow oxygen, if available
Acetazolamide 125–250 mg bid or dexamethasone 4 mg PO, IM, IV q 6 h
Hyperbaric therapy
or Immediate descent
High-altitude cerebral edema
Immediate descent or evacuation
Oxygen, 2–4 L/min
Dexamethasone 4 mg PO, IM or IV q 6 h
Hyperbaric therapy
High-altitude pulmonary edema
Minimize exertion and keep warm
Oxygen, 4–6 L/min until improving, then 2–4 L/min
Nifedipine 10 mg PO q 2–4 h by titration to response, or 20 mg extended-release q 6 h, if no oxygen or descent
Hyperbaric therapy
or Immediate descent
Periodic breathing
Acetazolamide 62.5–125 mg at bedtime as needed

Source: Ref. 44.

acetazolamide and dexamethasone for treatment of HAPE. Successful treatment of HAPE with nifedipine has been achieved in climbers in Alaska and the Alps [58,75].

E. Other Effects of High Altitude

In addition to the effects of high altitude on healthy, active persons previously described, we discuss here several special concerns at high altitude. These include reentry pulmonary edema, chronic lung disease, and advice for the elderly traveling to high altitude.

1. Reentry Pulmonary Edema

Residents of high altitude in the western United States and South America are able to travel quickly from their high-altitude homes to sea level and back. Some develop HAPE when they return to their high-altitude home. Children and adolescents are more susceptible than adults. In young people (age 1–20 years) the incidence of HAPE on reascent may be as high as 6%; in adults the risk seems similar between altitude residents and newcomers [76,77].

2. Chronic Lung Disease

Patients with chronic obstructive pulmonary disease (COPD) may have hypoxemia, pulmonary hypertension, disordered control of ventilation, and sleep-disordered breathing at sea level. These conditions may worsen on ascent to high altitude. Two studies on COPD patients report that they tolerate moderate altitude quite well [78,79]. Although it might be expected that altitude syndromes would be more frequent in this group, tolerance to moderate altitude may reflect the "acclimatization" to hypoxemia they have experienced at sea level. Many COPD patients venturing to altitude report reduced exercise ability.

Symptomatic pulmonary hypertension may be a contraindication to altitude exposure because of hypoxic pulmonary vasoconstriction, and enhanced susceptibility to HAPE. COPD patients with severe bullous disease may be at a theoretically increased risk for spontaneous pneumothorax, although there is no controlled study demonstrating an increased incidence. Patients with sleep apnea syndrome who become mildly hypoxemic at sea level may become severely hypoxemic at high altitude, contributing to altitude illness. Asthma is not a contraindication for ascent to altitude, but appropriate medications must be available [44].

3. The Elderly at High Altitude

It is generally safe for older active men and women to travel to moderate altitude for short visits. Nearly 100 older men and women were studied as they traveled from their sea-level homes to a convention at 2500 m in Colorado. The group included 25% with cardiovascular disease, 35% with hypertension, and 10% with pulmonary disease. All tolerated the altitude. Incidence of AMS was 16%, slightly lower than for younger persons at the same altitude. In spite of the prevalence of chronic illness (prevalence similar to that of a normal population of elderly at sea level), asymptomatic coronary artery disease, hypertension, or pulmonary disease were not exacerbated, did not result in any adverse medical consequences, and importantly, did not limit physical activity [78]. Similar results were found in a group of patients with known, symptomatic coronary artery disease [80].

REFERENCES

1. West JB. Acclimatization and tolerance to extreme altitude. J Wilderness Med 1993; 4:17–26.
2. Young AJ, Young PM. Human acclimatization to high terrestrial altitude. In: Pandolf KB, Sawka MN, Gonzalez RR, eds. Human performance physiology and environmental medicine at terrestrial extremes. Dubuque IA: Brown & Benchmark, 1986; 497–544.
3. Hackett PH, Rennie ID, Levine HD. The incidence, importance, and prophylaxis of acute mountain sickness. Lancet 1976; 2:1149–1154.
4. Singh I, Khanna PK, Srivastava MC, Lal M, Roy SB, Subramanyam CS. Acute mountain sickness. N Engl J Med 1969; 280:175–218.
5. Robinson SM, King AB, Aoki V. Acute mountain sickness: reproducibility of its severity and duration in an individual. Aerospace Med 1971; 42:706–708.
6. Hackett PH, Roach RC. High altitude pulmonary edema. J Wilderness Med 1990; 1:3–26.
7. Sophocles AM. High-altitude pulmonary edema in Vail, Colorado, 1975–1982. West J Med 1986; 144:569–573.
8. Muza SR, Fulco CS, Beidleman BA, Rock PB, Lyons T, Cymerman A. Ventilatory acclimatization to 4300 m is retained eight days after return to sea level. In: Sutton JR, Coates G, Houston CS, eds. Hypoxia and molecular medicine. Burlington VT: Queen City Press, 1993.
9. Lyons TP, Muza SR, Rock PB, Cymerman A. Prior acclimatization to 4300 m reduces acute mountain sickness symptomatology with reinduction. In: Sutton JR, Coates G, Houston CS, eds. Hypoxia and molecular medicine. Burlington VT: Queen City Press, 1993.
10. Schoene RB, Lahiri S, Hackett PH, et al. The relationship of hypoxic ventilatory response to exercise performance on Mount Everest. J Appl Physiol 1984; 56:1478–1483.
11. Weil JV, Byrne-Quinn E, Sodal IE, Filley GF, Grover RF. Evaluation of hypoxic ventilatory drive—findings at high altitude. Adv Cardiol 1970; 5: 132–138.
12. Moore LG, Harrison GL, McCullough RE, et al. Low acute hypoxic ventilatory response and hypoxic depression in acute altitude sickness. J Appl Physiol 1986; 60:1407–1412.
13. Roach RC. The role of the hypoxic ventilatory response in performance at high altitude. In: Wood SC, Roach RC, eds. Modern topics in sport medicine. New York: Marcel Dekker, 1994.
14. Severinghaus JW. Hypoxic respiratory drive and its loss during chronic hypoxia. Clin Physiol (Jpn) 1972; 2:57–79.
15. Klausen K. Cardiac output in man at rest and work during and after acclimatization to 3800 m. J Appl Physiol 1966; 21:609–616.
16. Saltin B, Grover RF, Blomqvist CG, Hartley LH, Johnson RL. Maximal oxygen uptake and cardiac output after 2 weeks at 4,300 m. J Appl Physiol 1968; 25:400–409.

17. Mazzeo RS, Brooks GA, Butterfield GE, Podolin DA, Wolfel EE, Reeves JT. Acclimatization to high altitude increase muscle sympathetic activity both at rest and during exercise. Am J Physiol 1995; 269:R201–207.
18. Reeves JT, Groves BM, Sutton JR, et al. Operation Everest II: preservation of cardiac function at extreme altitude. J Appl Physiol 1987; 63:531–539.
19. Antezana AM, Kacimi R, Le Trong JL, et al. Adrenergic status of humans during prolonged exposure to the altitude of 6,542 m. J Appl Physiol 1994; 76:3001–3005.
20. Stenberg J, Ekblom B, Messin R. Hemodynamic response to work at simulated altitude, 4000 m. J Appl Physiol 1966; 21:1589–1594.
21. Roach RC, Calbet JA, Olsen NV, Poulsen TD, Saltin B. Peak exercise heart rate at altitude. J Physiol (London) 1996; 491:60–61.
22. Smith EE, Crowell JW. Role of an increased hematocrit in altitude acclimatization. Aerospace Med 1967; 38:39–43.
23. Lenfant C, Ways P, Aucutt C, Cruz J. Effect of chronic hypoxic hypoxia on the O_2–Hb dissociation curve and respiratory gas transport in man. Respir Physiol 1969; 7:7–29.
24. Green HJ, Sutton JR, Cymerman A, Young PM, Houston CS. Operation Everest II: adaptations in skeletal muscle. J Appl Physiol 1989; 66:142–151.
25. Horstman DH, Gleser M, Wolfe D, Tyron T, Delehunt J. Effects of hemoglobin reduction on V_{O_2}max and related hemodynamics in exercising dogs. J Appl Physiol 1974; 37:97–102.
26. Kayser B, Hoppeler H, Claaseen H, Cerretelli P. Muscle structure and performance of Himalayan Sherpas. J Appl Physiol 1991; 70:1938–1942.
27. Kayser B, Hoppeler H, Desplanches D, Claasen H, Cerretelli P. Muscle ultrastructure and biochemistry of first generation lowland Tibetans [abstract]. In: Sutton JR, Houston CS, Coates G, eds. Hypoxia and the brain. Burlington VT: Queen City Press, 1995.
28. Hoppeler H, Kleinert E, Schlegel C, et al. Morphological adaptations of human skeletal muscle to chronic hypoxia. Int J Sport Med 1990; 11:S3–S9.
29. Hoppeler H, Desplanches D. Muscle structural modifications in hypoxia. Int J Sport Med 1992; 13:S166–S168.
30. Kronecker H. Mountain sickness. Med Magazine 1895; 4:651–666.
31. Lawler J, Powers SK, Thompson D. Linear relationship between V_{O_2}max and V_{O_2}max decrement during exposure to acute hypoxia. J Appl Physiol 1988; 64:1486–1492.
32. Young AJ, Cymerman A, Burse RL. The influence of cardiorespiratory fitness on the decrement in maximal aerobic power at high altitude. Eur J Appl Physiol 1985; 54:12–15.
33. Oelz O, Howald H, di Prampero PE, et al. Physiological profile of world-class high altitude climbers. J Appl Physiol 1986; 60:1734–1742.
34. Astrand PO, Rodahl K. Textbook of work physiology. New York: McGraw-Hill, 1977.
35. Maher JT, Jones LG, Hartley LH. Effects of high altitude exposure on submaximal endurance capacity of men. J Appl Physiol 1974; 37:895–898.

36. Pugh LG. Report of medical research project into effects of altitude in Mexico City. In: Astrand PO, Rodahl K, eds. Textbook of work physiology. New York: McGraw-Hill, 1977; 652.
37. Dick FW. Training at altitude in practice. Int J Sport Med 1992; 13: S203–S206.
38. Levine BD, Roach RC, Houston CS. Work and traning at altitude. In: Sutton JR, Coates G, Houston CS, eds. Hypoxia and mountain medicine. Burlington VT: Queen City Press, 1992.
39. Stray-Gundersen J, Levine B. Altitude acclimatization/normoxic training (high/low) improves sea level endurance immediately on descent from altitude [abstract]. Med Sci Sport Exerc 1994; 26:S64.
40. Laitinen H, Alopaeus K, Heikkinen R, et al. Acclimatization to living in normobaric hypoxia and training in normoxia at sea level in runners [abstract]. Med Sci Sport Exerc 1995; 27:S617.
41. Ravenhill TH. Some experiences of mountain sickness in the Andes. J Trop Med Hyg 1913; 1620:313–320.
42. Roach RC, Bärtsch P, Oelz O, Hackett PH. The Lake Louise acute mountain sickness scoring system. In: Sutton JR, Houston CS, Coates G, eds. Hypoxia and molecular medicine. Burlington VT: Queen City Press, 1993.
43. Honigman B, Theis MK, McLain J, et al. Acute mountain sickness in a general tourist population at moderate altitudes. Ann Intern Med 1993; 118: 587–592.
44. Hackett PH, Roach RC. High-altitude medicine. In: Auerbach PA, ed. Wilderness medicine. St. Louis: Mosby, 1995; 1–37.
45. Hultgren HN. High altitude pulmonary edema. In: Staub NC, ed. Lung water and solute exchange. New York: Marcel Dekker, 1978; 437–469.
46. Reeves JT, Wagner J, Zafren K, Honigman B, Schoene RB. Seasonal variation in barometric pressure and temperature in Summit County: effect on altitude illness. In: Sutton JR, Houston CS, Coates G, eds. Hypoxia and molecular medicine. Bulrington VT: Queen City Press, 1993.
47. Schoene RB. High altitude pulmonary edema: pathophysiology and clinical review. Ann Emerg Med 1987; 16:987–992.
48. Hamilton AJ, Cymerman A, Bloch M. High altitude cerebral edema. Neurosurgery 1986; 19:841–849.
49. Hackett PH. Mountain sickness: prevention, recognition and treatment. New York: American Alpine Club, 1980.
50. Dickinson JG, Heath J, Gosney J, Williams D. Altitude related deaths in seven trekkers in the Himalayas. Thorax 1983; 38:646–656.
51. Hackett PH, Rennie ID, Hofmeister SE, Grover RF, Grover EB, Reeves JT. Fluid retention and relative hypoventilation in acute mountain sickness. Respiration 1982, 43.321–329.
52. Bärtsch P, Shaw S, Wiedmann P, Franciolli M, Maggiorini M, Oelz O. Aldosterone, antidiuretic hormone and atrial natriuretic peptide in acute mountain sickness. In: Sutton JR, Coates G, Houston CS, eds. Hypoxia and mountain medicine. Burlington VT: Queen City Press, 1992.

53. Krasney JA. A neurogenic basis for acute altitude illness. Med Sci Sport Exerc 1994; 26:195–208.
54. Dickinson JG. High altitude cerebral edema: cerebral acute mountain sickness. Semin Respir Med 1983; 5:151–158.
55. Krasney JA, Curran-Everett DC, Iwamoto J. High altitude cerebral edema: an animal model. In: Sutton JR, Coates G, Remmers JE, eds. Hypoxia: the adaptations. Philadelphia: BC Dekker, 1990; 200–205.
56. Sutton JR, Bryan AC, Gray GW, et al. Pulmonary gas exchange in acute mountain sickness. Aviat Space Environ Med 1976; 47:1032–1037.
57. Anholm JD, Houston CS, Hyers TM. The relationship between acute mountain sickness and pulmonary ventilation at 2,835 meters (9,300 feet). Chest 1979; 75:33–36.
58. Hackett PH, Roach RC, Hartig GS, Greene ER, Levine BD. The effect of vasodilators on pulmonary hemodynamics in high altitude pulmonary edema: a comparison. Int J Sport Med 1992; 13:S68–S70.
59. Hultgren HN, Lopez CE, Lundberg E, Miller H. Physiologic studies of pulmonary edema at high altitude. Circulation 1964; 29:393–408.
60. Vock P, Brutsche MH, Nanzer A, Bärtsch P. Variable radiomorphologic data of high altitude pulmonary edema. Features from 60 patients. Chest 1991; 100:1306–1311.
61. Houston CS, Dickinson JG. Cerebral form of high altitude illness. Lancet 1975; 2:758–761.
62. Wilson R. Acute high altitude illness in mountaineers and problems of rescue. Ann Intern Med 1973; 78:421–427.
63. Kobayashi T, Koyama S, Kubo K, Fukushima M, Kusama S. Clinical features of patients with high altitude pulmonary edema in Japan. Chest 1987; 92:814–821.
64. Hackett PH, Yarnell PR, Hill R, Reynard K, Heit J, McCormick J. High altitude cerebral edema and MR imaging: clinical correlation and pathophysiology. JAMA 1997; in press.
65. Grissom CK, Roach RC, Sarnquist FH, Hackett PH. Acetazolamide in the treatment of acute mountain sickness: clinical efficacy and effect on gas exchange. Ann Intern Med 1992; 116:461–465.
66. Kamimori GH, Davis HQ, Ruocco M, Balkin TJ, Lawless N, Robles H. Effects of hypoxia (12% O_2) on cerebral edema and acute mountain sickness in men and women [abstract]. Med Sci Sport Exerc 28:S203, 1996.
67. Richalet JP, Hornych A, Rathat C, Aumont J, Larmignant P, Remy P. Plasma prostaglandins, leukotrienes and thromboxane in acute high altitude hypoxia. Respir Physiol 1991; 85:205–215.
68. Schoene RB, Swenson ER, Pizzo CJ, et al. The lung at high altitude: bronchoalveolar lavage in acute mountain sickness and pulmonary edema. J Appl Physiol 1988; 64:2605–2613.
69. Houston CS. Going higher: the story of man at high altitude. Boston: Little, Brown, 1987.
70. Larson EB, Roach RC, Schoene RB, Hornbein TF. Acute mountain sickness

and acetazolamide. Clinical efficacy and effect on ventilation. JAMA 1982; 288:328–332.

71. Levine BD, Yoshimura K, Kobayashi T, Fukushima M, Shibamoto T, Ueda G. Dexamethasone in the treatment of acute mountain sickness. N Engl J Med 1989; 321:1707–1713.
72. Bärtsch P, Maggiorini M, Ritter M, Noti C, Vock P, Oelz O. Prevention of high-altitude pulmonary edema by nifedipine. N Engl J Med 1991; 325: 1284–1289.
73. Kasic JF, Yaron M, Nicholas RA, Lickteig JA, Roach RC. Treatment of acute mountain sickness: hyperbaric versus oxygen therapy. Ann Emerg Med 1991; 20:1109–1112.
74. Hackett PH, Roach RC, Wood RA, et al. Dexamethasone for prevention and treatment of acute mountain sickness. Aviat Space Environ Med 1988; 59:950–954.
75. Oelz O, Maggiorini M, Ritter M, Noti C, Waber UV, Bärtsch P. Prevention and treatment of high altitude pulmonary edema by a calcium channel blocker. Int J Sport Med 1992; 13:S65–S67.
76. Hultgren HN. High altitude pulmonary edema. Adv Cardiol 1970; 5:24–31.
77. Scoggin CH, Hyers TM, Reeves JT, Grover RF. High altitude pulmonary edema in the children and young adults of Leadville, Colorado. N Engl J Med 1977; 297:1269–1273.
78. Roach RC, Houston CS, Honigman B, et al. How well do older persons tolerate moderate altitude? West J Med 1995; 162:32–36.
79. Graham WG, Houston CS. Short-term adaptation to moderate altitude. Patients with chronic obstructive pulmonary disease. JAMA 1978; 240: 1491–1494.
80. Levine BD, deFilippi CR, Zuckerman JH, McMinn SB, Beyer JR. High altitude exposure in the elderly [abstract]. In: Sutton JR, Coates G, Houston CS, eds. Hypoxia and molecular medicine. Burlington VT: Queen City Press, 1993.
81. Loeppky JA, Caprihan A, Luft UC. VA/Q inequality during clinical hypoxemia and its alterations. In: Shiraki K, Yousef MK, eds. Man in stressful environments. Springfield IL: CC Thomas, 1987; 199–232.
82. McFarland RA, Dill DB. A comparative study of the effects of reduced oxygen pressure on man during acclimatization. J Aviat Med 1938; 9:18–44.
83. Sutton JR, Reeves JT, Wagner PD, et al. Operation Everest II. Oxygen transport during exercise at extreme simulated altitude. J Appl Physiol 1988; 64:1309–1321.
84. Hurtado A. Animals in high altitudes: resident man. In: Dill DB, ed. Handbook of physiology: adaptation to the environment. Washington DC: American Physiological Society, 1964; 843–860.

17

The Role of Air Pollution in Exacerbating Exercise-Induced Asthma

David B. Peden
The University of North Carolina at Chapel Hill, Chapel Hill, North Carolina

I. INTRODUCTION

Air pollution is an important public health hazard, with a number of pollutants being monitored by the US Environmental Protection Agency (EPA), including total suspended particles, lead, carbon monoxide, nitrogen dioxide, sulfur dioxide, and ozone. Of these, ozone is likely the most frequently encountered pollutant, with over 50% of the population of the United States living in areas that exceed current National Ambient Air Quality Standards for ozone [1]. Of the pollutants currently regulated in the United States, ozone and sulfur dioxide have been the most extensively studied for their effect on lung function and bronchospasm. Acid aerosols, NO_2, and particulate matter may also influence lung function in asthmatics, but these effects have not been as extensively examined in controlled exposure studies of human volunteers [2]. Lead and carbon monoxide do not exert effects on airway function and are not likely to be a special risk for bronchospasm during exercise [2]. In general, the effect of air pollutants on lung function depends on the ambient concentration of the pollutant, the duration of pollutant exposure, and the total ventilation of exposed persons. Because exercise markedly increases ventilation, persons undergoing exercise in polluted environments are at increased risk for subsequent adverse effects on lung function.

According to recent estimates, 5–10% of the US population suffers from asthma. Asthmatics, even without pollutant exposure, often suffer increased bronchospasm as a consequence of exercise. Marked increases in asthma death and morbidity have been observed in the United States in recent years [3]. Epidemiological studies have demonstrated decrements in pulmonary function of both asthmatics and nonasthmatics associated with increased levels of ambient ozone [4–6]. Hospital admissions are also increased following increases in ambient ozone [4]. Sulfur dioxide is recognized to be a particularly potent inducer of bronchospasm in asthmatics [7–10]. Thus, those with asthma may be more susceptible to the effect of air pollution than those without, particularly when exercising. This chapter will review the effect of air pollutants on lung function during exercise, with emphasis on ozone and sulfur dioxide. Additional focus will be placed on lung function and inflammatory responses in persons with asthma following pollutant exposure.

II. OZONE

Ozone is the most significant component of photochemical smog, with over 50% of the US population living in regions that exceed the current National Ambient Air Quality Standard for this pollutant [1]. This standard allows exposure to no more than 0.12 ppm ozone averaged over 1 h on 1 day of the year. Although ozone levels have generally improved over the past decade, some cities still reach levels as high as 0.25 ppm at peak exposure times [1,8]. In the United States, the Los Angeles region has the highest levels of ozone as well as the greatest number of days in which the air standard is exceeded [1].

In persons without asthma, ozone causes a reproducible decrease of both forced vital capacity (FVC) and 1-s forced expiratory volume (FEV_1), increased nonspecific bronchial responsiveness, and substernal discomfort when taking a deep breath [11,12]. These effects are dependent on the concentration of ozone, duration of exposure, and the level of exercise (with corresponding increases in minute ventilation) [13]. Indeed, exposures to ozone without exercise generally reveal no effect on lung function at levels below 0.50 ppm [11,13]. With exercise, ozone induces increases in respiratory frequency, and the level of ozone required to cause decreases in FEV_1, FVC, airway resistance, and symptoms can be much lower [14].

The effect of exercise on pulmonary responses to ozone was initially reported by Bates et al. and Hazucha et al. [11,15]. Bates and colleagues demonstrated that mild, intermittent exercise sufficient to double resting ventilation over 2 hs markedly increased the effect of high levels of ozone on pulmonary function when compared with similar exposures performed without exercise [11]. The study by Hazucha and co-workers demonstrated that exposures to 0.37 and 0.75 ppm ozone caused a dose-related decrease in spirometric endpoints [15]. These studies were extended by others who revealed that, with low-intensity exercise, exposure to ozone at levels of 0.37, 0.50, and 0.75 ppm for 2 h caused decrements in lung function and increases in respiratory frequency that were dependent on the total effective dose of ozone, determined as the product of concentration, exposure time, and ventilation rate [16,17]. Thus, normal subjects experience reproducible impairment in lung function when confronted with ozone during exercise.

With more intense exercise, even smaller amounts of ozone may exert effects on lung function. Studies by several investigators examining the effect of ozone concentrations, ranging from 0.10 to 0.50 ppm, with varying levels of exercise, collectively demonstrate an effect of low levels of ozone when subjects perform heavier exercise, consistent with the observation that it is the total effective dose of ozone (concentration × time of exposure × ventilation rate) that determines the pulmonary response to this pollutant [13,18–21]. Dose–response studies by McDonnell et al. employing an alternating rest and exercise protocol over 2.5 h with a target ventilation rate of 67 L/min (normal resting ventilation being 15 L/min), at ozone concentrations of 0.12, 0.18, 0.24, 0.30, and 0.40 ppm, show that as little as 0.12 ppm ozone can cause significant decrements in FVC, FEV_1, and 25–50% forced expiratory flow (FEF25–75) [13]. Furthermore, FVC, FEV_1, FEF25–75 airway resistance, respiratory frequency, and symptoms, all were influenced in a concentration-dependent manner at levels over 0.24 ppm. Studies by others using comparable exercise regimens (ventilation rates of 68 and 70 L/min) confirm that ozone-induced changes in lung function occur at levels as low as 0.15 and 0.16 ppm [20,21].

Ozone also decreases exercise tolerance in well-trained athletes as well as in healthy subjects with average levels of fitness. Adams and Schelegle [22] reported that in ten trained distance runners, ozone levels of 0.20 and 0.35 ppm diminished both lung function and ability to perform exercise in a dose-dependent fashion. A second study by these investigators [23], involving a cohort of ten competitive cyclists, employed an exercise regimen of 30 min of moderate exercise (ventilation rate = 55 L/min) followed by 30 min of intense exercise (120 L/min) and ozone concentrations of 0.12, 0.18, and 0.24 ppm. Again, a dose-related effect of ozone on lung function and exercise tolerance was observed, with seven of the ten subjects failing to complete heavy exercise when exposed to 0.24 ppm [22,23].

Others have also examined the effect of ozone on lung function of exercising athletes. Foxcroft and Adams [24] reported that eight athletes subjected to 60 min of exercise (60 L/min) in 0.35 ppm ozone experienced decreases in FEV_1 and diminished exercise tolerance. Folinsbee et al. [25] demonstrated that exposure to 0.21 ppm ozone for 1 h, with an exercise ventilation rate of 90 L/min, caused a mean decrease in FEV_1 of 15% with a subjective assessment that exercise performance would be diminished in a cohort of seven competitive cyclists [25]. Ozone at a concentration of 0.18 also has a significant negative effect on lung function and endurance time in runners [23]. Gong et al. [26] examined the effect of 60-min exposures to 0.12 and 0.20 ppm ozone in 17 elite cyclists ventilating at a rate of 89 L/min and found minimally reduced FEV_1 with 0.12 ppm ozone, contrasted with a 22% decrease in FEV_1 after exposure to 0.20 ppm ozone [26]. The higher concentration also resulted in decreased exercise endurance time. Thus, persons vigorously exercising in ozone-enriched environments may be at substantially higher risk for impairment of lung function than those at rest or undergoing mild exercise.

Insight into possible mechanisms by which ozone exerts its effects has come from studies examining the effect of various pharmacological agents on respiratory responses to ozone. Beckett and colleagues [27] revealed that atropine inhibited ozone-induced decreases in airway resistance (although not spirometry), suggesting that vagally mediated influences on bronchial smooth muscle play a role in this response to ozone. An alternative possibility is that ozone causes direct increases in smooth-muscle sensitivity to acetylcholine. This idea is supported by the observation that sensitivity to inhaled methacholine, which may not require vagally mediated postganglionic release of acetylcholine to exert an effect on bronchial smooth muscle, is also increased by exposure to ozone [13,28,29].

In addition to cholinergically mediated responses, ozone may exert effects by cyclooxygenase-dependent mechanisms. Levels of prostaglandin E_2 (PGE_2; a cyclooxygenase pathway product) in bronchoalveolar lavage (BAL) fluid recovered from ozone-exposed individuals has been reported to have a positive correlation with their observed lung function decrements [30]. Additionally, cyclooxygenase inhibitors, such as ibuprofen and indomethacin, inhibit ozone-induced decreases in spirometry [31–34]. Interestingly, airway C fibers can be stimulated by PGE_2, suggesting that stimulation of bronchial C fibers, partly by arachidonic acid products, may also account for changes in lung function caused by ozone [35,36]. Animal studies in anesthetized dogs also suggest that ozone may act by C fiber-mediated mechanisms in the lung [36].

Lidocaine, when applied to the upper airway, also exerts a partial inhibition of ozone-induced decreases in spirometry. These results suggest that lidocaine-sensitive irritant receptors in the upper airway, when stimulated by ozone, exert a reflex-mediated decrease in inspiratory effort [2]. Other neurally mediated mechanisms involving effects on opiate receptors may also play a role in ozone-induced respiratory symptoms. This is supported by preliminary data in which sufentanyl (a short-acting narcotic) normalized lung function in subjects who have decreases in FVC and FEV_1 after ozone exposure [37]. Thus, those pain responses that are sensitive to opiates may partially account for the pulmonary response to ozone.

It would seem that alterations of β-adrenergic receptor function might also partially account for the effect of ozone. Beckett reported that β-adrenergic agonists did block ozone-induced bronchospasm. However, Gong and co-workers reported that albuterol has no effect on the deleterious effect of ozone on lung function [27,38]. Thus, the role of β-adrenergic receptors in the ozone response of normal subjects remains unclear.

Other studies of nonasthmatics have revealed that ozone causes neutrophilic inflammation of airways, as observed both in BAL fluid and in bronchial mucosal biopsy. Such inflammation has been observed after controlled exposures, ranging from 0.10 to 0.4 ppm ozone. Although the time course of ozone-induced inflammation has not been completely explored, neutrophil influx appears to be maximal between 1 and 6 h and persists to 18 h [39–43]. Other inflammatory changes occur as a result of ozone exposure, with increases in BAL levels of interleukin 6 (IL-6), PGE_2, leukotriene B_4 (LTB_4), thromboxane B_2 (TXB_2), fibronectin, plasminogen activator, and elastase having been reported [30]. In studies in which data are available 1 and 18 h after ozone exposure, changes in IL-6 and PGE_2 are maximal 1 h after exposure, whereas fibronectin and plasminogen activator are higher 18 h after exposure [30].

Studies of the effect of ibuprofen on BAL inflammatory endpoints demonstrate that ozone-induced increases in polymorphoneutrophils (PMNs), fibronectin, total protein, lactate dehydrogenase (LDH), LTB_4, and C3a were not inhibited, as were changes in IL-6, TXB_2, and PGE_2. It is notable that these subjects did have a blunted ozone effect on lung function following ibuprofen treatment, consistent with studies employing indomethacin [34]. Another preliminary study examining the effect of pretreatment with a combination of oral and inhaled glucocorticoids on ozone-induced changes in spirometry and lower airway inflammation shows that steroids have no significant effect on either PMN influx or lung function [44]. It is intriguing that oral glucocorticoids (in this case 40 mg of prednisone taken daily for 3 consecutive days before ozone exposure) which would logically cause decreased levels of arachidonic acid products by inhibition of phospholipase A_2 (PLA_2) had no effect on lung function. Taken together, these studies suggest that blockade of PLA_2 is not sufficient to inhibit ozone-induced changes in lung function. It is possible that, with ozone stimulation, arachidonic acid is released in a non–PLA_2-dependent fashion into the cytoplasm where it can be acted on by the cyclooxygenase cascade.

In vitro studies of epithelial cells or epithelial cell lines suggest possible mechanisms by which ozone may influence inflammation. Epithelial cell lines exposed to ozone generate the eicosanoids PGE_2, TXB_2, $PGF_{2\alpha}$, the proinflammatory cytokines interleukin (IL)-6 and IL-8, as well as the proinflammatory protein fibronectin. Nasal epithelial cells placed into culture respond to high-level (0.5 ppm) ozone by generating intracellular adhesion molecule-1 (ICAM-1), the major adhesion molecule for neutrophils and eosinophils in the airway, as well as the cytokines IL-1, IL-6, and tissue necrosis factor-α (TNF-α). Additionally, epithelial permeability in human subjects is increased after ozone exposure [45–47]. Thus, the effect of ozone on epithelial cells likely plays a major role in the inflammatory response to this pollutant, whereas neural responses (C fiber, pain fibers, and possibly cholinergic fibers) likely exert the major effect on lung function changes.

With the exception of PGE_2, none of the aforenoted markers of inflammation correlate with changes in lung function of normal subjects; nor has an association been made between ozone-induced inflammation and airway responsiveness in normal subjects. Thus, the clinical significance of ozone-induced inflammation in normal subjects remains unclear. It has been suggested that this proinflammatory effect of ozone could have a greater significance in asthma, a disorder partly characterized by an eosinophilic inflammation of the lower airways.

A number of epidemiologic studies suggest that increased ambient ozone is linked to asthma exacerbation [6]. Bates and Sizto examined hospital admission rates for asthma over a summer season and found a significant correlation between asthma admissions and increased ambient ozone and sulfate levels from the previous day [48]. The time lag between ozone exposure and increased evidence of disease exacerbation suggests that inflammatory changes, rather than immediate decreases in FVC, account for lung function changes in both normal subjects and asthmatics. An alternative possibility is that ozone primes the bronchial airways of asthmatics for increased responses to subsequently encountered allergens. The mechanisms by which ozone influences asthma are better addressed in controlled exposure studies.

Initial controlled exposure studies of asthmatics with mild disease found little increased sensitivity of these subjects to ozone above that of nonasthmatic subjects at concentrations of 0.25 ppm or less, employing exposure protocols that involved little or no exercise [49]. However, it is possible that experiments employing low levels of exercise likely underestimate the effect of ozone in asthma. Indeed, Kriet and co-workers have demonstrated that, with more rigorous exercise (ventilation of 30 L min^{-1} m^{-2}), exposure to 0.4 ppm ozone for 2 h causes greater changes in airway resistance of asthmatics than normal individuals [50]. Nonspecific airway hyperresponsiveness was also enhanced in asthmatic subjects after ozone exposure. Silverman et al. [49] also demonstrated that exposure to 0.25 ppm ozone for 2 h resulted in decreased pulmonary function in asthmatic subjects. Other studies indicate that ozone not only causes the well-described decrease in FVC, but also causes true bronchospasm in persons with asthma [50–52]. Thus, ozone has been demonstrated to have a direct effect on the impaired airflow in asthma.

However, although exposures employing exercise may result in true bronchospasm in persons with asthma beyond that of the baseline ozone effect observed in normal subjects, recent studies [53,54] have shown that ozone exposure before exercise exerts no effect on subsequent exercise-induced bronchospasm (EIB). This was studied by Weymer and colleagues [54], who exposed a cohort of mild asthmatics with EIB to 0.0, 0.1, 0.25, and 0.40 ppm ozone for 1 h with mild exercise (enough to result in V_E of 20–30 L min^{-1}). One hour later, an exercise challenge was then performed if the FEV_1 was back to 90% of preexposure baseline. Even though there was a dose-dependent effect of ozone exposure on both lung function and subjective symptom scores immediately after exposure, the resultant EIB was no greater after exposure to any ozone concentration than that which occurred following a control exposure to clean air. A separate study, examining the effect of exposure to 0.12 ppm ozone at rest for 1 h in asthmatics with EIB, also revealed no exacerbation of EIB attributable to ozone [53].

Ozone may also affect allergic asthmatic persons by augmenting airway responses to subsequently encountered allergens. This may be of special importance to those who may encounter both airborne allergens and ozone during exercise. Molfino and colleagues [55] examined seven seasonally allergic asthmatic patients after exposure to 0.12 ppm ozone at rest for 1 h and subsequent challenge with inhaled allergen. Six of the seven subjects required less inhaled allergen to induce a 15% decrease in FEV_1 after an ozone exposure than after a clean air exposure. However, a recent attempt to replicate this study, which enrolled 12 subjects, did not demonstrate an effect of this level of ozone exposure on responses to inhaled allergen [56].

Another study [57] describes increased sensitivity of 18 of 23 mild asthmatics to inhaled allergen after exposure to 0.25 ppm ozone for 3 h with intermittent exercise. Smaller changes were also noted in 11 subjects with allergic rhinitis. Both groups, as well as a cohort of normal subjects, had equivalent changes in methacholine responsiveness and lung function. Thus, asthmatic subjects were again shown to experience increased sensitivity to inhaled allergen after exposure to ozone. Examination of allergen-induced nasal inflammation in asthma reveals that ozone augments the late-phase eosinophilic response to allergen [58]. Taken together, these findings suggest that the effect of ozone exposure on classic allergen-induced bronchoconstriction may be more significant than the direct effect of ozone in persons with asthma. It is less clear what level of ozone is required to exert deleterious effects on lung function of these individuals.

Ozone induces an influx of neutrophils and increases in other inflammatory mediators in nonasthmatic subjects, suggesting a proinflammatory effect of this pollutant. In asthma, airway inflammation is characterized by mast cells and eosinophils and also involves other inflammatory cells, such as neutrophils. Such inflammation has been associated with increased disease severity as well as increased bronchial sensitivity to both nonspecific stimuli (methacholine, histamine, and cold, dry air) and specific allergen to which an asthmatic is already sensitized. Ozone has been reported to enhance nonspecific and specific allergic bronchial reactivity. It has been argued that in asthma, such changes may be due to increased airway inflammation.

To date, there are few studies that have examined the effect of ozone exposure on bronchial inflammation in allergic or asthmatic subjects. Nasal studies of subjects with allergic rhinitis and asthma suggest that ozone may induce eosinophilic influx onto airway mucosal surface. Bascom et al. [59] have reported that subjects with allergic rhinitis have increased nasal eosinophils after exposure to 0.5 ppm ozone for 4 h without exercise. However, allergen-induced eosinophil influx was not changed after ozone exposure. In asthmatics, ozone (0.4 ppm for 2 h without exercise) again induced nasal eosinophil influx [58]. Unlike those with allergic rhinitis, asthmatics also had enhanced numbers of eosinophils and eosinophil cationic protein following allergen challenge when allergen challenge was preceded by ozone exposure.

In two studies examining bronchial inflammation in asthmatics following ozone exposure, little effect on the number of eosinophils recovered in BAL fluid was observed. However, these samples did reveal a greater neutrophil influx into the lower airways of asthmatic subjects than that observed in BAL from normal volunteers following ozone exposure [60,63]. Taken together, these data suggest that ozone exposure enhances airway inflammation in persons with asthma, perhaps to a greater extent than in those without. Such changes could account for some of the effects of ozone in asthma. However, one must be cautious in concluding that ozone-induced inflammation causes increased bronchial reactivity and bronchospasm in asthma, because such a relation has not been found in nonasthmatic subjects.

III. SULFUR DIOXIDE

Sulfur dioxide (SO_2) is released into the atmosphere primarily as a result of industrial combustion of high–sulfur-containing coal and oil. Common sources of SO_2 include paper, steel, and cement manufacturing plants. Controlled exposure studies clearly reveal the ability of SO_2 to induce exacerbations of asthma. Whereas controlled exposure studies fail to demonstrate an effect of SO_2 on pulmonary function of normal subjects at levels as high as 0.6 ppm, several investigators have demonstrated bronchoconstriction in asthmatic patients at concentrations as low as 0.25 ppm [62–68].

Unlike other pollutants, SO_2 exerts a rapid effect on lung function of asthmatic patients with significant responses occurring within 2 min and maximal response noted in 5–10 min. Spontaneous recovery has been reported as soon as 30 min after challenge, with a refractory period of up to 4 h. Repeated exposure to low levels of SO_2 results in tolerance to subsequent exposure. In one study, repeated exercise during an SO_2 exposure resulted in diminished airway responsiveness to SO_2. However, initial responsiveness was restored within 6 h after exposure was complete [69–72].

Responses to SO_2 include decreases in FEV_1 and increases in airway resistance. Decreases in FEV_1 as high as 60% have been observed after exposure to SO_2. Persons with asthma have a modest variation in sensitivity to SO_2, with some experiencing lung function decrements at levels of 0.25, whereas others have no response at levels of 2.0 ppm. However, levels higher than 0.50 ppm will usually induce bronchospasm in asthmatics. Exercise augments bronchial responses to SO_2, with the combined effect of exercise and SO_2 being additive in those with asthma. Symptoms associated with SO_2 inhalation include wheezing, chest discomfort, and dyspnea.

Interestingly, nasal breathing greatly protects against the effect of SO_2 on pulmonary function because this highly water-soluble gas is absorbed very efficiently by the nasal mucosa. This feature of SO_2 may explain why exercise increases the effect of this gas, as most persons shift from strictly nasal breathing to oronasal respiration with exercise sufficient to cause a ventilation rate of 35 L min^{-1}. However, even with heavy exercise, up to 60% of inspired air passes by the nasal mucosa. This may be important because asthmatics frequently suffer from allergic rhinitis or sinusitis, both of which cause decreased nasal airflow and increased oral breathing, increasing the percentage of inspired air that is not exposed to nasal tissue [73].

Several pharmacological agents attenuate the effect of SO_2 in asthma, including β-agonists, antimuscarinic agents, cromolyn sodium, and necdromil. Indeed, β-agonists have the most potent effect in mitigating SO_2-induced bronchospasm. Interestingly, prolonged use of methyl xanthines and inhaled corticosteroids as well as brief use of antihistamines have not affected the sensitivity of asthmatics to SO_2. Many investigators currently believe that SO_2 acts as a nonspecific bronchoconstricting agent, analogous with the action of inhaled histamine and methacholine, other agents to which asthmatic patients have increased sensitivity over normal subjects [74,75].

These pharmacological studies, coupled with those demonstrating development of tolerance to SO_2, the rapid onset of bronchoconstriction after exposure, and increased sensitivity of asthmatics to SO_2 when compared with nonasthmatics, suggest a cholinergically mediated neural mechanism of action for SO_2. However, recent observations [76] demonstrate that very mild airway inflammation may also be induced by SO_2 exposure. Thus, the mechanisms by which SO_2 may influence asthma remain incompletely explained.

Sulfur dioxide exposure also augments responses to other environmental agents that exacerbate bronchospasm. Exposure to ozone before exposure to SO_2 increases bronchial sensitivity to SO_2 in asthmatics [77]. Exposure to cold, dry air also exacerbates the bronchospastic effect of SO_2 in asthmatics [71]. However, unlike ozone, SO_2 exposure has not exacerbated allergen-induced bronchospasm. The question of whether there is a relation between sensitivity to SO_2 and asthma severity has not been resolved, although some studies suggest that SO_2 causes similar effects in mild and moderate asthma.

IV. OTHER POLLUTANTS

Other pollutants, although less potent relative to bronchospasm than sulfur dioxide or ozone, could also cause decreases in lung function and consequently pose a risk to persons with asthma or others involved in exercise. Nitrogen dioxide (NO_2), a precursor of photochemical smog, is found in ambient outdoor air in urban and industrial regions and, in conjunction with sunlight and hydrocarbons, results in the production of ozone. Automobile exhaust is the most significant source for outdoor NO_2, although power plants and other industrial sources that burn fossil fuels also release it into the environment. However, the most significant exposure to NO_2 occurs indoors in conjunction with the use of gas-cooking stoves and kerosene space heaters.

Controlled chamber studies reveal no consistent effect of NO_2 on airway function of either normal subjects or those with asthma. Some investigators report that low levels of NO_2 induce increased airway reactivity to pharmacological or cold air challenge in asthmatics, but others find no such effect on methacholine reactivity in another cohort of asthmatic subjects [62,71,78–80]. Higher levels of NO_2 (4.0 ppm) have been reported to alter airway function in asthma. The mechanism by which NO_2 may alter airway function is also unclear. In studies of normal subjects, NO_2 was much less potent than ozone in inducing airway PMN influx [81]. NO_2 increases proinflammatory cytokine production in epithelial cells after in vitro pollutant exposure [82]. Overall, these data suggest that NO_2 could influence airway function of asthmatic patients and demonstrate the need for more research on the effect of NO_2 in asthma.

Acid aerosols may also have an effect on lung function. Epidemiological studies suggest that asthmatic symptoms are increased on days in which increased levels of aerosolized acid are observed [48,83]. Acid (H^+) concentrations of over 100 mmol m^{-3} (5 $\mu g\ mL^{-1}$ H_2SO_4 equivalent) have been observed over 24-h periods, and 12-h concentrations over 500 nmol m^{-3} (25 $\mu\ mL^{-1}$ H_2SO_4 equivalent) have been observed. Repeated studies in normal adults demonstrate that brief exposure to H_2SO_4 as high as 2000 $\mu g\ m^{-3}$ for 1 h does not cause decreases in lung function [62,71,83]. However, some controlled exposure studies of acid aerosols indicate that asthmatics may be more sensitive than nonasthmatics to the bronchocontrictive effect of such exposure [10,84]. This may be particularly true for adolescents with asthma, who have had some lung function decrements at acid levels as low as 100 $\mu g\ m^{-3}$ and appear to be more sensitive that adult asthmatics to acid aerosol. However, substantial controversy exists over the significance of acid aerosol exposure on lung function of asthma.

High levels of oral respiratory ammonia may counter the effect of inhaled acid aerosols owing to the resulting formation of NH_4 salts, which are much less effective in causing changes in lung function [83,85]. One explanation for the difficulty in establishing a dose range for the effect of acid on lung function may lie in differences in experimental techniques that could allow different exposure of the inhaled acids to oral NH_3. Additionally, inhaled acids are buffered in the airway fluids as well as by oral NH_3, also adding to potential differences between these studies. However, in studies of nonasthmatics in whom efforts to minimize the action of oral NH_3 on inhaled acid were employed, little difference was seen in the effect of inhaled acid on lung function. In studies of asthmatic subjects, it has been suggested that the effect of inhaled aerosolized acid on lung function may roughly correlate with baseline levels of airway hyperresponsiveness.

Combinations of acid aerosols and ozone may be more significant than the effect of acid alone. One report indicated mildly enhanced decreases in lung function and increased airway reactivity in asthmatics exposed to 0.12 ppm ozone and 100 $\mu g\ m^{-3}$ H_2SO_4 when compared with the effect of ozone alone; H_2SO_4 alone had no effect on lung function of these subjects. Exposures occurred over 6.5 h with exercise such that ventilation was 29 L min^{-1}. However, other studies examining the effect of combined exposures of ozone, H_2SO_4, or HNO_3 have shown no effect of acid aerosols on lung function of asthmatics, either alone or in combination with ozone [9,77,86,87].

Recent studies of particulate matter smaller than 10 mm (PM10; that which can be deposited in the lower airway) indicate that ambient exposure to such particles may be a very underappreciated factor in exacerbation of respiratory disease. Examination of data from Stubenville, Ohio, collected over an 11-year period, revealed a relation between increased daily mortality and increased particulate levels occurring the previous day [88]. A similar examination of mortality rates and particulate exposure in Philadelphia revealed increased respiratory and cardiovascular deaths associated with increased ambient particulate levels on the preceding day [89]. Increased requirement for asthma medication in a cohort of asthmatics in Utah was correlated with increased particulate levels [90,91]. Another study in the Seattle area also suggests that hospitalization because of increased asthma morbidity occurs in conjunction with increases in airborne particulate matter [92]. These data demonstrate the important role that particulates could play in asthma morbidity.

The current data on the effect of particulate matter is based on only particle size. It is likely that the chemical and biological character of these particulates is a key factor in their effect in the airway. Studies of normal human volunteers show neutrophil influx 48 h after instillation of inert particles into the lower airway [93]. These data suggest that particles may enhance inflammation of the bronchial mucosa. However, other more biologically active particles could have a greater effect in asthma. Data on the effect of nonacid particulate matter on lung function of either normal or asthmatic subjects is currently lacking and further study of the effect of particulate matter on lung function of persons who are asthmatic, especially when exercising, is needed to clearly establish the risk to asthmatics from this pollutant.

V. SUMMARY

Air pollution is a significant problem in the United States, with certain pollutants, such as ozone and sulfur dioxide, clearly having marked effects on lung function that are exacerbated by exercise. Additionally, other pollutants, such as NO_2, PM10, and acid-aerosols, are also likely to influence lung function. As with ozone, the effect of these pollutants will likely be increased by exercise. The effect of pollutants on lung function, with subsequent influence on performance, is likely to be greater in persons with asthma than on those without. Because asthma is an inflammatory disease and airway responses to allergen are mediated largely through increases in mucosal inflammation, it is especially important to determine how pollutants influence baseline airway inflammation in asthma. Extrapolation of data from normal subjects is not adequate because asthma is characterized by an eosinophilic inflammation that does not occur in normal subjects. Other mechanisms by which pollutants may act, including stimulation of neurally mediated airway reflexes, also need to be fully investigated.

If possible, exercise should be avoided when conditions favorable for increased ambient pollutant exposure are present. Areas in which large amounts of automobile exhaust remain trapped in the atmosphere and are acted on by UV light will likely have elevated levels of ozone and NO_2. This is especially likely in valleys in which air inversions are possible. In areas such as Los Angeles, peak ozone levels are reported in the late morning through the afternoon. Areas in which coal-burning industries are prevalent, usually found in large metropolitan areas in the northeastern regions of the United States, are more likely to have increased levels of sulfur dioxide and particulate matter.

However, when pollutant avoidance is not possible, certain currently available medications may be useful in preventing adverse effects on lung function. Anticholinergics may be useful in mitigating the effects of ozone, and β-agonists, anticholergics, and cromolyn attenuate the effects of SO_2 in asthma. Of note, corticosteroids do not protect specifically against the effects of either ozone or SO_2 in either asthmatics or nonasthmatics. However, use of such medications should not be discontinued when used for other indications, including treatment of moderate or severe chronic asthma or a marked exacerbation of asthma. Lack of understanding of the mechanisms by which other pollutants (acid aerosols, particulate matter, or NO_2) influence lung function preclude any rational recommendation for prophylactic intervention strategies other than avoidance of these agents.

REFERENCES

1. Gong H, Linn WS. What we don't understand about ozone effects. Chest 1995; 107:594–595.
2. Folinsbee LJ. Human health effects of air pollution. Environ Health Perspect 1993; 100:45–56.
3. Woolcock AJ. Epidemiology of asthma. Am Rev Respir Dis 1992; 1465: 1358–1359.
4. Bates DV. Sizto R. Air pollution and hospital admissions in Southern Ontario: the acid summer haze effect. Environ Res 1987; 43:317–331.
5. Ostro BD, Lipsett MJ, Mann JK, et al. Air pollution and respiratory morbidity among adults in Southern California. Am J Epidemiol 1993; 137:691–700.
6. Balmes JR. The role of ozone exposure in the epidemiology of asthma. Environ Health Perspect 1993; 101:219–224.
7. Koenig JQ, Morgan MS, Horike M, et al. The effects of sulfur oxides on nasal and lung function in adolescents with extrinsic asthma. J Allergy Clin Immunol 1985; 76:813–818.
8. Pierson WE, Koenig JQ. Respiratory effects of air pollution on allergic disease. J Allergy Clin Immunol 1992; 90:557–566.
9. Koenig JQ, Pierson WE. Air pollutants and the respiratory system: toxicity and pharmacologic interventions. Clin Toxicol 1991; 29:401–411.
10. Koenig JQ, Pierson WE, Korike M. The effects of inhaled sulfuric acid on pulmonary function in adolescent asthmatics. Am Rev Respir Dis 1983; 128: 221–225.
11. Bates DV, Hazucha MJ. The short-term effects of ozone on the human lung. US Government Printing Office 1973; 93–15:507–540.
12. Hazucha MJ, Bates DV. Combined effect of ozone and sulphur dioxide on human pulmonary function. Nature 1975; 257:50–51.
13. McDonnell WF, Horstman DH, Hazucha MJ, et al. Pulmonary effects of ozone exposure during exercise: dose–response characteristics. J Appl Physiol Respir Environ Exerc Physiol 1983; 54:1345–1352.
14. McDonnell WF, Kehrl HR, Abdul Salaam S, et al. Respiratory response of humans exposed to low levels of ozone for 6.6 hours. Arch Environ Health 1991; 46:145–150.
15. Hazucha MJ, Silverman F, Parent C, et al. Pulmonary function in man after short-term exposure to ozone. Arch Environ Health 1973; 27:183–188.
16. Silverman F, Folinsbee LJ, Barnard J, et al. Pulmonary function changes in

ozone—interaction of concentration and ventilation. J Appl Physiol Respir Environ Exerc Physiol 1976; 41:859–864.
17. Folinsbee LJ, Silverman F, Shephard RJ. Exercise responses following ozone exposure. J Appl Physiol Respir Environ Exerc Physiol 1975; 38: 996–1001.
18. Adams WC, Savin WM, Christo AE. Detection of ozone toxicity during continuous exercise via the effective dose concept. J Appl Physiol Respir Environ Exerc Physiol 1981; 51:415–422.
19. Folinsbee LJ, Drinkwater BL, Bedi JB, et al. The influence of exercise on the pulmonary function changes due to exposure to low concentrations of ozone. Environ Stress 1978; pp 125–145.
20. Kulle TJ, Sauder LR, Hebel JR, et al. Ozone response relationships in healthy nonsmokers. Am Rev Respir Dis 1985; 132:36–41.
21. Linn WS, Avol EL, Shamoo DA, et al. A dose–response study of healthy, heavily exercising men exposed to ozone at concentrations near the ambient air quality standard. Toxicol Ind Health 1986; 2:99–112.
22. Adams WC, Schelegle ES. Ozone and high ventilation effects on pulmonary function and endurance performance. J Appl Physiol Respir Environ Exerc Physiol 1983; 55:805–812.
23. Schelegle ES, Adams WC. Reduced exercise time in competitive simulations consequent to low level ozone exposure. Med Sci Sports Exerc 1986; 18: 408–414.
24. Foxcroft WJ, Adams WC. Effects of ozone exposure on four consecutive days on work performance and VO_2max. J Appl Physiol Respir Environ Exerc Physiol 1986; 61:960–966.
25. Folinsbee LJ, Bedi JF, Horvath SM. Pulmonary function changes after 1 h continuous heavy exercise in 0.21 ppm ozone. J Appl Physiol Respir Environ Exerc Physiol 1984; 57:984–988.
26. Gong H Jr, Bradley PW, Simmons MS, et al. Impaired exercise performance and pulmonary function in elite cyclists during low-level ozone exposure in a hot environment. Am Rev Respir Dis 1986; 134:726–733.
27. Beckett WS, McDonnell WF, Horstman DH, et al. Role of the parasympathetic nervous system in acute lung response to ozone. J Appl Physiol Respir Environ Exerc Physiol 1985; 59:1879–1885.
28. Holtzman MJ, Fabbri LM, O'Byrne PM, et al. Importance of airway inflammation for hyperresponsiveness induced by ozone. Am Rev Respir Dis 1983; 127:686–690.
29. Folinsbee LJ, Horstman DH, Kehrl HR, et al. Respiratory responses to repeated prolonged exposure to 0.12 ppm ozone. Am J Respir Crit Care Med 1994; 149:98–105.
30. Koren HS, Devlin RB, Becker S, et al. Time-dependent changes of markers associated with inflammation in the lungs of humans exposed to ambient levels of ozone. Toxicol Pathol 1991; 19:406–411.
31. Ying RL, Gross KB, Terzo TS, et al. Indomethacin does not inhibit the ozone-induced increase in bronchial responsiveness in human subjects. Am Rev Respir Dis 1990; 142:817–821.

32. Schelegle ES, Adams WC, Siefkin AD. Indomethacin pretreatment reduces ozone-induced pulmonary function decrements in human subjects. Am Rev Respir Dis 1987; 136:1350–1354.
33. Eschenbacher WL, Ying RL, Kreit JW, et al. Ozone-induced lung function changes in normal and asthmatic subjects and the effect of indomethacin. Atmos Ozone Res Policy Implications 1989; pp. 493–499.
34. Hazucha MJ, Madden MC, Pape C, et al. Effects of cyclooxygenase inhibition on ozone-induced respiratory inflammation and lung function changes. Eur J Appl Physiol 73:17–27, 1996.
35. Coleridge HM, Coleridge JCG, Ginzel KH, et al. Stimulation of "irritant" receptors and afferent C-fibers in the lungs by prostaglandins. Nature 1976; 264:451–453.
36. Coleridge JCG, Coleridge HM, Schelegle ES, et al. Acute inhalation of ozone stimulates bronchial C-fibers and rapidly adapting receptors in dogs. J Appl Physiol 1993; 74:2345–2352.
37. Passannante A, Hazucha MJ, Seal E, et al. Nociceptive mechanisms modulate ozone-induced human lung function decrements [abstract]. Anesth Analg 1995; 80:S371.
38. Gong H Jr, Bedi JF, Horvath SM. Inhaled albuterol does not protect against ozone toxicity in nonasthmatic athletes. Arch Environ Health 1988; 43: 46–53.
39. Aris RM, Christian D, Hearne PQ, et al. Ozone-induced airway inflammation in human subjects as determined by airway lavage and biopsy. Am Rev Respir Dis 1993; 148:1363–1372.
40. Koren HS, Devlin RB, Graham DE, et al. Ozone-induced inflammation in the lower airways of human subjects. Am Rev Respir Dis 1989; 139:407–415.
41. Schelegle ES, Siefkin AD, McDonald RJ. Time course of ozone-induced neutrophilia in normal humans. Am Rev Respir Dis 1991; 143:1353–1358.
42. Devlin RB, McDonnell WF, Mann R, et al. Exposure of humans to ambient levels of ozone for 6.6 hours causes cellular and biochemical changes in the lung. Am J Respir Cell Mol Biol 1991; 4:72–81.
43. Seltzer J, Bigby BG, Stulbarg M, et al. O_3-induced change in bronchial reactivity to methacholine and airway inflammation in humans. J Appl Physil 1986; 60:1321–1326.
44. Bottei GM, Devlin RB, Bromberg PA, et al. The effect of corticosteroids on lower airway inflammation and pulmonary function after ozone exposure [abstract]. Am J Respir Crit Care Med 1995; 151:A29.
45. McKinnon KP, Noah T, Madden M, et al. Cultured human bronchial epithelial cells release cytokines, fibronectin, and lipids in response to ozone exposure. Chest 1992; 101:22S.
46. McKinnon KP, Madden MC, Noah TL, et al. In vitro ozone exposure increases release of arachidonic acid products from a human bronchial epithelial cell line. Toxicol Appl Pharmacol 1993; 118:215–223.
47. Beck NB, Koenig JQ, Luchtel DL, et al. Ozone can increase the expression of intercellular adhesion molecule-1 and the synthesis of cytokines by human nasal epithelial cells. Inhalation Toxicol 1994; 6:345–357.

48. Bates DV, Sizto R. Relationship between air pollutant levels and hospital admissions in Southern Ontario. Can J Public Health 1983; 74:117–122.
49. Silverman F. Asthma and respiratory irritants (ozone). Environ Health Perspect 1979; 29:131–136.
50. Kreit JW, Gross KB, Moore TB, et al. Ozone-induced changes in pulmonary function and bronchial responsiveness in asthmatics. J Appl Physiol Respir Environ Exerc Physiol 1989; 66:217–222.
51. Ball B, Horstman D, Folinsbee L, et al. Pulmonary responses in asthmatics performing light exercise in clean air (air) and 0.16 ppm ozone (O_3) [abstract]. Am J Respir Crit Care Med 1993; 147:A640.
52. Horstman D, Roger LJ, McDonnell W, et al. Increased specific airway resistance (SRaw) in asthmatics exercising while exposed to 0.18 ppm ozone (O_3). Physilogist 1984; 27:212.
53. Fernandes ALG, Molfino NA, McClean PA, et al. The effect of pre-exposure to 0.12 ppm of ozone on exercise-induced asthma. Chest 1994; 106: 1077–1082.
54. Weymer AR, Gong H, Lyness A, et al. Pre-exposure to ozone does not enhance or produce exercise-induced asthma. Am J Respir Crit Care Med 1994; 149:1413–1419.
55. Molfino NA, Wright SC, Katz I, et al. Effect of low concentrations of ozone on inhaled allergen responses in asthmatic subjects. Lancet 1991; 338: 199–203.
56. Ball BA, Folinsbee LJ, Peden DB, et al. Response to allergen bronchoprovocation of mild allergic asthmatics following low level ozone exposure [abstract]. Am J Respir Crit Care Med 1995; 151:A27.
57. Jorres R, Nowak D, Magnussen H. The effect of ozone exposure on allergen responsiveness in subjects with asthma or rhinitis. Am J Respir Crit Care Med 1996; 153:56–64.
58. Peden DB, Setzer RW Jr, Devlin RB. Ozone exposure has both a priming effect on allergen-induced responses and an intrinsic inflammatory action in the airways of perennially allergic asthmatics. Am J Respir Crit Care Med 1995; 151:1336–1345.
59. Bascom R, Naclerio RM, Fitzgerald TK, et al. Effect of ozone inhalation on the response to nasal challenge with antigen of allergic subjects. Am Rev Respir Dis 1990; 142:594–601.
60. Basha MA, Gross KB, Gwizdala CJ, et al. Bronchoalveolar lavage neutrophilia in asthmatic and healthy volunteers after controlled exposure to ozone and filtered purified air. Chest 1994; 106:1757–1765.
61. Scannell CH, Chen LL, Tager I, et al. Ozone-induced pulmonary function changes and airway inflammation in asthmatic and non-asthmatic subjects [abstract]. Am J Respir Crit Care Med 1995; 151:A28.
62. Molfino NA. Effect of air pollution on atopic asthma. Medicina 1992; 52: 363–367.
63. Boushey HA. Bronchial hyperreactivity to sulfur dioxide: physiologic and political implications. J Allergy Clin Immunol 1982; 69:335–338.

64. Witek TJ, Schachter EN. Airway responses to sulfur dioxide and methacholine in asthmatics. J Occup Med 1985; 27:265–268.
65. Hackney JD, Linn WS, Bailey RM, et al. Time course of exercise-induced bronchoconstriction in asthmatics exposed to sulfur dioxide. Environ Res 1984; 34:321–327.
66. Horstman D, Roger LJ, Kehrl H, et al. Airway sensitivity of asthmatics to sulfur dioxide. Toxicol Ind Health 1986; 2:289–298.
67. Kehrl HR, Roger LJ, Hazucha MJ, et al. Differing response of asthmatics to sulfur dioxide exposure with continuous and intermittent exercise. Am Rev Respir Dis 1987; 135:350–355.
68. Folinsbee LJ, Bedi JF, Horvath SM. Pulmonary response to threshold levels of sulfur dioxide (1.0 ppm) and ozone (0.3 ppm). J Appl Physiol Respir Environ Exerc Physiol 1985; 58:1783–1787.
69. Roger LJ, Kehrl HR, Hazucha MJ, et al. Bronchoconstriction in asthmatics exposed to sulfur dioxide during repeated exercise. J Appl Physiol Respir Environ Exerc Physiol 1985; 59:784–791.
70. Horstman DH, Seal E Jr, Folinsbee LJ, et al. The relationship between exposure duration and sulfur dioxide-induced bronchoconstriction in asthmatic subjects. Am Ind Hyg Assoc J 1988; 49:38–47.
71. Pierson WE, Koenig JQ. Respiratory effects of air pollution on allergic disease. J Allergy Clin Immunol 1992; 90:557–566.
72. Gong H Jr. Health effects of air pollution. A review of clinical studies. Clin Chest Med 1992; 13:201–214.
73. Linn WS, Shamoo DA, Spier CE, et al. Respiratory effects of 0.75 ppm sulfur dioxide in exercising asthmatics: influence of upper-respiratory defenses. Environ Res 1983; 30:340–348.
74. Heath SK, Koenig JQ, Morgan MS, et al. Effects of sulfur dioxide exposure on African–American and Caucasian asthmatics. Environ Res 1994; 66:1–11.
75. Bigby B, Boushey H. Effects of nedocromil sodium on the bronchomotor response to sulfur dioxide in asthmatic patients. J Allergy Clin Immunol 1993; 92:195–197.
76. Sandstrom T, Stjernberg N, Andersson M. Cell response in bronchoalveolar fluid after exposure to sulfur dioxide: a time response study. Am Rev Respir Dis 1989; 140:1828–1831.
77. Koenig JQ, Covert DS, Hanley QS, et al. Prior exposure to ozone potentiates subsequent response to sulfur dioxide in adolescent asthmatic subjects. Am Rev Respir Dis 1990; 141:377–380.
78. Bauer MA, Utell MJ, Morrow PE, et al. Inhalation of 0.30 ppm nitrogen dioxide potentiates exercise-induced bronchospasm in asthmatics. Am Rev Respir Dis 1986; 134:1203–1208.
79. Linn WS, Shamoo DA, Spier CE, et al. Controlled exposure of volunteers with chronic obstructive pulmonary disease to nitrogen dioxide. Arch Environ Health 1985; 40:313–317.
80. Anto JM, Sunyer J. Nitrogen dioxide and allergic asthma: starting to clarify an obscure association. Lancet 1995; 345:402–403.

81. Sandstrom T, Stjernberg N, Eklund A, et al. Inflammatory cell response in bronchoalveolar lavage fluid after nitrogen dioxide exposure of healthy subjects—a dose–response study. Eur Respir J 1991; 4:332–333.
82. Devalia JL, Campbell AM, Sapsford RJ, et al. Effect of nitrogen dioxide on synthesis on inflammatory cytokines expressed by human bronchial epithelial cells in vitro. Am J Respir Cell Mol Biol 1993; 9:271–278.
83. Bates DV, Utell MJ, Dockery DW, et al. Health effects of atmospheric acids and their precursors: report of the ATS workshop on the health effects of atmospheric acids and their precursors. Am Rev Respir Dis 1991; 144: 464–467.
84. Utell MJ, Morrow PE, Speers DM, et al. Airway responses to sulfate and sulfuric acid aerosols in asthmatics. Am Rev Respir Dis 1983; 128:444–450.
85. Utell MJ, Margiglio JA, Morrow PE, et al. Effects of inhaled acid aerosols on respiratory function: the role of endogenous ammonia. J Aerosol Med 1989; 2:141–147.
86. Aris R, Christian D, Sheppard D, et al. Lack of bronchoconstrictor response to sulfuric acid aerosols and fogs. Am Rev Respir Dis 1991; 143:744–750.
87. Koenig JQ, Covert DS, Pierson WE. Effects of inhalation of acidic compounds on pulmonary function in allergic adolescent subjects. Environ Health Perspect 1989; 79:173–178.
88. Schwartz J, Dockery D. Particulate air pollution and daily mortality in Steubenville, Ohio. Am J Epidemiol 1992; 135:12–19.
89. Schwartz J, Dockery DW. Increased mortality in Philadelphia associated with daily air pollution concentrations. Am Rev Respir Dis 1992; 145: 600–604.
90. Pope CA, Dockery DW, Schwartz J. Review of epidemiological evidence of health effects of particulate air pollution. Inhalation Toxicol 1995; 7:1–18.
91. Pope CA III. Respiratory illness associated with community air pollution in Utah, Salt Lake and Cache Valleys. Arch Environ Health 1991; 46:90–97.
92. Schwartz J, Slater D, Larson TV, et al. Particulate air pollution and hospital emergency room visits for asthma in Seattle. Am Rev Respir Dis 1993; 147: 826–831.
93. Lay JC, Bennett WD, Bromberg PA, et al. Particle instillation in human lungs: a method for measuring lung response to inert particles. Inhal Toxicol 1995; 7:819.

18

Scuba Diving: Asthma and Respiratory Diseases

Frank J. Twarog
Harvard Medical School, Boston, Massachusetts

I. BACKGROUND

Scuba diving is an increasingly popular leisure sport activity in the United States, with an estimated 2.5–3 million divers involved [1]. Although it is most popular in coastal states where opportunities for diving abound, this activity is not limited to ocean areas alone. Opportunities to scuba dive also exist in other bodies of water, such as lakes, quarries, abandoned mines, and caves. Scuba divers may be involved either in recreational- or commercial-diving enterprises. In recent years, some divers have extended the usual limits of diving and have developed a subspecialty sometimes referred to as "technical diving," for which the depth and complexity of diving is extreme.

Physicians are often asked to certify that individuals are physically fit to participate in scuba (self-contained underwater-breathing apparatus) diving and it is essential to recognize that some medical conditions may place a diver at increased risk for diving-related injury. For individuals with asthma, this presents somewhat of a dilemma, because there is considerable controversy over the degree of risk caused by underlying asthma. Of concern is whether those with asthma are at an increased risk for developing decompression illnesses, including arterial-gas embolism (AGE) or decompression sickness (DCS). Because the severity of asthma varies considerably among individuals, the degree of airway obstruction or airway hyperreactivity present at the time of diving must almost certainly affect the likelihood of complications. Data concerning the risk related to the degree of asthma activity with diving accidents unfortunately is as yet difficult to obtain.

Decompression illnesses were first described in workers who, during the mid-19th century, were engaged in tunnel or bridge work [2]. Laborers who returned to the surface after working in an atmosphere of compressed air oftentimes developed a variety of symptoms. These included neurological manifestations, such as weakness and seizures, joint pains, and in the most severe forms, death. Workers with decompression illnesses often walked with a slightly bent-over posture. This stooped-over posture resembled a style of walking which was popular among some women at the time and was called "the Grecian bend." This observation resulted in the term "the bends" when referring to individuals with decompression illness.

II. SYMPTOMS

Complications associated with diving are related to the behavior of gases under the conditions of changing pressure during diving. Boyle's law states that at constant temperature, volume is inversely related to pressure. During ascent, the volume of air in the lungs expands dramatically by a factor of two to three times. If a diver is unable to exhale properly, expanding gas in the lungs may result in lung rupture, causing pneumothorax, pneumomediastinum, or AGE [3]. Barotrauma describes the injury that may result from failure to equalize internal pressures to changes in ambient pressure in a variety of organs, such as the lungs, middle ear, and sinuses.

Arterial-gas embolism occurs when airways are obstructed and prevent expanding intrapulmonary gases from easily escaping. The airway obstruction may either be generalized, as may occur in active asthma, or the obstruction may be localized to a single lobe or segment secondary to a mucous plug, anatomical abnormality, asthma, or other etiologies. The expanding gas can result in lung rupture, or it may escape into the bloodstream. Gas embolism subsequently obstructing arterial flow into vital organs, especially the brain and spinal cord, causes paralysis, seizure, loss of consciousness, or death. In fact, AGE is the second most common cause of death in divers, exceeded only by drownings [4]. Those who do survive an episode are often left with severe, lifelong disability.

Decompression sickness, in contrast, refers to symptoms that occur when dissolved nitrogen or helium, at elevated pressures, enters tissues directly and forms bubbles in these tissues, with a decrease in ambient pressure during rapid ascents. Occurring in the brain, DCS may result in personality change, seizures, impaired consciousness, or paralysis. In the spinal column, these bubbles result in decreased sensation or strength in the lower extremities, as well as loss of bladder or bowel control. In joint tissues or muscles, this may cause the joint or muscle pains typical of the bends. The tissues involved depend on the degree of arterial perfusion as well as the degree of gas exchange with vigorous activity.

III. CONCERNS

Diving injuries associated with pneumothorax, AGE, or both occur most often for reasons other than asthma. The most common cause of lung overexpansion is a rapid or panicky ascent with breath-holding [3]. Limiting the depth of diving would not preclude this risk, as pressure changes are greatest at more shallow depths. Physicians unfamiliar with risks of diving and asthma may feel comfortable recommending that their patients dive, but restrict diving to shallow depths. In fact, recently two cases of gas embolism in asthmatic scuba divers practicing in swimming pools illustrate the potential dangers of even shallow dives [5].

Divers rely on tables or computers to help them determine safe depth and duration of a dive. It has been estimated that between 500 and 900 cases of DCS or AGE are reported in the United States each year, resulting in an overall risk for diving of 0.017–0.2% [2,6]. Many of these cases, unfortunately, are reported in divers who have used computer or table calculations, and the etiology of their problem is not readily apparent.

Physiological data suggest that active asthma should be a strong contraindication to scuba diving [7–11]. Patients with airway obstruction are at increased risk of pulmonary barotrauma and AGE, even in normal ascents without complications, such as panic, out-of-air conditions, or breath-holding. Airway obstruction and decreased lung compliance have been associated with AGE [3,12–14]. Melamed et al. [14] in their review of the physiological consequences of diving discuss whether conditions, such as asthma, may predispose divers to barotrauma, nitrogen narcosis, and DCS.

At least 7% of the United States' population has a diagnosis of asthma [15]. Some diving surveys indicate that 7% of divers also consider themselves to have a diagnosis of asthma [8]. This is not surprising, in view of the popularity of diving as a recreational activity. What remains unclear is whether patients with asthma or allergic disorders are overrepresented in the statistics of those experiencing adverse events. In addition, the severity or activity of airway disease in those reporting a diagnosis of asthma is usually uncertain in most surveys.

To illustrate the controversy, one authoritative source has stated: "Considering the potential catastrophic consequences of air embolism, it seems appropriate to recommend that asthmatics not dive" [13]. This conservative view is not held by all authorities, however. In fact, the author continued to say, "In the future, should data become available that define the risk of asthma and diving more clearly, more liberal recommendations might be possible."

Available data on asthma and scuba diving suffer from limitations on our ability to assess disease activity in divers with asthma preceding recreational or professional dives, either in those who have engaged in routine dives, or in those who have experienced some form of barotrauma. Not surprisingly, there have been no prospective studies in which measures of airway hyperreactivity either by methacholine, histamine, or cold air challenge have been used in scuba divers with asthma to quantitate risk. Bidaily peak flow measurements to measure airway lability, or even basic spirometry measurements before diving accidents, have not been available. Our understanding of the pathophysiology of asthma has evolved over the last few years, and we are now aware that significant airway inflammation and, in turn, presumably airway hyperreactivity often exist in relatively asymptomatic individuals and even in the early course of their disease [16]. Because of this, many of the stresses encountered during diving could trigger bronchospasm, even in relatively asymptomatic individuals. Some measure of airway reactivity, such as methacholine challenge or bidaily peak flow rates, would be helpful to quantitate the degree of asthma activity. In turn, these data could be used to evaluate their effect on diving-related injuries if they were measured in a large number of active asthmatic divers.

In spite of these limitations for diving accidents, the same authority, after review of more recently available statistics on asthma and accident data, has altered his recommendations. He now states: "Despite these limitations, careful review indicates the risks of serious morbidity or mortality during scuba diving appears to be inconsequentially elevated in subjects whose asthma was not characterized" [17].

Because of concerns over possible risks of diving accidents in asthmatic scuba divers, it has generally been advised against training these individuals for recreational or professional diving activities [18]. Many of the potential risks related to asthma were well outlined in a recent article by Neuman et al. [17]. First, is that bronchospasm may develop rather abruptly in an individual with asthma. They point out that an asthmatic may be asymptomatic at the onset of a dive, but may develop obstruction during the course of diving activities. Exercise, anxiety, and any number of factors could be responsible for this occurrence. Second, although an individual may be asymptomatic, airway obstruction still may be present and localized to small areas of the lungs. This could lead to obstruction and secondary hyperexpansion of these areas, with resulting barotrauma. Lastly, they note that asthmatic divers are exposed to various potentially asthmagenic stimuli during diving. In addition to vigorous exertion, airway drying or aspiration of small quantities of cold water may occur, potentially triggering airway reactivity and subsequent obstruction. This would increase the chance of lung overexpansion and development of the complications previously discussed.

IV. AVAILABLE DATA

Several attempts have been made to quantify the risk of pulmonary diving injuries in patients with asthma. In theory, patients with airway hyperreactivity should experience diving accidents more frequently. Available data, however, although incomplete, do not seem to confirm the impression that asthmatic divers have more frequent difficulties.

A questionnaire survey of divers in 1988 attempted to quantitate risk [8]. Of 1745 questionnaires distributed, 443 were completed and returned. Thirty-one of these divers reported a history of asthma. When questioned further, 19 of the asthmatic divers reported making 100 dives without experiencing a case of either AGE or DCS.

A survey of scuba divers with asthma in the United Kingdom was completed by 104 individuals who had performed 12,864 dives [19]. Suspected precipitants of asthma in this group included upper respiratory infections, pollen allergy, exercise, and cold air. Twenty-two of the respondents reported wheezing on a daily basis. Of these, 9 felt they could dive within an hour after experiencing symptoms of bronchospasm. In fact, 96 took β-adrenergic agents prophylactically or symptomatically just before diving. In spite of what should have been a significant risk in this population, only 1 diver reported having DCS on two occasions, but none had more severe symptoms such as pneumothorax or AGE.

The investigators, based on these data, suggest that diving should be prohibited within 48 h of any wheezing symptoms. They did not encourage monitoring peak flow rates or comment on the degree of bronchospasm that should prohibit an asthmatic from diving. Perhaps of some interest, a physician, with what he described as "extremely mild asthma," responded to the journal article. He reported experiencing a sudden severe asthma episode during his first deep-sea dive, although he was asymptomatic at the onset of this dive [20].

Several reports have been published in which the frequency of asthma diagnosis can be evaluated in fatal diving accidents. Of 11 fatalities reported from New Zealand for the years 1981 and 1982, only one person was determined to have asthma [21]. The circumstances surrounding this accident suggested that factors, other than the asthma, played a role in this fatality. Data collected over 20 years by the University of Rhode Island for diving fatalities in the United States identified only 1 with asthma of 2132 deaths reported [4] These limited data do not support the concept that asthmatic divers are at a significantly greater risk for death than the normal healthy diver.

The Divers Alert Network (DAN) is a national organization with headquarters at Duke University in North Carolina. This group has reviewed diving accidents from 1987 through 1990 [9]. In 1213 cases of DCS, asthmatic divers constituted 6 of the 119 cases of AGE and 3 of the 755 cases of type II (more severe) DCS. Seven divers with AGE and 16 with type II DCS were said to have currently active asthma. In contrast, in a control group of 696 divers with no history of diving-related accidents, 37 subjects had a history of asthma and 13 had current symptoms of reactive airway disease. Odds ratio assessment of these data did not attribute an increased risk to asthma. These investigators performed a subsequent survey of asthmatic divers by questionnaire [10]: 279 questionnaires were completed and returned. There were 11 reported cases of DCS from a total of 56,334 dives. Eighty-eight percent of those with asthma symptoms used some type of asthma medications. Nearly 56% took this medication in preparation for diving. Further evidence that a significant number had ongoing airway reactivity is supported by the fact that 30% reported daily or weekly wheezing and 26.4% had been admitted to the hospital on at least one occasion with a diagnosis of asthma. In this group, the risk of DCS (1:5100 dives) exceeded prior estimated risks in recreational divers with an odds ratio of 4:16. In neither of these studies, however, are specific details about cases or pulmonary function data reported.

Some of the data reported concerning asthma and risks of diving may be biased, as individuals with asthma who wish to be certified may not report their underlying condition. In another direction, the data may also be affected by "healthy worker" bias, because asthmatic individuals with more severe disease may elect to avoid diving activities altogether. It remains uncertain, however, whether individuals with a history of asthma, but normal pulmonary functions or normal assessment of airway hyperresponsiveness, would have an increased risk of complications from diving. If, in fact, asthma is a risk factor for diving, the interval of 48 h after the most recent episode of wheezing, as recommended in Britain [19], certainly does not allow sufficient time to permit airway hyperreactivity to normalize.

Current data on the risk for diving complications related to underlying asthma are, in summary, inadequate, and there is honest difference of opinion among physicians caring for those with asthma. If we accept that there is an increased risk of injury, the question is whether the degree of this risk is acceptable. Until more data concerning the nature and degree of risk associated with asthma are further clarified, the decision of whether to certify an individual to dive remains with that individual and his or her physician. The physician, however, must assume the responsibility to clearly discuss the available data and the theoretical increased risk that this person is undertaking by diving. This discussion can take place only if the physician herself or himself is aware of the possible problems.

In addition to asthma, other respiratory diseases may pose potential problems to the scuba diver. Upper airway disease, including chronic sinus and ear disease, may cause difficulties. Both of these are common causes of symptoms in divers. It has been stated that barotrauma to the middle ear and sinuses is the most common disorder experienced by scuba divers [22]. Because it is necessary for pressure changes across the tympanic membrane to equalize during diving, eustachian tube dysfunction and otitis significantly predispose to barotrauma. Those who have had ear surgery (including tympanoplasty or middle-ear surgery) or tympanic membrane perforation, are at increased risk of injury. These individuals should probably have a full otolaryngology evaluation before diving. A complete ear examination that demonstrates ability to autoinsufflate and that includes a normal tympanogram should be included in the examination. One conservative recommendation suggests that diving should be limited for 3 years after having an episode of otitis [23].

Nasal congestion and rhinitis related to allergic upper respiratory congestion, anatomical abnormalities such as septal deviation, or upper respiratory illnesses may also result in eustachian tube dysfunction. Sinusitis is also a relative contraindication to diving until the sinus disease has been appropriately treated. However, unlike complications that may be related to asthma, barotrauma to the sinuses rarely leads to life-threatening complications.

Divers frequently use decongestants, either orally or topically, before diving to establish adequate eustachian tube function. These are often employed after upper respiratory illnesses or during periods when allergic rhinitis is being experienced. The safety related to this practice has not been tested.

The data presented here clearly indicate that there is some concern over a variety of respiratory symptoms and diving safety. Physicians should make themselves aware of these considerations and discuss them frankly with their patients before approving or recommending participation in scuba diving. In particular, the potential risks of serious consequences when an individual has asthma should be recognized to allow a patient who is unaware of these risks to make informed decisions.

The DAN, in review of various medically related areas and the risk of diving, has stated: "Ultimately, however, making the decision to accept the risks involved in diving is each individual's responsibility" [24].

REFERENCES

1. Wachholz C. What is the incidence of non-fatal diving injuries? Alert Diver 1988; 4:1.
2. Moon RE, Vann RD, Bennett PB. The physiology of decompression illness. Sci Am 1995; 273:70.
3. Neuman TS. Pulmonary considerations. In: Vorosmarti J Jr, ed. Fitness to dive: Proceedings of the 34th Undersea and Hyperbaric Medical Society Workshop. 1987; 70:49.
4. McAniff JJ. US underwater diving fatality statistics. University of Rhode Island Report, URI-SSR 90–21, 1988.
5. Weiss LD, Van Meter KW. Cerebral air embolism in asthmatic scuba divers in a swimming pool. Chest 1995; 107:1653.
6. Twarog FJ, Weiler JN, Wolf SI, et al. Discussion of risk of scuba diving in individuals with allergic and respiratory diseases. J Allergy Clin Immunol 1995; 96:871.
7. Davis JC. Medical examination of sport SCUBA divers. San Antonio TX: Medical Seminars, 1986; 35.
8. Corson KE, Moon RE. Risk of diving injuries in asthmatics. Alert Diver 1991; Sept/Oct:12.
9. Corson KE, Dovenbarger JA, Moon RE, et al. Risk assessment of asthma for decompression illness. Undersea Biomed Res 1991; 18(suppl):16.
10. Corson KE, Moon RE, Nealen NL, et al. A survey of diving asthmatics. Undersea Biomed Res 1992; 18(suppl):18.
11. Bove AA, Neuman T, Kelsen J, et al. Observations on asthma in the recreational diving population. Undersea Biomed Res 1992; 19(suppl):18.
12. Shaefer KE, McNulty WI, Care C, et al. Mechanisms for development of interstitial edema and air embolism on decompression from depth. J Appl Physiol 1958; 13:15.
13. Neuman TS. Pulmonary disorders in divers. In: Bove AA, Davis JC eds. Diving medicine. 2nd ed. Philadelphia: WB. Saunders, 1990; 233.
14. Melamed Y, Shupak A, Bitterman H. Medical problems associated with underwater diving. N Engl J Med 1992; 236:30.
15. Turkeltaub PC, Gergen PJ. Prevalence of upper and lower respiratory conditions in the US population by social and environmental factors: data from the Second National Health and Nutrition Examination Survey, 1976–1980 (NHANES II). Ann Allergy 1991; 67:147.

16. Laitenan LA, Laitenan A, Haahtela T. Airway mucosal inflammation even in patients with newly diagnosed asthma. Am Rev Respir Dis 1993; 147:697.
17. Neuman TS, Bove AA, O'Connor RD, et al. Asthma and diving. Ann Allergy 1994; 73:344.
18. Hickey D. Outline of medical standards for divers. Undersea Biomed Res 1984; 11:407.
19. Farrell PJS, Glanvill P. Diving practices of SCUBA divers with asthma. Br Med J 1990; 300:166.
20. Martindale JJ. Scuba divers with asthma. Br Med J 1990; 300:609.
21. Walker D. New Zealand diving-related fatalities 1981–1982. J South Pac Underwater Med Soc 1984; 14:12.
22. Neblett LM. Otolaryngology and sport SCUBA diving update and guidelines. Anna Otolaryngol Rhinol Laryngol Suppl 1985; 115:1.
23. Farmer JC Jr. ENT considerations: otolaryngologic standards for diving. In: Vorosmarti J Jr, ed. Fitness to dive: Proceedings of the 34th Undersea and Hyperbaric Medical Society Workshop. 1987; 70:70.
24. Dovenbarger J. DAN's Top-10 questions. Alert Diver 1992; Nov/Dec:4.

19
Football

Arthur E. Varner and Robert K. Bush
University of Wisconsin—Madison, and William S. Middleton Memorial Veterans Hospital, Madison, Wisconsin

Gregory L. Landry
University of Wisconsin—Madison, Madison, Wisconsin

I. INTRODUCTION

Football is truly the all-American sport. It is the only remaining sport in the world for which participants and fans are predominantly from the United States. The sport embodies all qualities considered all-American: teamwork, loyalty, preparation, precision, cunning, strength, and power. Football requires all 11 players to work together for proper execution of an offensive play or defensive scheme. The game itself requires individual and team skills over a long time period: hours. Yet each play generally lasts less than 10 s of actual playing time. Short bursts of speed, power, agility, and strength define great players and make up great teams. These anaerobic bursts are needed from the first quarter to the fourth, so endurance plays a role as well. That is why it is so surprising that recent studies have shown that football players at several colleges and at the middle school and high school level have an increased number of participants with asthma and exercise-induced asthma (EIA) compared with most other sports.

Football would seem to discourage athletes with asthma from participation. Preparation for football begins in August, generally a very symptomatic period for individuals with ragweed-induced allergic rhinitis or extrinsic asthma. "Two-a-day" (twice-daily) practices at this time maximize exposure to the allergen. Hot, humid days also promote symptoms in those with mild sensitivity. Later in the season players are exposed to cool, crisp, dry autumn air—the type of air known to be the best stimulant of EIA.

Perhaps it is the nature and flow of the sport itself that allows players with asthma to excel and draws individuals with asthma to the sport initially. In this chapter the epidemiology of asthma in football, speculations on its high frequency, and approaches to diagnosis and management will be discussed.

II. SCOPE OF ALLERGIC DISEASES AND ASTHMA IN PARTICIPANTS

A. Underrecognition

Much publicity has been given recently to asthma and its increasing mortality rate over the last several years. Although the cause of this concerning trend is not fully known, it is felt that the prevalence of asthma, the number of people actually diagnosed with asthma, is increasing as well. It may be a matter of better detection of asthma, or the disease may be becoming more common owing to a variety of factors—indoor and outdoor air pollution, exposure to tobacco smoke, and increased frequency of respiratory infections in childhood. About 5–9% of the population of the United States has asthma, and another 3–4% has EIA. Fifty to eighty percent of asthmatic patients have EIA as well. Twenty percent of the population has atopic, or allergic, disease—either asthma, hay fever, or eczema. Up to 40% of patients with allergic rhinitis have EIA [1].

With this epidemiological information in mind for the general population, the 1984 Olympic Games in Los Angeles gave medical researchers the opportunity to evaluate the frequency of asthma and EIA in highly trained athletes [1]. Given answers to a survey, 11.2% of the US Olympic athletes had exercise-induced bronchoconstriction: 58% were male; there was a 2:1 male/female ratio up to 30 years of age. In all, 67 of 597 athletes were felt to have EIA—26 had a history of physician-diagnosed asthma (4%), 41 used β-agonist inhalers for asthma symptoms, 13 made a formal request to the IOC for approved use of asthma medications, and 42 (7%) had a history of symptoms compatible with EIA. [Note: 33 had more than one positive response.]

Thus, asthma and EIA are present in even the most highly trained athletes. It is doubtful that any cases of asthma were missed in this select group, yet several studies demonstrate undiagnosed asthma is very common. In a study of young adults (an age group comparable with collegiate football players) preparing for US Air Force Basic Training [2], 30% diagnosed with asthma had never had the diagnosis even considered despite complaints of shortness of breath, mainly with or after exertion. These researchers concluded that undiagnosed asthma, particularly EIA, is common in this age group.

Another study that supports the high rate of undiagnosed asthma and EIA involves adolescent athletes [3]: 1241 middle school and high school athletes were studied. Four percent had a diagnosis of EIA and were receiving treatment. By screening questionnaire and then exercise challenge for those with positive risk factors for EIA, 66 more students had EIA by positive exercise challenge tests, with drops of forced expiratory volume in 1–S (FEV_1) of more than 15%. Thus, another 6% of the total athletes had EIA, yet only one-third of these players had been diagnosed previously. These data, along with data from the University of Wisconsin and University of Iowa (discussed in the following section) show that asthma and EIA are greatly underrecognized in athletes and young adults, and especially in football players.

B. Epidemiology

For the last several years, medical faculty at the University of Wisconsin at Madison have evaluated incoming freshman athletes [4]. The evaluation has included complete history and physical examination, specific history concerning asthma and exercise-induced asthma symptoms, prick skin testing with common aeroallergens, and a methacholine challenge study if baseline pulmonary function tests were normal. A total of 304 male collegiate athletes were studied, 205 of whom were football players. Only 8 (<3%) had a history of diagnosed asthma or EIA and were currently using inhaled β-agonist therapy before exercise. These subjects were excluded from the evaluation.

Specific symptoms investigated included personal history of asthma, hay fever, bronchitis, sinusitis, urticaria, or drug allergy, and a family history of asthma, hay fever, or bronchitis was obtained. Specific symptoms pertaining to asthma and rhinitis were elicited. These included rhinorrhea, nasal congestion, nasal itch, postnasal drip, sneezing, nocturnal cough, cough with or after exercise, cough with cold air exposure, chest tightness, and shortness of breath after exercise. Physical examination included complete head, eyes, ears, nose, and throat evaluation as well as lung and cardiac auscultation. Two hundred ninety-five athletes underwent this evaluation and completed an abbreviated methacholine bronchial challenge. Eight athletes with previously diagnosed asthma and one with a viral upper respiratory infection and abnormal baseline spirometry were excluded from methacholine challenge.

Of the 245 who had a negative methacholine challenge, only 5 had any type of the aforementioned respiratory or allergic symptoms. However, 50 (17%) had a positive response with a drop in FEV_1 of 15% and 34 and had a drop in FEV_1 of 20% or more. Of these 50 positive responses, 46% had no lower or upper respiratory symptoms, 22% had symptoms of only rhinitis, 18% had symptoms consistent with asthma, and 14% had symptoms consistent with asthma and rhinitis. If one includes all the athletes with symptoms of asthma and a positive methacholine challenge or previous diagnosis of asthma, 9% of the total athlete study population had asthma. The diagnosis was present in only one-third before the study, consistent with the report of Rupp [3]. The screening history revealed 21 with asthma or EIA symptoms, 16 of whom went on to have positive methacholine challenges. Thus, this inclusive history was fairly specific in detecting asthma and EIA.

Another aspect of this study was the addition of prick skin testing for common aeroallergens. Studies have shown that young adults (early third decade) have the highest rate of positive skin tests compared with other age groups, occurring in approximately 50% [5]. Data from the Wisconsin athletes was in line with this, for 49% had positive skin tests to at least one allergen [4]. Over half of these with positive skin tests had symptoms of allergic rhinitis, whereas fewer than 3% with negative skin tests had rhinitis symptoms. Twenty-four percent of athletes with positive skin tests had positive methacholine challenge tests, whereas only 11% with negative skin tests had positive challenges. Of those with positive methacholine challenges, 36% had a history of rhinitis symptoms. The high rate of atopy and rhinitis in this population increases the risk of those athletes developing EIA. In one study [6] individuals with positive skin tests had a risk of developing allergic rhinitis or asthma proportional to the amount of reactivity of the skin testing; furthermore, younger adults with positive tests had more of an increased risk of developing wheezing than did older subjects with positive skin tests.

The University of Iowa's experience with asthma in football players began in December 1981, when their team was preparing for the Rose Bowl in California. A large number of players developed symptoms consistent with asthma, prompting further study [7]: 12% of the football players studied had asthma, whereas none of the basketball players and 7% of age-similar control subjects had asthma.

Their evaluation included a history of nasal and respiratory or asthma symptoms as well as a modified methacholine bronchial provocation (MBP) test. Overall, a remarkable 50% of the football players had a positive MBP test (defined as a drop in FEV_1 to less than 80% baseline). Of the football players with symptoms, 76% had a positive MBP test. In players with nasal symptoms, consistent with allergic rhinitis, 70% had a positive MBP test. For nasal symptoms, 40 players had MBP tests done in January and August (ragweed season) and there was no statistical difference in the rate of positive MBP tests. Overall there was a 45% rate of positive MBP tests in all players and control subjects, a rate somewhat higher than previously described for the test.

At the University of Washington [8], 983 athletes were surveyed, of which 155 were football players. Each athlete received a medical questionnaire concerning symptoms, risk factors, medications, or diagnosis of EIA. Positive responses prompted referral to a physician for evaluation and decision to pursue exercise challenge by treadmill. Only 1%, 9 of 983 athletes, had a history of currently diagnosed EIA. Fifty with positive results of questionnaire were referred for exercise testing and 41 underwent the challenge. Of these 46% had EIA, as shown by a drop of more than 10% in FEV_1. Thus, this survey and testing revealed another 18 athletes with EIA, tripling the original number in the population. This provides additional evidence that only one-third to one-half of athletes or young adults with EIA are actually diagnosed under usual circumstances.

As for the football players in this study, none of the 155 had previously been diagnosed with EIA. Yet 9 gave a history positive for EIA symptoms. This rate of 5.8% was third behind basketball (6.3%) and track–cross country (6.1%) among prevalence of male athletes with EIA symptoms by sport. Unfortunately, no other rates of diagnosed EIA by sport were provided.

C. Speculations on High Frequency

Asthma and EIA are present in even highly trained athletes at a rate of about 5–10% and appear to be even more frequent in football players when compared with other sports' athletes. If one examines the demographics of football players, the vast majority are male. Before puberty boys have a higher rate of asthma than girls, this equalizes at puberty, however. Thus, any influence the age of onset of asthma has on children's selection of sports and activities occurs before the age of the athletes we have been discussing. Football may attract younger boys with asthma symptoms more so than other sports. The rate of atopy and allergic rhinitis, which may predispose development of EIA, is also slightly more prevalent in males.

Young adults in their early third decade have a higher rate of skin test positivity than other age groups [5], increasing the risk for allergic rhinitis. Skin test positivity also portends a greater risk of wheezing in the future [6]. With preseason conditioning and two-a-day practice sessions occurring during peak ragweed season (for which 75% of the population with allergic rhinitis is sensitive [9] it would seem football players would be even more susceptible to develop asthma symptoms than other athletes.

Most football is played outdoors, thereby increasing exposure not only to airborne allergens, but also to pollution. This concern prompted the research [1] involving the US Olympic athletes in the 1984 summer games at Los Angeles. Safety of athletes with respiratory difficulties in the hot summer months of Los Angeles with its increased intensity of atmospheric pollution was worrisome. It is well known that sulfur dioxide and ozone can exacerbate airway hyperresponsiveness [10]. Football players, by playing mostly outdoors, are certainly exposed to various climates and environments during the course of a season, some of which may be more polluted than others.

The football season is long and football players are also exposed to virtually all weather conditions. Hot, humid, or dry, summer conditions occur during preseason practice and two-a-days. During fall and winter the most asthmogenic of air—cold and dry—occur on autumn afternoons and nights. This is yet another reason why athletes with asthma should not be drawn to football.

Young adults are prone to viral and bacterial upper and lower respiratory infections. Viral infections and bacterial sinus infections are well known to exacerbate or even initiate asthma symptoms in previously asymptomatic individuals. Most members of football teams spend many hours together in practice, meetings, travel, and games, making them particularly susceptible to epidemics of infections. Many collegiate football teams live together in the same dormitory, further increasing this risk. All are exposed to the rest of the student body population during the school day as well. Athletes are more prone to infections simply by their higher risk of transmission of infections from close contact, increasing the risk of developing asthmatic symptoms [11].

Competitive athletes, by definition, are the segment of the population most likely to experience EIA. No other age group has as many athletes or individuals that consistently exert themselves to the point where EIA symptoms may be precipitated. So why does football, with all these provocative factors for asthma, seem to have a higher rate of asthmatic players than other sports?

There are several reasons that allergic rhinitis may increase the risk of having EIA. Atopy alone may explain the increase risk. Or perhaps allergic rhinitis or rhinitis [12] from other etiologies (vasomotor, polyps, infections, or anatomical abnormalities) promote mouth breathing, which increases the amount of bronchial hyerresponsiveness in those with asthma and EIA. Rhinitis may even precipitate EIA in those without asthma.

Of all the protective equipment football players wear, the mouthpiece is one that athletes from other sports did not use regularly until recently, when more emphasis on preventative dental concerns expanded the use of mouthpieces worn by all athletes. Despite all the adverse factors football players endure, perhaps wearing a mouthpiece offers protection against asthma and EIA by promoting nasal breathing over mouth breathing.

Exercise testing with nasal breathing (mouth closed) has shown decreased postexercise bronchoconstrictive response, compared with oral breathing only (nose clipped) in asthmatic patients with EIA [13]. Interestingly, in two control groups (asthma without EIA and normal controls without asthma or EIA), all had better FEV_1 at all time periods after exercise with nasal rather than oral breathing. However, this study was not controlled for matched exertion by heart rate or measure of exercise intensity. Another study [14], which did demonstrate equivalent exercise workloads by heart rate and exercise protocol, also showed decreased bronchial responsiveness with nasal versus oral breathing.

The reasons for beneficial effects of nasal breathing on asthma and EIA are not fully known. It is postulated that nasal breathing allows filtering of polluted air, irritant gases, and allergens from inspired air and prevents their entrance to the lower respiratory tract where they initiate hyperresponsiveness. Sulfur dioxide, a potent stimulus for bronchial hyperresponsiveness and a common pollutant, is highly water soluble; with nasal breathing much SO_2 is absorbed in the upper airway, thereby preventing lower tract exposure [10]. Much research has also focused on the etiology of EIA as the result of changes in airway temperature. Nasal breathing, which warms and humidifies inspired air, may attenuate EIA. The athlete who relies primarily on nasal breathing may also have the advantage of exercise's effects on the nasal mucosa. Exercise increases sympathetic nervous system discharge and, by sympathetic-induced vasoconstriction of mucosal vessels, improves nasal patency and decreases nasal airflow resistance [15].

No studies have shown that football players wearing mouthpieces have less risk of asthma and EIA symptoms, but if mouth pieces increase nasal breathing, this may be a significant factor in reducing EIA. It is also unknown how much nasal breathing occurs or what percentage of inspired air is from nasal breathing in football players, but at least during the actual play and moments preceding, all players are wearing mouthpieces and, presumably, doing some nasal breathing. Of recent popular interest are nasal dilator strips (Breathe Right®) worn by several highly successful and visible professional football players. Their method of action is touted to be by stenting open the nasal airway in such a manner that improved nasal airflow is promoted. No study has supported this, but if it does stimulate players to use more nasal breathing, it may indeed aid pulmonary performance in athletes with EIA.

Probably the most convincing argument on why asthmatics are able to excel at football is based on the type of exertion the sports requires. Most articles on EIA and sports note that activities that require intermittent running of short duration are better tolerated than sports requiring more constant running [16–18]. Swimming and walking are often cited as perhaps the least asthmogenic of activities perhaps because of humidity and work load, Godfrey states, "The worst type is sustained exercise lasting some 6 to 8 minutes, at a constant and moderately severe power output. Brief exercise, even if it is quite severe, does not usually cause much EIA and types of intermittent exercise (e.g., playing football) is often well tolerated" [17].

Several studies have compared the properties of different types of running and their asthmogenic potential as well as their ability to prevent exercise-induced bronchoconstriction or induce a refractory period. One study [19] had athletes with EIA perform seven 30-s sprints, 2½ min apart, 20 min before a standard 6-min exercise challenge. This group did not experience significant bronchoconstriction after the sprints, but still demonstrated induction of a refractory period with a smaller decrease in FEV_1 after exercise challenge, when compared with the same exercise without the sprints beforehand. This finding could partly explain the non-asthmogenic nature of football, in that intermittent strenuous activities lessen the severity of hyperresponsiveness while still inducing a refractory period.

A more convincing argument comes from a study in Australia comparing five differing running regimens [20]. The data, from 27 asthmatic patients, showed that compared with continuous running for 6 min at a slow pace, 20 repetitions of high-intensity running for 10 s, with a 30-s rest period between sprints, was associated with an overall 14% less total drop in FEV_1 (38 to 25%). Also only three subjects reached their maximal FEV_1 reduction with the repetitive sprint pattern, as opposed to 19 with the continuous 6-min run. This pattern of sprints very closely resembles the situation of a sustained drive in a football game and may explain why asthmatics tolerate football.

III. APPROACHES TO DIAGNOSIS

A. History and Questionnaire

Asthma and EIA are common in football players and are diagnosed less than half the time. A simple history or questionnaire can be useful in eliciting responses that would prompt further investigation of possible asthma or EIA. A history of asthma, EIA, or using medications for asthma (prescription or over-the-counter) is a good starting point. Family history of allergic (atopic) diseases, asthma, or bronchitis is helpful. One should include questions about the player's personal history of atopic associated diseases—allergic rhinitis; hayfever; urticaria or angioedema; anaphylaxis; eczema; dust, pollen, or animal hair sensitivity; and environmental and drug allergies. Symptoms of sneezing, postnasal drip, nasal discharge, sinus congestion, decreased sense of taste and smell, frequent throat clearing, nocturnal cough, ocular or palatal itching, snoring, or skin rash and itching should be elicited. Prescribed antihistamines or decongestants or similar over-the-counter type medication use for these symptoms should be ascertained. To increase the sensitivity of the questionnaire, ask about cough during or after exercise, wheezing, dyspnea after exercise out of proportion to usual or others, chest pain or tightness, cough, shortness of breath, or wheezing with cold air exposure, or chest symptoms after exposure to airborne irritants. A recent history of upper or lower respiratory viral illness or sinusitis symptoms may predispose the player to bronchial hyperresponsiveness as well.

The sensitivity and specificity of these questionnaires is not well documented. In the Iowa study, the number of asthma and nasal symptoms did correlate with the risk of a positive methacholine challenge test. Yet in a study by Rupp [21] on EIA in high school athletes, questionnaire results put 37 of 166 athletes at risk, of whom only 8 had EIA documented by exercise challenge. With exercise challenge as the gold standard, the questionnaire had a sensitivity of 36% and specificity of 85%. The authors concluded that routine screening with their questionnaire was not efficient in detecting the number of high school athletes with EIA. Their questionnaire, when compared with Iowa's questionnaire and Wisconsin's history on asthma symptoms and exercise-induced symptoms, did not include as many specific chest symptoms associated with EIA and, therefore, may not have been as sensitive.

More study into questionnaire-directed evaluation of EIA by specific provocation testing is needed to optimize sensitivity, specificity, and cost-effectiveness in screening populations of football players. Also with the outdoor and seasonal venue of the sport, locally directed questionnaires may be needed relative to allergens and climate.

B. Exercise Testing

Standard exercise testing is the gold standard for diagnosing EIA. There are several protocols that can be used. The test should be performed without any recent use of medications for EIA. Most involve at least 6 min of high-intensity (> 85% maximum heart rate or 50–60% predicted maximal oxygen consumption [$\dot{V}O_2$ max]) exercise on treadmill or cycle. The FEV_1 should be more than 75% predicted value pretest. FEV_1 is measured 2 min after testing and at regulate intervals up to 30 min after exercise [22]. A drop in FEV_1 of more than 15% or of peak expiratory flow rate (PEFR) of more than 10% is diagnostic [23,24]. A common reason for false-negative results includes exercise intensity of insufficient duration or intensity to mimic the exertion the athlete experiences in training or competition. Different environmental conditions may also cause a false-negative test; cold dry air is the best stimulus. A peak flow meter and a free run may be used for an inexpensive screening test.

C. Methacholine Testing

If standard exercise testing fails to diagnose EIA, then a methacholine provocation challenge can be useful. As shown by the University of Iowa study, the methacholine bronchial provocation (MBP) challenge may be positive in a large number of subjects, with and without EIA, especially younger ones. Those researchers note [7] that a positive MBP indicates only nonspecific bronchial hyperresponsiveness and is not diagnostic of EIA.

The studies at the Universities of Iowa and Wisconsin defined a positive MBP challenge as a drop in FEV_1 of 20% or more. Eliason [25] notes that positive tests are derived from arbitrarily defined thresholds to improve the test's sensitivity and specificity. In his study, four different bronchial provocation challenges (BPC) were compared in diagnosing EIA. Of 20 normal control subjects and 20 subjects with EIA, a fall in FEV_1 of more than 15% at 188 cumulative breath units (BU) [Iowa used 150 BU maximum, Wisconsin 125 BU] was 100% specific for airway hyperesponsiveness, but had a sensitivity of only 55%. Other methods used included exercise challenge with stationary bicycle, eucapnic voluntary hyperventilation (EVH) with cold gas, and EVH with dry gas. These three tests were less sensitive than MBP.

Shapiro [26] states that "methacholine provocation is more sensitive than exercise challenge for diagnosis of hyperreactive airways. If the allergic athlete complains of exercise related symptoms, such as cough, dyspnea, or chest pain, and an exercise tolerance test fails to reproduce these symptoms, a methacholine challenge should be performed before the possibility of EIA is dismissed." Because the expense and need for referral to a specialized center, the MBP's place in evaluating EIA appears to be as a second-line test should an exercise challenge test be negative in an athlete with strong clinical evidence of EIA.

IV. APPROACHES TO MANAGEMENT

A. Peak Flow Monitoring

Once the diagnosis of EIA is made, there are several treatment options and issues. Response to therapy can generally be judged clinically from the athlete's symptomatic response. If symptoms persist, peak flow monitoring can be done before exercise and serially after exercise to see objectively if airflow obstruction truly persists in the presence of subjective symptoms. It can also be used to follow clinical response to medication changes if they are needed. Peak flow monitoring is also important in the athlete with chronic asthma. An increase in exercise-induced symptoms in these athletes should alert the physician to evaluate the overall effectiveness of the athlete's asthma mediation regimen.

B. Nonpharmacological

Although medications are effective treatment for EIA, there are several nonpharmacological techniques that have been demonstrated to reduce its severity. Many involve decreasing the amount of airway cooling and dehydration, felt to be responsible for EIA. While playing in ideal conditions (warm, humid air) would be desirable, football players are exposed to a wide range of climatic conditions during the season, much of which involves cold, dry air. The beneficial effects of nasal, rather than oral, breathing were discussed earlier [13–15]. The required use of mouthpieces for football players on most levels may increase nasal breathing and is potentially a mechanism of protection for some athletes with EIA. The nasal dilators worn by several professional football players may also help. Several studies have shown that wearing a protective mask [27] prevents drops in FEV_1 after exercise challenge in a cold environment in asthmatics with EIA. The masks (or scarves) may be more feasible for certain positions than others.

In approximately 50% of patients with EIA it is possible to induce a refractory period in which the athlete experiences less bronchial hyperresponsiveness than with the initial bout of exercise. Much study [19] has been done into which type of exercise regimen produces the most complete refractoriness. Currently, recommendations are for a continuous warm-up at 60% $\dot{V}O_2max$ (roughly 60% maximum heart rate) for 15 min, approximately 45–60 min before the game or practice. This protective effect can last up to 2 h. It may be of benefit to use peak flow monitoring to see if the player benefits objectively from this type of regimen.

Most researchers investigating the pathogenesis of EIA believe that exercising in cold, dry air is the most asthmogenic environment. But some note that if the athlete "cools off" in an environment warmer than where the exertion took place it may worsen the severity of exercise-induced bronchoconstriction by means of more rapid airway rewarming [28]. Although this observation is not uniformly accepted, it may be of relevance to football players, mainly at halftime and at the end of games when the players go indoors.

C. Pharmacological

Nonpharmacological measures as outlined in the foregoing are important, but physicians should not hesitate to use medical therapy for EIA. Treatment is discussed in detail in Chapters 8 and 9. Briefly, for football players, a simple regimen of a short-acting β-agonist by inhaler (two to four puffs 15 min before exercise) is extremely effective in most individuals. β-agonists are safe in these doses, but not all are approved by all athletic governing bodies. Inhaled cromolyn sodium and nedocromil are good second-line agents. Each can be used alone or in combination with β-agonists. Theophylline, inhaled and oral corticosteroids, and long-acting β-agonists play a role in treating the player with underlying asthma to stabilize lung function and reduce further exercise-induced bronchoconstriction [1,18]. They may also be needed in players with severe EIA not responsive to first- and second-line treatment. Players with well-controlled chronic asthma may still need preventative treatment with β-agonists before the game.

D. Other Factors

Other medical conditions that increase airway hyperresponsiveness should also be evaluated and treated. Players with atopic disease may have worsening of EIA during the peak of the ragweed season with preseason conditioning and practices. The mechanism may be extrinsic asthma, triggered specifically by allergen exposure or allergic rhinitis leading to a generalized increase in bronchial hyperresponsiveness to nonspecific stimuli. Appropriate therapy of allergic rhinitis can decrease symptoms of nasal congestion and discharge. Most antihistamines and topical medications are approved by athletic governing bodies, but the decongestants are banned for international competition.

Allergic rhinitis may also predispose players to sinus infections that can also exacerbate asthma. Nasal polyps are well known to worsen nasal symptoms and allow development of sinusitis. A history of nasal or facial trauma and subsequent anatomical changes (i.e., septal deviation) also could lead to nasal symptoms and recurrent sinusitis, worsening EIA.

Other infections, particularly viral, of the upper and lower airways can increase airway reactivity. Team physicians and trainers should be aware that these infections may unmask players with EIA or exercise-induced cough. This airway hyperresponsiveness could be present for up to 2 months, even in players without previous history of asthma.

Other medical problems should not be overlooked as contributing to respiratory symptoms. A player at Ohio State University had a recent diagnosis of histoplasmosis infection, with resultant chronic constrictive pericarditis. His original complaint included chest pain and shortness of breath, both worsened with exertion. Other medications may also contribute to symptoms. β-blockers used for migraine headache prophylaxis and use of nonsteroidal anti-inflammatory agents in aspirin-sensitive players are common examples of medication-provoked "asthma."

Environmental factors, such as pollution, may vary depending on location and time of year. Sulfur dioxide, ozone, and other constituents of atmospheric pollution increase airway reactivity [10]. Of recent concern is the increase in smoking rates among teenagers and its contribution to asthma and EIA. Second-hand exposure in children will exacerbate asthma and pulmonary symptoms and probably has similar effects on athletes. In surveys of athletes, most will deny smoking when asked in a medical setting, especially if coaching staff is present. This makes attempts at studying the effect of smoking on EIA in athletes very difficult.

V. SUMMARY AND CONCLUSIONS

Many issues are raised in discussing asthma and football. Three studies [4,7,8] demonstrated a higher prevalence of asthma symptoms, positive provocation tests for asthma, or diagnosis of asthma itself, in collegiate football players than in athletes in most other sports. A study of middle school and high school athletes [3] also found football players were more likely to have asthma or EIA than any other group, except softball players. One could conclude that, even at an early age, athletes with asthma are more likely to participate in football than in other sports, perhaps because running in short bursts, although at high intensity, followed with short periods of rest provoke less bronchoconstriction than continuous running of even moderate intensity [20].

Do children with asthma learn at an early age that they can exert themselves for short, powerful bursts as well as others, but only experience symptoms with more prolonged exertion? Males, having a higher prevalence of asthma before adolescence, may have more of a predisposition to learning this behavior pattern of intermittent exertion. By repetition of this activity, it may then enhance their bodies' and musculatures' ability to perform quick powerful anaerobic movements, thus promoting participation in sports such as football.

Interestingly, one study found no difference in the prevalence of asthma by position (i.e., running or defensive backs versus linemen) [7]. Perhaps it is not just the physical requirement of each position in football on game day that allows players with asthma and EIA to succeed, but the physical requirements of preparing for football in general. Again, football is a sport of strength, quickness, and explosive movements. Preparation involves weight training, sprints, and repetitive drills of short duration, all ideally suited for the athlete with any type of asthma to participate equally with nonasthmatic players.

The mandatory use of mouthpieces at all levels of football, but especially in younger players, could promote enough nasal breathing to reduce symptoms of EIA [13–15]. The refractory period of EIA may also play a role because platooning separates active time on the field with periods of rest, thereby promoting this protective phenomenon throughout the game. Yet football also has several characteristics that make it undesirable to those with asthma—exposure to peak seasonal allergens, cold air exposure, and environmental pollution. These factors must not play a large enough role, however, to dissuade athletes with asthma from participating, as demonstrated by the prevalence of asthma and EIA in football players compared with other sports.

There is little scientific evidence to explain why asthma is more common in football players than participants in other sports. Data are limited on the asthmogenic potential of all sports by objective measure. Most is based on intuition and perception of how much continuous running is required by each sport. Nevertheless, the message for physicians and trainers taking care of football players is that asthma and EIA are more common in their athletes than in other sports' participants. Recognizing symptoms as well as precipitating and associated factors may lead to an earlier diagnosis of asthma and EIA and earlier initiation of treatment for this eminently treatable disease.

REFERENCES

1. Voy RO. The US Olympic Committee experience with exercise induced bronchospasm. Med Sci Sports Exerc 1986; 18:328–330.
2. Nish WA, et al. Underdiagnosis of asthma in young adults presenting for USAF basic training. Ann Allergy 1992; 69:239–242.

3. Rupp NT, et al. Unrecognized exercise-induced bronchospasm in adolescent athletes. Am J Dis Child 1992; 146:941–944.
4. Huftel MA, et al. Finding and managing asthma in competitive athletes. J Respir Dis 1991; 12:1110–1122.
5. Barbee RA, et al. Immediate skin-test reactivity in general population sample. Ann Intern Med 1976; 84:129–133.
6. Burrows B, et al. Respiratory disorders and allergy skin-test reactions. Ann Intern Med 1976; 84:134–139.
7. Weiler JM, et al. Prevalence of bronchial hyperresponsiveness in highly trained athletes. Chest 1986; 90:23–28.
8. Rice SG, et al. Identification of EIA among intercollegiate athletes. Ann Allergy 1985; 55:790–793.
9. Rickett AJ. Allergic rhinitis. In: Patterson R, Grammer LC, Greenberger PA, Zeiss CR, eds. Allergic diseases: diagnosis and management. Philadelphia: JB Lippincott, 1993; 225–253.
10. Pierson WE, et al. Implications of air pollution effects on athletic performance. Med Sci Sports Exerc 1986; 18:322–327.
11. Douglas D. Upper respiratory infections in the conditioned athlete. Med Sci Sports Exerc 1978; 10:55.
12. Katz RM. Rhinitis in the athlete. J Allergy Clin Immunol 1984; 73:708–711.
13. Mangla PK, et al. Effect of nasal and oral breathing on EIA. Clin Allergy 1981; 11:433–437.
14. Shturman-Ellstein R, et al. The beneficial effects of nasal breathing on exercise-induced bronchoconstriction. Am Rev Respir Dis 1978; 118:65–73.
15. Olson LG. The response of the nasal airway to exercise. Am Res Respir Dis 1987; 135:356–359.
16. Katz RM. Asthma and sports. Ann Allergy 1983; 51:153–160.
17. Godfrey S. Exercise induced asthma—clinical, physiological, and therapeutic implications. J Allergy Clin Immunol 1975; 56:1–17.
18. Cypcar D, et al. Asthma and exercise. Clin Chest Med 1994; 15:351–368.
19. Schnall RP, et al. Protective effects of repeated short sprints in EIA. Thorax 1980; 35:828–832.
20. Morton AR. Continuous and intermittent running in the provocation of asthma. Ann Allergy 1982; 48:123–129.
21. Rupp NT. The value of screening for risk of EIA in high school athletes. Ann Allergy 1993; 70:339–342.
22. Brudno PS. Length of post-exercise assessment in the determination of exercise-induced bronchospasm. Ann Allergy 1994; 73:227–231.
23. McFadden ER Jr. Exercise induced asthma. N Engl J Med 1994; 330: 1362–1367.
24. Anderson SD. Exercise-induced asthma. In: Middleton E Jr, et al., eds. Allergy: principles and practice. St Louis: CV Mosby, 1993; 1343–1367.
25. Eliason AH. Sensitivity and specificity of bronchial provocation testing. Chest 1992; 102:347–355.

26. Shapiro GG. Methacholine challenge—relevance for the allergic athlete. J Allergy Clin Immunol 1984; 73:670.
27. Schachter EN. The protective effects of a cold weather mask on EIA. Ann Allergy 1982; 46:12–16.
28. McFadden ER Jr. Post exertional airway rewarming and thermally induced asthma. J Clin Invest 1986; 78:18–25.

20

Skiing and Other Winter Sports

William S. Silvers
Greenwood Medical Center, Englewood, Colorado

I. SKIING AND ASTHMA

A. Nordic or Cross-Country Skiing

Because airway obstruction is maximized when the inspirate is cold or dry [1,2], cross-country skiing is often considered the most asthmagenic exercise, given the prolonged duration of high-ventilation rates in the cold and dry air, thereby increasing the respiratory heat and water loss.

Whereas the prevalence of asthma in the general population may be near 5%, the prevalence of exercise-induced bronchospasm in the elite athlete has been reported as higher than 11%, as seen with the 1984 Summer Olympic Games [3–5]. However, asthma-like symptoms and bronchial hyperreactivity have been reported as much more common in cross-country skiers than in the general population and nonskiers [6]. In studying the prevalence of asthma in 42 elite Swedish cross-country skiers, bronchial responsiveness was significantly greater, and asthma symptoms more prevalent in the skiers than in the nonskiing referents. Interestingly, there was no difference in bronchial responsiveness within either group between winter and summer. Strenuous exercise at low temperatures entailing breathing large volumes of cold air was described as the most probable explanation of persistent asthma in skiers. However, other factors such as humidity, hypocapnia, and hypoxia, may also play a role in bronchoconstriction [7]. With skiers competing at high altitudes, their hypoxic ventilatory responses might cause further hyperventilation and a greater degree of hypocapnia. Absolute humidity is depressed at reduced temperatures. Thus, even if the air is fully saturated with water vapor, the actual amount of water will be small at low temperatures, making cold air exposure also dry air exposure. In contrast with skiing in the northeastern United States, the ambient conditions in the Rocky Mountains are naturally very dry (leading to the description of snow conditions as "champagne powder"). Given that hypoxia causes an acute increase in airway resistance in humans breathing a normocapnic hypoxic gas mixture, the effect of higher altitudes and the relative associated hypoxia may contribute to more bronchoconstriction than found with cold air sports at lower altitudes.

Koshela et al. assessed the effect of subfreezing temperature and wind on lung function in asthmatic patients; 19 stable asthmatic subjects who were exposed to subfreezing temperature at rest, received a moderate exercise challenge at subfreezing temperature, and a similar exercise challenge at room temperature in an environmental chamber with an artificial wind [8]. The two challenges at subfreezing temperature caused statistically significant changes in 1-S forced expiratory volume (FEV_1), but the exercise challenge at room temperature had no effect. These results indicate that even moderate exercise can cause severe bronchoconstriction in certain asthmatic subjects at climatic conditions similar to the Scandinavian winter.

The diagnosis of exercise-induced asthma in Nordic or cross-country skiing requires, first and foremost, the inclusion of bronchospasm in the differential diagnosis of exercise intolerance in the cold air. Thereafter, a sport-specific exercise challenge should be performed in cold air to confirm the presence and degree of bronchospasm. This is best done by performing a spirometry or peak flow meter recording before and after a Nordic or cross-country skiing run. Otherwise, a trial of β-agonists, given by inhalation before skiing or for acute symptoms, giving subjective or objective improvement would help confirm the suspicion of exercise-induced bronchospasm in cold air. An exercise pulmonary stress test performed in the warm air, such as with cycle, treadmill, or free running, may not confirm bronchospasm in cold air sports.

Therapeutically, nonpharmacological measures would include a gradual warm-up to attenuate the degree of bronchospasm, or the use of a scarf or gator over the mouth and nose to warm and humidify the inspired air.

Pharmacological approaches are similar to regimens for warm air sports in preventing and attenuating the exercise-induced bronchospasm. These include use of β-agonists, both short-acting and long-acting, cromolyn sodium or nedocromil, and perhaps the use of maintenance inhaled steroids for greater airway stabilization.

1. The Story of Bill Koch

America's top cross-country ski racer in the 1970s and early 1980s was Bill Koch. Eight time US National Champion, Silver Medalist of the 1976 Olympics, and World Cup Champion in 1982, he established world speed records in the 15-, 30-, and 50-km distances. As a teenager in 1974, after a series of streptococcal throat infections, he noticed that his lungs hurt a lot when he raced. After nearly a year of his lungs "burning" when he raced, he finally went to a pulmonary specialist who diagnosed exercise-induced asthma. He was placed on a medication program that he discontinued in 1980 without his physician's consent. From 1980 to 1984 he skied without medication and tried other approaches to overcoming his asthma. He developed a special warm-up program for 30–45 min before every race, slowly getting his pulse up to the race pace without tiring out. He found that this would attenuate his breathing difficulty. In this way, he was still able to become World Champion in 1982. However, he became sick before the 1984 Winter Olympic Games in Sarajevo and knew that he "burned" his lungs badly and would not recover for several weeks. He did not think it was appropriate to talk about this openly, for he suspected that other competitors might consider his health problem a "sour grapes" excuse. From this experience, he is now more attentive to his asthma, on a medication program preexercise, and has become an inspirational speaker to children with asthma, encouraging skiers of all levels to recognize their asthma, pay appropriate attention to personal triggers, work with their physicians, and take medications appropriately to maximize their performance [9].

B. Alpine and Downhill Skiing

Asthma may not be considered as significant a problem during alpine skiing as with cross-country skiing because the duration of the downhill run is usually less than 1–2 min; therefore, the respiratory heat and water loss would be less than that with the prolonged duration of exercise in cross-country skiing. However, the potential for impaired training given the prolonged cold exposure should be considered by downhill skiers as well as coaching personnel.

Diagnostically, knowledge of the bronchospastic potential in cold air and improvement with inhaled bronchodilators is clinical confirmation of exercise-induced asthma, as seen and discussed in the previously section (Nordic or Cross-Country Skiing). Therapeutically, considerations are the same as for Nordic skiing and cold air sports. Additionally, it may be advisable to keep the metered-dose inhaler on the inside of the ski suit, closer to the body warmth, to assure proper functioning.

1. Asthma Ski Day

Children and adults with asthma should be encouraged to fully participate in outdoor winter sports, given proper precautions and pretreatment. Many children with asthma may have experienced an exacerbation while playing outside in the cold weather. This may have discouraged these patients, or their parents, from pursuing or enjoying winter sports. To establish a safety profile for an ongoing Colorado Asthma Ski Day, peak expiratory flow rates (PEFR) were measured before skiing and at the end of the day's events, with pretreatment and as-needed use of regularly prescribed medications. Results demonstrated that, with medical supervision, PEFR monitoring, and properly administered medications, peak flow rates can be stabilized and even improved during cold weather exercise, to an extent that safety concerns need not restrict children with asthma from engaging in exercise or winter sports [10].

C. Other Sports and Considerations

Ice skating and hockey, outdoors or indoors, can certainly have an asthmagenic potential, given the prolonged duration of vigorous exercise in cold air. Bronchospasm may clinically manifest during rests in the action after skating for several minutes. Children, their parents, and coaches, should recognize this potential with ice skating. Pretreatment, and inhalers readily available for immediate use, should be encouraged. Ice skating or hockey performed on an indoor rink may have less asthmagenic potential than outdoors, given the climate control.

The increasing popularity and ease of recreational snowshoeing has allowed many more people to enjoy walking and hiking during the winter. As with other winter outdoor aerobic exercises, including running and cycling, a potential for asthma, given the cold dry air exposure and exercise, should be considered, and precautions should be taken with pretreatment or immediate-acting bronchodilators available.

Cold-induced urticaria has generally been associated with cold water lake swimming, not with skiing or other winter sports [11]. Exercise-induced anaphylaxis has to date generally been associated with warm air sports [12].

1. The Liz McIntyre Story

Liz McIntyre was the 1994 Olympic Women's Freestyle Silver Medalist. Although she had never felt she could breathe fully and freely, she had not had a seriously concerning episode of shortness of breath or wheezing. However, in spring of 1993, she began cross-training by mountain biking near her home in Winter Park, Colorado. During this pollen season, she experienced chest tightness and wheezing while mountain biking, prompting her to relate this to the trainers at US Skiing and, thereafter, she was referred to a local allergist. Although results of her pulmonary function tests were normal at rest, she was given a trial of inhaled β-agonists, and then pretreatment with β-agonists and cromolyn sodium, which were not significantly helpful. Thereafter, she was placed on a maintenance regimen of inhaled steroids and did not return for follow up—until after she won a silver medal at the 1994 Olympics at Lillehammer, Norway. She said she felt so well on her maintenance program that she was able to increase her training and endurance and did not feel need for more follow-up. Now, she too, is an inspirational speaker for young children with asthma in programs such as Asthma Ski Day.

II. THE "SKIER'S NOSE": COLD-INDUCED RHINORRHEA

Cold-induced rhinorrhea is a commonly experienced discomfort in cold weather, especially evidenced by skiers [13]. This is fondly referred to as the "skier's nose," which is an aesthetic clinical problem, with increasing numbers of tissue boxes appearing in ski lift lines as a testament to its prevalence. There are even cross-country ski gloves made with absorbent terry cloth to capture this rhinorrheic release. However, it may also be seen in people with any exposure to cold air. In an epidemiological survey at the Vail Mountain Medical Clinic, 96% of general medical patients reported some degree of cold-induced rhinorrhea, with 48% describing moderate to severe cold-induced rhinorrhea. Fifty percent had some degree of nasal congestion and 33% reported sneezing. Allergic and nonallergic patients described similar degrees of rhinorrhea. In an effort to moderate this mucous hypersecretion, the use of atropine sulfate, administered intranasally, was evaluated. Atropine has been used clinically by nebulization in the lower airways for obstructive airways disease, with reversibility; therefore, it was introduced for use in the nasal airways. With the Vail Ski Patrol volunteering as subjects in a double-blind, placebo-controlled crossover protocol, pretreatment with a 0.005% solution of atropine sulfate in saline nasal spray effectively blocked the cold-induced rhinorrhea with only minimal short-term side effects.

Secretion from the anterior serous and small seromucous glands in the nose constitutes nasal discharge [14]. The presence of parasympathetic innervation to the submucous glands, therefore, supports the use of anticholinergics to block the mucocilliary nasal discharge. Further studies have demonstrated an improvement with ipratropium bromide administered intranasally [15], as had been demonstrated for the control of hypersecretion of vasomotor rhinitis [16]. Although laboratory cold air nasal challenge studies have demonstrated that the mediators released in the mucus are the same as those seen with antigen-induced rhinorrhea [17], selective H_1-antihistamines have no effect on the cold air mucous secretion, thereby further substantiating the primary cholinergic pathway of cold air-induced rhinorrhea, or the skier's nose [18].

REFERENCES

1. Strauss RH, McFadden ER, Ingram RH, Jaeger J. Enhancement of exercise-induced asthma by cold air. N Engl J Med 1977; 297:743–7.
2. McFadden ER, Gilbert IA. Exercise-induced Asthma. N Engl J Med 1994; 330:1362–67.
3. Voy RO. The US Olympic Committee experience with exercise-induced bronchospasm. Med Sci Sports Exerc 1984; 18:328–30.
4. Katz RM. Rhinitis in the athlete. J Allergy Clin Immunol 1984; 73:708–11.
5. Weiler JM, Metzger WJ, Donnelly AL, Crowley ET, Sharath MD. Prevalence of bronchial hyperresponsiveness in highly trained athletes. Chest 1986; 90:23–8.
6. Larsson K, Ohlsen P, Larsson L, Malmberg P, Rydström P-O, Ulriksen H. High prevalence of asthma in cross country skiers. Br Med J 1993; 307: 1326–1329.
7. Pollard RC, Pollard AJ. Asthma in cross country skiers. Br Med J 1994; 308.
8. Koskela H, Tukiainen H, Kononoff A, Pekkarinen H. Effect of whole-body exposure to cold and wind on lung function in asthmatic patients. Chest 1994; 105:1728–31.
9. A skier's story. The Proventil Advisor 1991; vol 1 No 1, Sept/Oct.
10. Silvers WS, Morrison M, Wiener M. Asthma Ski Day: cold air sports safe with peak flow monitoring. Ann Allergy 1994; 73:105–8.
11. Wanderer AA. Cold urticaria syndromes: historical background, diagnostic classification, clinical and laboratory characteristics, pathogenesis, and management. J Allergy Clin Immunol 1985; 85:965–81.
12. Silvers WS. Exercise-induced allergies: the role of histamine release. Ann Allergy 1992; 68:58–63.

13. Silvers WS. The skier's nose: a model of cold-induced rhinorrhea. Ann Allergy 1991; 67:32–35.
14. Mygind N. Mediators of nasal allergy. J Allergy Clin Immunol 1982; 70: 149–59.
15. Silvers WS, Wiener MB, Wood CC, et al. The "skier's nose": a randomized double-blind placebo controlled study of ipratropium bromide (Atrovent) administered intranasally for the prevention of cold-induced rhinorrhea (CIR) [abstract]. J Allergy Clin Immunol 1988; 81:255.
16. Dolovich J, Kennedy L, Vickerson F, et al. Control of hypersecretion of vasomotor rhinitis by topical ipratropium bromide. J Allergy Clin Immunol 1987; 80:274–8.
17. Togias AG, Naclerio RM, Proud D, et al. Nasal challenge with cold, dry air results in release of inflammatory mediators. J Clin Invest 1985; 76:1375–81.
18. Silvers WS, Morrison MR, Wiener MB. The skier's nose: evaluation of terfenadine in cold-induced rhinorrhea (CIR) [abstract]. Ann Allergy 1992; 68: 87.

21

Case Studies of Asthma in Elite and World-Class Athletes: The Roles of the Athletic Trainer and Physician

Margaret M. Peter
United States Olympic Committee, Colorado Springs, Colorado

William S. Silvers
Greenwood Medical Center, Englewood, Colorado

Faye L. Thompson and John M. Weiler
University of Iowa, Iowa City, Iowa

I. INTRODUCTION

A certified athletic trainer-based (ATC-based) sports medicine system is an ideal model for providing health care services to athletes at every level. The scope of this system may range from a small core of individuals to a large, multidisciplinary network, with multiple outreach clinics. Regardless of size and complexity, the system is typically organized to deliver prompt, professional assistance for medical problems and injuries encountered by the athlete. The goals of the service are to recognize problems early and then to review the case with advanced care providers to determine the desired course of action.

Within the ATC-based system, the typical health care team comprises the following members: athlete, certified athletic trainer, primary care physician, specialty care physician, parents, and coaches. Health care team members bear responsibility and have roles in maintaining and maximizing the health and well-being of the athlete. Therefore, strong and continuing relationships must be established to provide full-service sports medicine management. The major focus for this chapter is the role of the athletic trainer in the on-site, daily management of exercise-induced asthma (EIA) and other respiratory diseases commonly seen in athletes.

II. MANAGEMENT OF EXERCISE-INDUCED ASTHMA

As the primary, on-site health care provider, the athletic trainer performs four activities in the management of exercise-induced asthma: (a) screening and recognition, (b) triage referral, (c) education, and (d) follow-up monitoring. These activities require regular communications between the trainer and the primary and specialty care (usually internal medicine, pulmonary, or allergy specialist) physicians.

A. Screening and Recognition

When an athlete officially becomes a team member, the team athletic trainer, in consultation with the team physician or family physician, conducts a thorough and systematic review of the athlete's previous medical background. The review process typically begins as the athlete completes a preparticipation medical history questionnaire. Musculoskeletal, respiratory, gastrointestinal, cardiovascular, and neurological systems are surveyed to determine past history and positive findings. The health history questionnaire that is used should be designed to elicit the following information about respiratory illness: (a) previous diagnoses of asthma, exercise-induced asthma, or other respiratory disorders; (b) current diagnoses of asthma, exercise-induced asthma, or other respiratory disorders; (c) family history of respiratory conditions or diagnoses; (d) history of "allergies"; (e) respiratory-related symptoms experienced by the athlete during or after exercise; (f) recent and current medications; (g) nonpharmacological therapies or treatments; (h) respiratory problems or limitations with exercise or performance; and (i) course and status of respiratory illnesses to date. This written self-report should provide the athletic trainer with sufficient information to permit recognition of potential problem(s). Further information is then gathered through personal interview to make a proper referral. It is important to determine (a) nature, timing, frequency, intensity, and duration of symptoms; (b) previous treatments attempted; (c) physical limitations; and (d) course and present status of the disorder. Following a detailed interview, or when respiratory symptoms are present, the athletic trainer may elect to perform a brief assessment of the athlete's eyes, nose, face, throat, and chest. The athlete's self-report, combined with the interview and physical evaluation, formulate the basis of a clinical impression and plan of action for the athletic trainer.

B. Triage Referral

The next step is to make a proper triage referral. The referral may be to a designated team physician, a family physician, or a specialty physician, and will follow established institutional protocols for medical referral. At the time of referral, it is crucial that the athletic trainer accurately and fully communicate the pertinent historical and physical findings, as well as practical concerns and impressions about the problem. Direct transfer of athletic training room records (or copies) is mandatory.

C. Education

The athletic trainer may provide important educational information to the athlete about exercise-induced asthma before and after the referral is initiated. The trainer explores and documents pertinent factors surrounding symptomatic episodes, including (a) environmental variables, such as air temperature and humidity; (b) temporal factors, such as time of year and day; (c) nutrition factors, such as food allergies and types, amounts, and timing of foods taken before an episode; (d) sport or activity selection factors, such as interval sprint training, distance running, or freestyle swimming; (e) intensity of exercise and type and duration of warm-up; and (f) pharmacological factors, such as timing, dosage, and influence of medications. These should be recorded, as should specific details about nature, type, timing, duration, and resolution of symptoms. Thus, the athlete and the trainer jointly define the problem. This helps the athlete cooperate with preventive health measures, as well as enhances compliance with therapy (such as the use of a peak flow meter and medications). Regular communication between the athlete and athletic trainer are necessary to maximize the quality of care and to minimize exercise-induced asthma's effect on the athlete's ability to exercise and to perform athletic skills.

D. Follow-up Monitoring

Following referral and medical testing, the athlete will usually return to team participation with more information about exercise-induced asthma, with instructions about the use of flow meters, and with directions for administering oral and inhaled medications. Some athletes may tend to feel overwhelmed, confused, or impatient at this point. The athletic trainer has an opportunity to establish intervention strategies and promote better understanding by interpreting and reinforcing directions, by giving the athlete reminders, and by reinterpreting instructions and information. Additionally, the athletic trainer may monitor and inform physicians about responses to medications and other modifications, and inform and educate coaches and parents by disseminating relevant information about exercise-induced asthma and instructions for treatment. In this manner, ongoing communication among athletes, athletic trainers, physicians, other health care providers, coaches, and parents fosters high-quality follow-up and management.

III. CASE STUDIES

Case 1

An 18-year-old female intercollegiate field hockey player presented to her athletic trainer for evaluation. The athlete had been active in several indoor and outdoor sports throughout her teen years. Her primary competitive field hockey seasons were played outdoors during the months of August, September, October, and November. During her season, she spent 2–6 h daily on the field performing intense drills, interval sprints, endurance running, and actual game play. Although she was still quite active during the winter, her exercise level decreased considerably when she worked out indoors. During the months of April, May, June, and July, she undertook weight training and sport-specific conditioning programs in preparation for the fall season.

As a freshman she was required to provide a medical history and to undergo a physical examination. At that time she disclosed that in the past she had sustained a variety of minor injuries and illnesses all categorized as aches, pains, sprains, strains, and contusions. She denied or failed to recall any previous history of respiratory symptoms, and her physical examination failed to demonstrate any abnormalities.

She was also required to perform a 12-min run test, in which the goal was to pace herself for maximal distance running in 12 min. This was conducted on a 400-m track, multipurpose rubber surface, at 244 m (800 ft) above sea level. She completed the run without obvious difficulty, but later reported that she had noticed some respiratory difficulties with the run. Three days following this run, during the interval-running–conditioning portion of practice, she again developed respiratory symptoms, described as chest tightness and wheezing, and was unable to continue. At this time, athletic-training staff became aware of this problem for the first time. The athlete again denied any prior episodes of respiratory difficulty except for very recent episodes of wheezing.

The athlete was immediately referred to an allergy specialist, who obtained a history of respiratory difficulty for the past year. At this time, the athlete admitted having been prescribed albuterol inhaler in the past and had taken 2 puffs before exercise as needed. A physical examination and laboratory studies were performed showing that the athlete had no obvious findings of asthma. Pulmonary function tests revealed a 1–S forced expiratory volume (FEV_1) of 3.26 L (92% of predicted) and a forced vital capacity (FVC) of 3.83 L (96% of predicted). By history, it was likely that she had exercise-induced bronchospasm, and she was instructed to use albuterol inhaler 2 puffs before exercise and 1–2 puffs as needed during exercise. She was to record peak flow meter values twice daily, and to return to the clinic in 2–3 months.

Through the remainder of this athlete's first collegiate season, several mild episodes of similar symptoms of chest tightness, wheezing, and dyspnea were encountered. Only one of these was significant enough to trigger the filing of a formal injury report. None resulted in significant (more that a few minutes on the sideline) loss of participation time. The athlete was always able to recover quickly with a brief period of rest and supplemental puffs from the albuterol inhaler. She was, in fact, sufficiently satisfied with her comfort and performance levels that she entirely failed to comply with recommended use of the peak flow meter and with meeting the 2-month follow-up appointment in the allergy clinic. Her activities through the rest of the school year included moderately intensive indoor conditioning workouts, four to five times a week, consisting of weight lifting, interval and distance running, as well as an 8-week indoor spring field hockey season with three 2-h practices each week. The athlete was faithful with her albuterol inhaler treatment regimen, and completed the year uneventfully as far as symptoms were concerned.

She had a similar pattern of symptoms during the early weeks of the following season. When she began to participate in two and three practices a day during the preseason in mid-August, she was briefly forced to the sidelines three to four times each week, complaining of dyspnea, wheezing, and chest tightness, in spite of the usual albuterol inhalation routine. Weather conditions were variable, with temperatures ranging from 75° to 90°F.

Four weeks into the season, the athlete was again referred by the athletic trainers to the allergy clinic for reevaluation and management recommendations. She again described that she experienced problems only during the fall season, and that exercise was the only trigger for her symptoms. Results of her physical examination at this time were again entirely negative, with the exception of mild rhinitis. Pulmonary function tests demonstrated an FEV_1 of 3.82 L (106% of predicted) and an FVC of 4.49 L (110% of predicted). This "normal" pulmonary function test suggests that her levels a year earlier were actually significantly lower for her than were obvious at that time. The allergist recommended the addition of sodium cromolyn metered-dose inhaler 5 puffs before exercise. She was to return to clinic in 4 to 6 weeks, or sooner if this did not control her symptoms.

The athlete did return to the clinic for what was to be her final follow-up visit during this second of her 4-year collegiate career. At this time, she noted much improvement in her symptoms and her exercise tolerance. A thorough physical examination was once again completely negative. Pulmonary function tests showed an FVC of 4.14 L (102% of predicted) and an FEV_1 of 3.51 L (97% of predicted). The allergist concluded that she was able to control the symptoms of exercise-induced asthma with a regimen of cromolyn (5 puffs) and albuterol (1–2 puffs) before exercise. She was told to continue this regimen and to return to the clinic in 6 months, or sooner if symptoms were to recur. This athlete fulfilled the remaining 2½ years of her field hockey career without significant incident and never returned for follow-up care.

Comment

This is a case of apparent mild exercise-induced asthma and demonstrates the difficulties of obtaining follow-up visits in athletes with this disorder. Even during her regular visits, owing to time constraints on her part, it was not possible to obtain skin testing, methacholine bronchoprovocation challenge, or exercise testing. The main concern for this athlete was that she be able to perform at her peak level. She was generally satisfied with her overall performances and was unwilling to participate in the evaluation process sufficiently to allow physicians and trainers to provide her complete follow-up and optimal care. On several occasions, her coaches indicated that they believed her level of physical-conditioning improved during the course of each season and distinctly over the course of her career. It was clear that season-by-season she was able to tolerate the same or more exercise with less distress. Thus, it is likely that her symptoms diminished as she aged.

Case 2

A 27-year-old world-class athlete who participated in a contact, anaerobic sport moved from the Midwest United States to begin training at the Colorado Springs Olympic Training Center (CSOTC). Colorado Springs is an arid region, located at an altitude of 1890 m (6200 ft) above sea level. Resident athletes live and train at the Colorado Springs Olympic Training Center full-time. The normal resident-training schedule consisted of two sessions daily of 2–3 h of training, 5 days/week, as well as 2 h on Saturdays. Training sessions variably consisted of aerobics, plyometrics and weight-lifting, and technique work.

The athlete presented to the training room on seven separate occasions from March 1992 to April 1993, with symptoms of bronchitis and upper respiratory infection. Symptoms often included rales and rhonchi. Each time the athlete was referred by a staff athletic trainer to a family practice physician at the Colorado Springs Olympic Training Center for evaluation, and the athlete was treated with a course of erythromycin or amoxicillin, as well as over-the-counter medications. Notably, these referrals were to different physicians, owing to the rotating volunteer physician schedule of the Colorado Springs Olympic Training Center.

In June 1993, the athlete reported to a staff athletic trainer after completing a vigorous training session of running on a treadmill. He presented with a rash covering his chest, arms, and back. He also reported difficulty breathing while running. During the examination, his breathing pattern and respiratory rate were normal. The athlete attributed his shortness of breath to being out of shape, although he had been training regularly. The athlete was referred to the attending physician for evaluation. His diagnosis was exercise-induced urticaria, and he was advised to increase his vitamin C intake to 800–2400 mg on training days.

The athlete did not report another episode of shortness of breath or exercise-induced urticaria until September 1993. Again, he presented with an urticarial rash over his trunk and arms, as well as shortness of breath during exercise. Following this episode, he was evaluated by an attending physician, who identified wheezing. At this time the patient's diagnosis was exercise-induced urticaria and asthma. He was prescribed an albuterol inhaler (2 puffs every 4 h). Results of a blood test showed a high eosinophil level of 16.4% (normal range 0–4%), a low neutrophil level of 30.0% (normal range 52–76%), and a high basophil level of 4.9% (normal range 0–2%). The athlete was advised to follow-up with a local allergist within the month.

During the appointment with the allergist, a complete allergy history was taken that revealed the athlete had been experiencing symptoms of itchy nose and eyes, and sneezing since April or May of 1993. The allergist also discovered that the athlete had noticed symptoms of wheezing, shortness of breath, and chest tightness, all of which were brought on by exercise, since the summer of 1993. The athlete reported that the symptoms were worse when he returned to his home in the Midwest United States. He also complained of fatigue, but attributed this to his heavy-training schedule.

His previous history indicated lactose intolerance and one episode of pneumonia as an adult. A family history did not identify any family members with hay fever or asthma.

Pulmonary function testing was performed on his initial visit to the allergist. His FEV_1 was 3.65 L (72% of his predicted) and his FVC was 4.74 L (76% of his predicted). After inhaling 2 puffs of albuterol inhaler his FEV_1 was 3.99 L (78% of predicted value—a 10% increase from baseline), and FVC was 4.90 L (78% of predicted value). The results of the tests indicated a mild impairment in pulmonary functions, and substantiated the diagnosis of an obstructive pulmonary disease that was only modestly responsive to bronchodilators.

Treatment was to consist of albuterol (2 puffs) and cromolyn sodium (2 puffs) before exercise. He was also prescribed loratadine tablets, 1/day, as needed for itching or rash. If lower respiratory symptoms worsened, he was to begin using triamcinolone acetonide, 3 puffs, three times per day. The athlete was to return to the allergist's office in 1 month for follow-up to report responsiveness to this therapy and perhaps to substantiate the diagnosis of exercise-induced asthma.

On return to the sports medicine clinic from his appointment with the allergist, the athlete verbally informed sports medicine staff of the results of his visit. Between September 1993 and April 1994, the athlete returned to the sports medicine clinic five times complaining of cold symptoms. These symptoms ranged from runny nose and productive cough to rhonchi and rales. During an examination in April by a local primary care practitioner, he had a diagnosis of bronchitis. Again he was given erythromycin as well as a steroid inhaler. It was assumed at this time that he was using his albuterol correctly.

In June 1994, he again presented with mild bronchitis. During follow-up visits to the sports medicine clinic pertaining to this episode, it was discovered that he was neither taking his medication properly nor regularly. He was instructed in the proper technique of using the albuterol inhaler and given antibiotics and expectorants. No mention was made in the follow-up note of the previously prescribed medications (cromolyn sodium or inhaled or nasal steroids). It was assumed that he was not taking any of these medicines at that time.

During training sessions, and during pre- and posttraining treatment sessions in the sports medicine clinic, the athlete often expressed concern about his performance level, which did not seem to satisfy his coach. He felt pressure from his coach to achieve a higher level of fitness. Asthma was an unacceptable excuse for being unable to keep up. The athlete felt that his dependence on the inhaler was viewed by coaches and teammates as an excuse for not being well conditioned. The athlete wanted to avoid this pressure from coaches and peers, so he often avoided using his medications when in their presence. The athlete continued to struggle through his workouts, even when prompted by the staff athletic trainers to use his inhalers properly and to take the other medications.

More than a year after the initial examination, the athlete participated in a local asthma seminar. During this seminar he explained his reasons for not returning for follow-up testing. He was concerned about the time commitment and cost of each appointment. Even though he was told that there would be no cost to him, he was still unwilling to return for reevaluation by the allergist because he felt "guilty" for taking up the physician's time when he could not compensate him for his work. Consequently, the allergist was unable to document reversible airway obstruction. Because the athlete never had a 15% change in FEV_1, exercise-induced asthma was presumed but never definitively diagnosed.

The athlete also described a feeling of being "experimented on." He voiced a concern that he was asked to "just try" medications, but he wanted definitive care that would end his problem. The athlete indicated he had no way to differentiate between a day of feeling poorly (because he was tired), and a day when he was suffering from exercise-induced asthma. He then openly admitted he was noncompliant with his asthma medications.

The allergist was present at the seminar and said that the diagnosis had been explained to the athlete and treatment options were clearly described. The allergist also told the athlete that not everybody responds to all medicines the same and, therefore, the allergist wanted the athlete to see which medication worked best. The athlete said that this was not acceptable when he was in the middle of a competitive season. He wanted to be healthy, and was worried that these new medications could make him worse or unchanged. He wanted medication that was effective, without any trial-and-error approach.

Following the seminar, the athlete told the staff athletic trainers and the allergist that he was interested in following up on his initial examination and having a reevaluating of his current medication protocol. In December 1994, the athlete returned to the allergist's clinic for a follow-up examination. Pulmonary function tests resulted in findings similar to the initial pulmonary test. The FEV_1 was 3.88 L (76% of predicted value), and FVC was 5.0 L (80% of predicted value). Chest examination revealed occasional rhonchi in the lungs. Chest and sinus x-ray films were normal. Sputum smears showed many eosinophils. Skin tests were negative.

The physician and athlete discussed the results and the treatment plan. Treatment was to consist of 2 puffs of albuterol and 4 puffs of nedocromil sodium before exercise. Three to four puffs of triamcinolone acetonide were to be used three times a day. An expectorant, guaifenesin, was to be used on an as-needed basis. The athlete was also advised to perform peak flow tests twice a day as well as before and after exercise. He was to return in 1 month.

The athlete never returned to the physician's office for a follow-up appointment and also never reported to the sports medicine staff complaining of respiratory illness in the ensuing months. The athlete left the Colorado Springs Olympic Training Center during the spring of 1995 for other than medical reasons.

Comment

Many factors contributed to this athlete's overall health and to the treatment of his asthma. Training at the Colorado Springs Olympic Training Center is similar to many college and university athletic programs. The athletes residing at the Colorado Springs Olympic Training Center receive room, meals, and most medical care at no personal cost. The sports medicine facility is operated by five full-time certified athletic trainers and four 1-year position certified athletic trainers. The staff is supplemented during peak Colorado Springs Olympic Training Center attendance periods, primarily the summer months, by volunteer certified athletic trainers, chiropractors, and physicians. At times, the rotation of staff and volunteers contributes to a breakdown of communication between the athletes and full-time staff. It is not uncommon for physicians to have varying treatment plans for illnesses, especially exercise-induced asthma. Occasionally, breakdowns occur somewhere along the communication loop of the athlete, athletic trainer, and physician. This is not unlike many large athletic-training rooms around the country. The importance of complete and accurate documentation and availability of past records is apparent.

Another communication problem that occurred among this athlete, the local referral physician, and the Colorado Springs Olympic Training Center sports medicine staff was that the athlete was unaccompanied by athletic-training staff for his appointments. The athlete failed to understand what he was told and did not communicate all that he knew to the Colorado Springs Olympic Training Center staff. The Olympic Training Center received no report from the physician to whom the athlete was referred. These problems are easily resolved by having a trainer accompany the athlete, when possible, phone calls between the health care providers, or paper communication.

It is not unusual for any athlete to misunderstand physician recommendations and instructions concerning an injury or illness. It is also common for an athlete to remember only the first or last pieces of information told to him or her. The Colorado Springs Olympic Training Center sports medicine staff has found it helpful to ask the athlete to repeat the information and directions given before allowing him or her to leave the examination area.

This particular athlete may have been unique in his feelings of guilt, because not everyone feels badly about receiving free services. Had he expressed this concern early, the process could have been explained to him. Perhaps it is also easier for athletes to accept certain procedures if they are performed in a familiar environment, such as the training room or sports medicine clinic. General practitioners and orthopedists routinely visit training rooms for "sick call" or "ortho hours." Because of the increasing numbers of athletes with diagnoses of exercise-induced asthma, it may be an appropriate policy to implement bimonthly or monthly "asthma/allergy hours" in training rooms in an attempt to minimize miscommunication and increase compliance.

Case 3

Amy Van Dyken, a 23-year-old Olympic athlete, represented the United Sates at the 1996 Summer Games in Atlanta, won four gold medals in swimming, an Olympic record, despite having had lifelong severe asthma. Her parents first enrolled her in a swimming program at age 6 because her severe asthma did not allow her to participate in other athletic activities. At that time, she could not swim across the pool. She tried dance, soccer, and gymnastics, but found that swimming caused fewer problems with asthma. She continued to swim, despite active asthma, and by 12 years of age completed her first 100-m butterfly race, finishing last. At age 14 she was selected to be a member of the Cherry Creek High School swimming team, but continued to suffer asthma attacks. She was limited in her ability to compete and found it difficult to complete workouts because of recurrent asthma exacerbations. However, she persisted in her efforts to participate and was selected as a substitute for the 50-m–freestyle race at the Colorado State Championships. She won the consolation heat and the next year won the event. During her junior year of high school, she was hospitalized for 5 days owing to an asthma exacerbation, 2 weeks before the state finals. Soon after discharge she swam in the Junior Nationals and won both the 50-m–freestyle and 100-m–butterfly competitions. In her senior year of high school, she set Colorado State records in the 50-m–freestyle and 100-m–butterfly.

Next, she enrolled at the University of Arizona and was chosen to be the first alternate for the 1992 Summer Olympics. As a freshman, competing in the NCAA Championships, she was the second leading scorer. After her sophomore year, she transferred to Colorado State University and was named "swimmer of the year" during her junior year. She set American records in the 50-m–freestyle and swam the second fastest time in history in the 100-m–freestyle. She then qualified for the World Championships, but because of another asthma attack, was unable to perform well.

In late 1994, she became an athlete-in-residence at the Colorado Springs Olympic Training Center, and remained there until the 1996 Summer Olympic Games in Atlanta. During that time in Colorado Springs she had multiple flares of asthma while in the swimming pool, requiring visits to a local emergency room, where she was prescribed nebulizer treatments and parenteral glucocorticosteroids. Staff athletic trainers at the Colorado Springs Olympic Training Center worked with her to supervise her use of a peak flow meter (which she had used for many years) and her medication use. As the trainers became more familiar with her, they developed an understanding of her need for rapid therapy at the onset of asthma flares. Early recognition and treatment of flares, manifested by symptoms and by a decrease in her peak flows, improved her ability to perform. Staff athletic trainers and pool personnel learned that the low ceiling at the indoor aquatic center at the Colorado Springs Olympic Training Center caused an increase in airborne irritants; air quality was particularly poor if she swam in the center lane. Thus, she learned to swim in the outside lane of the pool to improve her ability to complete the workouts.

At the 1996 Summer Games she won gold medals in the 4 × 100-m freestyle relay, the 100-m–butterfly (the event she considered her weakest), the 4 × 100-m medley relay (as the anchor), and the 50-m freestyle. She became the first American woman to win four gold medals in a single summer or winter Olympics. At the time of her Olympic competition, she was using high-dose inhaled steroids, theophylline, nedocromil sodium, albuterol by metered-dose inhaler (2 sprays before exercise as well at other times when required), and nasal steroids. She was also using salmeterol, the long-acting β2-agonist, which had been approved for Olympic athletes in January of 1996.

Throughout her life, she was hospitalized or required emergency room treatments at least once a year, and in many years considerably more often. More remarkably, her pulmonary function test results were never entirely within the normal range, whereas most swimmers have supernormal pulmonary function test results. One week before participating in the 1996 Summer Olympic Games, her FVC was 95% of predicted, her FEV_1 was 69% of predicted, her FEV_1/FVC ratio was 73%, and her 25–75% forced expiratory flow ($FEF_{25/75}$) was 35% of predicted normal values.

Following completion of her participation in the 1996 Summer Games she has focused on lecturing and working with patients with asthma to help them pursue their athletic dreams as she has done. Even before her Olympic participation, she was willing to take time to counsel young patients with asthma.

Comment

Amy Van Dyken became an elite, highly successful swimmer despite requiring high doses of bronchodilators and anti-inflammatory medications. She achieved success as a result of a close collaboration with her physicians and with the athletic trainers who worked with her at the Colorado Springs Olympic Training Center. Her case is a clear contrast to other athletes who might have failed to seek adequate medical care or to follow suggested treatment regimens. Clearly, her desire to perform *at her personal best* drove her to compete at levels never before achieved by any American athlete, with or without a chronic disorder.

Perhaps her achievements are best captured on the souvenir Wheaties cereal boxes that feature her picture with the following caption:

> The crowning moment for Amy Van Dyken's swimming career came at the 1996 Olympic Games. Van Dyken, in winning the 50-meter freestyle, set an American record time of 24.87 seconds and defeated the Chinese world champion for the gold medal. Most amazingly, this was the fourth gold medal Van Dyken won, making her the only U. S. woman to win four gold medals in a single Olympic Games. That's not all. Van Dyken was an improbable champion. She suffers from severe asthma and could not swim the length of the pool until the age of 12. Her championship performance has made Olympic history. Wheaties salutes this American champion for letting us know that all dreams are possible.

IV. CONCLUSION

Educating athletes, as well as coaches, has always been a priority in sports medicine. Education is a two-step approach: presentation and comprehension. Finding a way to address and approach many groups of athletes and coaches has always been a challenge. Readily available flyers or pamphlets describing the signs, symptoms, and treatments of exercise-induced asthma are concrete ways of presenting the information. Personal communication and question and answer periods should also be encouraged and promoted, whether this is through individual, small groups, or team approaches.

Finally, the athlete needs to be aware that he or she is ultimately responsible for his or her health. It is up to the athlete to attend appointments and communicate problems. Only then will the athlete receive optimal evaluations and treatments for asthma that will allow full participation at maximal levels of performance.

22
Management of the Elite Athlete Who Has Exercise-Induced Asthma

Roger M. Katz
UCLA School of Medicine, Los Angeles, California

I. OVERVIEW

Exercise-induced asthma (EIA) in elite, competitive athletes presents unique problems [1]. The athlete who is well conditioned may experience difficulties only during maximal effort, while exercising in polluted environments, such as in smog with high SO_2 concentrations [2], or with exposure to chlorine in swimming pools [3]. Others will experience EIA on exposure to cold air, fog, high humidity, or with inhalant allergen exposure to pollens, molds, mites, and feathers, as well as to particular ingested foods.

Physicians caring for elite athletes may not realize that a problem exists because the athlete may not properly recognize symptoms such as shortness of breath, chest tightness, chest heaviness, and breathlessness. The athlete often attributes these symptoms to lack of proper conditioning, or "a weakness" in the athlete. In some cases the athlete will not want others to realize that he or she may have a physical problem such as asthma. Other athletes may even vomit to relieve the tightness feeling in the chest and abdomen during EIA. Still others seem to experience lightheadedness when experiencing EIA. Occasionally, the athlete will complain of chest pain, which needs to be further elucidated as to what "pain" is really experienced. I have seen one case of apparent laryngospasm with exercise that mimicked EIA.

Elite athletes vary in age from young children to adults. In the young athlete, growth and development play an important role, as demands for weight gain or loss, replacement of fluids, heat loss, and proper eating during training and before events need special attention. The asthmatic child who has a fluid imbalance during exercise presents another challenge. Fluid imbalance is particularly important because an athlete may lose 2–8 cups of water per hour (1.0 FL m^{-1} h^{-1}) [4] in the form of sweat (perspiration). It is conceivable that this may exacerbate EIA. The American Academy of Pediatrics and the American College of Sports Medicine recommend that the adolescent take 4–8 oz of fluid every 10–15 min during exercise (16 oz of fluid for every pound lost after the event) [5,6].

Another clinical problem for the athlete may be food allergy, as discussed in Chapter 15. If an athlete eats a food to which he or she is allergic, an immediate or a late-phase reaction may occur that involves the respiratory track with subsequent bronchospasm. I have seen athletes experience ongoing symptoms for several days after such an eventful occurrence. At other times an athlete may eat a food that may result in a reaction only if the athlete exercises within 2 h of the food ingestion. This latter form of reaction often diagnosed as exercise-induced anaphylaxis is described in Chapter 15.

It is important to communicate with athletes, parents, coaches, and trainers so that in their relationship with the athlete, fluid replacement and proper timing of the events to eating will be provided. As reported in Chapter 5 both heat and water loss may be the primer events in causing EIA. Children tend to produce more heat per square meter of body surface area during exercise. They are also less capable of transferring heat from muscles to the skin; thus excess heat loss within the lungs by rapid breathing adds to EIA considerations.

EIA is characterized by a decrease in pulmonary function tests (PFT) occurring after 5–6 min of hard or near maximal exercise. The decrease in PFT often occurs during the next 7–10 min, even while resting. Recovery then occurs over the next 20 min. In most adult elite athletes these symptoms are experienced as chest tightness, and breathlessness (often with cough or wheeze). Elite athletes may have the ability to perform during this time and may "run through" the episode. Additionally, the athlete who experiences EIA finds that after repeated exercise within 40–60 min, asthma symptoms are less likely to occur or are milder (the refractory period).

Studies suggest that highly trained athletes with asthma have even more bronchial hyperresponsiveness when they exercise in polluted air (see Chap. 17) or in cold air. Hypercapnea, especially in dry, cool air, or with sulfate concentrations higher than 0.04 ppm can exacerbate EIA. It is often thought by athletes, their trainers, and coaches that physical training will reduce EIA occurrences. In general, training and conditioning may not help the asthmatic athlete [7] as much as pharmacological and nonpharmacological techniques as described in Chapter 10. Pulmonary function testing on elite athletes, as well as those persons who play wind instruments, may show normal values, as based on a normal population; however, most of these individuals have super normal PFT values that will still show a significant 15% improvement in the FEV_1 after bronchodilators are given.

Both medications and nonpharmaceutical therapies can be used by the athlete to control EIA. The latter includes a warm-up that does not induce EIA; breathing through the nose, rather than through the mouth; warm moist air; and controlling polluted air intake. It is important to assure that patency of the nose is maximized as described in Chap. 11. A study in two Olympic athletes with EIA revealed that the nasal cavity increases resistance to airflow almost at the same time that lower airway obstruction was measured [8,9]. Another study in asthmatic children who were recreational athletes showed that the obstruction of the nose often occurs during exercise [9]. This, in turn, may prevent the conservation of water and heat loss from the lungs. Nasal breathing can also be a problem when concomitant sinus infections exist in the athlete. Again the athlete resorts to mouth breathing and increases the likelihood of EIA occurrence.

Athletes, particularly highly competitive athletes, often will not allow others to discover that they are taking medications for their physical problems. Thus, metered-dose inhalers and tablets are hidden and are not taken at the optimum time intervals. However, these athletes may not view over-the-counter preparations as medications; hence, frequently, less effective medication may be taken to prevent EIA. Furthermore, if a medication has a side effect, such as bad taste, or causes any perceived impairment in well-being, then the athlete may simply not take it. When in doubt, ask the athlete about drug compliance. Conversely, many nonasthmatic athletes will attempt to take medication, such as metered-dose inhalers, because they perceive a benefit, even if they do not have asthma. The use of most antiasthmatic drugs does not affect performance in nonasthmatic athletes [10].

In many situations a careful history, including questions that specifically address EIA symptoms should identify the patient with EIA. Other questions that suggest EIA include those related to hay fever (allergic rhinitis), allergic conjunctivitis, recurrent sinusitis, urticaria, and a family history of atopy and asthma. A history of childhood asthma or bronchitis should also lead one to suspect reactive airways associated with exercise.

The history form used by the USOC in 1984 for identifying athletes with the potential for EIA or chronic asthma is quite useful (Fig. 1).

USOC EIB QUESTIONNAIRE

RECENT = within past 2 months EXERCISE = before, during, after	NO	YES	RECENT	WITH COLDS/ INFECTION	EXERCISE
1.* EYES					
A. ITCHY					
B. WATERY					
C. PUFFY					
2.* NOSE					
A. ITCHY					
B. STUFFY					
C. SNEEZING					
D. RUNNY					
E. HAY FEVER					
F. POST NASAL DRIP					
3.* SINUS INFECTION					
A. YELLOW/GREEN NASAL DISCHARGE					
B. TENDER SINUSES/ HEADACHE					
4.* EARS					
A. POPPING SENSATION					
B. EARS FEEL FULL/ CONGESTED					
C. SENSATION OF BEING IN RISING ELEVATOR					
5.* CHEST					
A. COUGH					
B. WHEEZING					
C. NOISY BREATHING					
D. CHEST CONGESTION					

Fig. 1.

RECENT = within past 2 months EXERCISE = before, during, after	NO	YES	RECENT	WITH COLDS / INFECTION	EXERCISE
E. CHEST TIGHTNESS					
F. UNABLE TO GET DEEP BREATH					
G. ASTHMA					
* Questions 1-5 relate to symptoms after exercise					
6. SKIN REACTIONS					
A. HIVES					
B. ITCHY SKIN					
C. DRY SKIN					
D. SWELLING OF SKIN					
E. ECZEMA					
F. ATOPIC DERMATITIS					
7. CONTACT DERMATITIS - Skin reacts to things which touch the skin					
A. UNDERWRAP					
B. TAPE					
C. SWEAT BANDS					
D. DEODORANTS					
E. AFTERSHAVE LOTION					
F. ELASTIL					
G. OTHER					
8. FOOD & MEDICATION					
A. ASPIRIN					
B. PENICILLIN					
C. SULFA DRUG					
D. OTHER MEDICATION					
E. FOOD ALLERGY					

Occasionally the sports practitioner will encounter an athlete who has an unusual presentation. In these cases, it is important to consider the athlete's sport. For example, if the patient wears a helmet, be sure you are not dealing with pressure on the carotids that leads to anoxia, which can mimic some of the symptoms of EIA. If the athlete complains of chest pain during exercise, it may be appropriate to consider cardiovascular disease [11], although chest pain in children usually is more consistent with EIA. Many athletes will hyperventilate as part of their training process. This may increase the water and heat loss from the lungs and increase the EIA response. If recognized, then teaching a slower, nonhyperventilation technique may help control the problem of EIA.

RECENT = within past 2 months EXERCISE = before, during, after	NO	YES	WITH COLDS/ INFECTION	EXERCISE
9. ALLERGIC OR SENSITIVE TO THE FOLLOWING:				
A. DUST				
B. ANIMALS/PETS				
C. MOLD/MILDEW				
D. POLLEN/GRASS				
E. AIR POLLUTION				
10. LIFE-THREATENING (SYSTEMIC) REACTIONS REQUIRING HOSPITAL TREATMENT				
A. SHOCK FROM BEE STING				
B. DIFFICULTY BREATHING				
11. IF YOU WERE SENT OUT TO RUN 1 MILE, CAME BACK AND RESTED FOR 15 MINUTES:				
A. WOULD YOUR CHEST FEEL TIGHTER?				
B. WOULD YOU EXPERIENCE A COUGH?				
IF YOU ANSWERED YES TO A OR B ABOVE, ARE YOU *MORE LIKELY* TO HAVE THESE SENSATIONS OF COUGH CHEST TIGHTNESS IN:				
A. COLD WEATHER				
B. CERTAIN SEASONS OF THE YEAR				
C. DURING PERIODS OF AIR POLLUTION				
12. HAVE YOU HAD SKIN TESTS FOR ALLERGIES IN THE PAST?				
13. HAVE YOU HAD ALLERGY SHOTS? (IMMUNOTHERAPY)				
14. RECENT COLDS/ CHEST COLDS?				
15. HEADACHE AFTER EXERCISE?				
16. STOMACH ACHE AFTER EXERCISE				

Fig. continues

Not all athletes respond to usual treatments. Some athletes will require treatment with a β-adrenergic agent (sometimes orally, rather than inhaled) along with ipatropium bromide and perhaps additional inhalers such as cromolyn sodium or nedecromil, as well as oral theophylline. Other athletes have chronic asthma that occasionally requires short bursts of corticosteroids before events. I have treated some patients who do best after inhaled corticosteroids when these were given at high doses before events.

RECENT = within past 2 months EXERCISE = before, during, after	NO	YES	RECENT	WITH COLDS / INFECTION	EXERCISE
17. HAVE YOU TAKEN ANY OF THE FOLLOWING MEDICATIONS?					
A. ANTIHISTAMINE					
B. DECONGESTANT/ COLD MEDICATION					
C. ANTIBIOTICS					
D. BRONCHODILATORS (To open breathing passages)					
E. OTHER					
F. ARE YOU TAKING ANY OF THESE MEDICATIONS NOW?					
18. HAVE YOU EVER BEEN HOSPITALIZED FOR:				DATES	
A. PNEUMONIA					
B. ASTHMA					
C. BRONCHITIS/					
BRONCHIOLITIS					
D. OTHER LUNG PROBLEM					
19. HAVE YOU EVER SMOKED?					
20. HAVE YOU EVER USED SMOKELESS TOBACCO?					

In general, athletes have fewer and milder symptoms when they participate in water sports, and more problems in crew, in field and track, and in heavy-energy events such as polo and wrestling. In sporting events that are more likely to induce EIA, the athletes may learn to use the refractory period or to breathe through the nose to control EIA. In world class competition, there are many restrictions on what medications are permitted [12]. Rules change annually, and many medications require preapproval. Some highly effective medications are banned (see Chap. 23).

II. CASE HISTORY

As a young child JB was told that her asthma, diagnosed in infancy, prevented her from "playing, running and swimming." At age 9 she realized that she could run and she began to participate in athletic events even though she was limited by her breathing disability. She had chronic symptoms throughout the year and needed to take medications on a regular basis. Some of the medications made her quite nervous, so she relied only on theophylline for major relief of her symptoms, despite ridicule from her peers for needing medication because she was "out of shape." She learned to depend on a treatment that controlled her symptoms. At age 13, she learned that swimming was less asthmogenic than running, but continued to participate in field and track events. At age 14, she was first treated with albuterol metered-dose inhaler, which allowed her to control symptoms without the side effects of earlier medications. This allowed her to participate, to be competitive, and ultimately, allowed her to win a gold medal in Olympic competition.

JB also noted that if she could breathe through her nose she had less difficulty in controlling her asthma. Unfortunately, when she worked-out she would experience nasal blockage and, subsequently, would have to rely on mouth breathing. Oral breathing increased her need for medication to control asthma associated with exercise. She learned that when training for her events, she could "warm-up" and would have less asthma after exercise. However, she found that before events she would have to wait more than 2 h after warming up and needed to adjust her use of the metered-dose inhaler. She required more than one administration of medication and increased the theophylline dosage to add protection from developing exercise-related asthma. She also noticed that while traveling she was experiencing episodes of severe wheezing unassociated with exercise. Many of these episodes were related to exposure to allergens, such as feather pillows, seasonal pollens, and the ingestion of fish. She was reevaluated and told to avoid exposure to these substances and was given additional medications to block the allergic reaction from occurring.

This patient now is a field and track coach at a major university. She understands asthma and relates to those on her team who suffer from the same infliction. She also supervises a summer program by the Asthma and Allergy Foundation of America for asthmatic children that teaches the child to participate in sports with nonpharmacological methods and with the proper use of medications as prescribed by the child's physicians.

REFERENCES

1. Update on Exercise Induced Asthma—A Report of the Olympic Asthma Conference, Phys and Sports Med 1997; in press.
2. Pierson WE, Covert DS, Koenig JQ. Air pollutants, bronchial hypersensitivity and exposure. J Allergy Clin Immunol 1984; 73:717–721.
3. Drobuic F. Centre d'Alt Rendiment, Barcelona (personal communication, 1994).
4. Costill DL, Krammer WF, Fisher A. Fluid ingestion during distance running. Arch Environ Health 1970; 21:520.
5. Costill DL. Water and electrolyte requirements during exercise: Clin Sports Med 1984; 3:639.
6. Primos WA, Landry GL. Fighting the fads in sports nutrition. Contemp. Pediatr 1989; 6:14–50.
7. Clark CJ. The role of physical training in asthma. Chest 1992; 101:293S–298S.
8. Katz RM. Rhinitis in the athlete. J Allergy Clin Immunol 1984; 73:708–711.
9. Ohki M, Hasegawa M, Sakuma A. Exercise-induced nasal obstruction in patients with allergic rhinitis. Am J Rhinol 1989; 3:1–4.
10. Fitch KD. The use of anti-asthmatic drugs. Do they affect performance? Sports Med 1986; 3:136–145.
11. Beoclaqun F, Schicchi JS, Haas F, Axen K, Levin N. Aortic arch anomaly presenting as exercise-induced asthma. Am Rev Respir Dis 1989; 140: 805–808.
12. United States Olympic Committee Drug Education and Doping Control Program: USOC Hot Line 1-800-233-0393.

23

Doping Rules and the Treatment of Respiratory and Allergic Disease

Wade F. Exum and Joan M. Price
United States Olympic Committee, Colorado Springs, Colorado

I. INTRODUCTION

The hallmark of exercise induced bronchospasm (EIB)—a shortness of breath after exercise—was noted by Hippocrates, the Greek physician of 5th–4th century BC, and by Aretaeus the Cappadocian in 200 AD.

EIB is a common problem that affects athletes and nonathletes alike. Especially at risk are those with asthma and respiratory infection. There continues to be concern about doping rules surrounding treatment of athletes with asthma and other bona fide respiratory diseases. It is the pharmacological, rather than the nonpharmacological treatment that is of concern by those who regulate drug use in sport. The various organizations governing athletic participation have different regulations on banned and permitted medications.

It is difficult at best for the treating physician to stay within the boundaries of various protocols while providing sound medical care. Along with the risk of disqualification and loss of awards, the athlete is faced with the threat of sanctions and penalties after the detection of a banned substance. The physician's contribution to an athlete's success is the full utilization of appropriate medications. The best way for a physician to avoid problems and potential litigation is to be informed. This chapter addresses the philosophy of regulating drugs and provides information on the United States Olympic Committee (USOC) and National Collegiate

Athletic Association (NCAA) guidelines on medications commonly prescribed for treatment. Resources for obtaining current information on policies of major sports organizations are listed in Appendix C.

II. HISTORY

The act of doping by athletes is condemned on both the principle of fair play and concerns for the athlete's health and safety. *Doping* is simply the use of drugs or chemical substances or specifically defined methods solely for the purpose of gaining a competitive advantage in sports. The abuse and misuse of drugs is among the most sorrowful issues of today. Historical precedents of athletes seeking an unfair advantage are not unknown. Gladiators were boosted by stimulants, Greeks experimented with mushrooms, Romans added strychnine to their wine, and 19th century athletes tried alcohol, caffeine, nitroglycerin, and opium [1]. Following distribution of anabolic steroids to German troops during World War II, and treatment of postwar wasted and castrated prisoners, athletes began experimentation seeking an artificial means to heightened aggression and muscular development. The abuse of stimulants in modern-day sports became pointedly clear with the death of Denmark's elite cyclist, Knud Jensen, and the publicized amphetamine scandals within American football in the mid-1900s [2].

With the increase of drug abuse among athletes, drug control programs blossomed. In an effort to eliminate the edge of enhancement from ergogenic aids, the guardians of the ideal of fair play persevered. The introduction of drug testing took place at the Summer and Winter Olympic Games in 1968. The Munich Games of 1972 brought comprehensive testing [3]. At these games an asthmatic, Rick DeMont, tested positive for ephedrine and was stripped of his gold medal [4]. The 1988 International Olympic Committee Charter Against Doping in Sport outlined the vast scope of the problem, noting that potential for doping is present in every sport. The charter stated concerns for the health and safety of the athlete; the integrity of sport; the rights and roles of the athlete, and the desire for fair play. It presented a plan for an ideal program guaranteeing ethical behavior in sport [5]. In its definition of doping, the IOC Medical Commission states that doping contravenes the ethics of both sport and medical science, and bans the administration of substances belonging to selected classes of pharmacological agents, as well as the use of various doping methods [6].

The purpose of drug control programs is to prevent any unfair advantage by a competitor, as well as to protect the health and safety of the athlete. Of importance is the assertion that evidence exists that a substance does indeed elevate performance. Also of consideration is a relation between drugs and an adverse effect on performance and health and the desire to provide a fair and equal contest [7].

An important consideration in doping regulations and the treatment of asthma is evidence that permitted medications are not ergogenic. Drugs that are not prohibited do not provide an advantage to the athlete with asthma over the nonasthmatic. They are seen as a means to eliminate the handicap under which the athlete competes.

III. MEDICATIONS

For the 1968 Winter Olympics the International Olympic Committee (IOC) published a list of banned drugs [8]. That list has evolved into a framework used for reference by many other sports organizations throughout the world. The USOC adopted the IOC concept and list into its Drug Control Program in 1983 (see Appendix A). In 1986 the NCAA founded their program, based on this model. Throughout the years both organizations have continued to change and perfect their programs. Because regulations (see Appendix B) are in a continuous state of flux, it is not advisable to administer any medication to an athlete without first confirming acceptability with the governing authority. The USOC doping control program is used as a basis for this text, with the caution that no two organizations follow the same rules.

The USOC program applies to the US Olympic Festivals, US Pan American Team Trials, and US Olympic Team Trials. By agreement, the various sports national governing bodies (NGBs) also comply at their sponsored competitions. Many have additional regulations as dictated by their international federations (IFs).

When treating the athlete with asthma, the intent of the physician is to prevent or limit the advent of EIB to allow competition without major respiratory complication [9]. When the words athlete and asthma are mentioned together, the EIB study on the 1984 US Olympic Team is often referenced. Of the 597 athletes tested, 67 were identified with EIB, and medications approved for use in these conditions by the IOC were prescribed. Of this group 41 members earned medals: 15 gold, 21 silver, and 5 bronze [10]. This success rate is held out to athletes as an encouragement that treatment within doping regulations can provide a level playing field.

What has not been taken into consideration is that doping regulations of the IOC have changed since 1984. Two β_2-agonist medications were allowed in both aerosol and oral forms at that time. Albuterol and terbutaline are now limited to inhaled administration, and only with written notification sent from the prescribing physician to the USOC before competition. Similar products, developed in recent years, await a nod of approval from the IOC. Glucocorticosteroids, once permitted for use in all forms, are now restricted.

Asthmatic athletes should continue to pursue their goals in spite of respiratory handicaps. A present-day example of overwhelming success is seen in the many awards earned by world-class athletes such as US track and field star, Jackie Joyner-Kersee [11].

IV. DOPING CLASSES AND METHODS

A. Stimulants

Decongestants are prohibited as central nervous system stimulants, with the exception of aerosol forms of naphazoline, oxymetazoline, phenylephrine, tetrahydrozoline, and xylometazoline. However, antihistamines are allowed. The NCAA permits decongestants in certain cough and cold remedies.

B. β_2-Agonists

Considered to be powerful stimulants, oral and injectable administration of β-agonists is banned. Only aerosol forms of albuterol, terbutaline, and salmeterol are permitted. The treating physician must provide written notification to the USOC before athlete competition. The NCAA does not restrict use.

C. Street Drugs

Cocaine and heroin are the only two substances that have been identified in every doping control program to date as prohibited.

D. Narcotic Analgesics

The only exception in this class made by the USOC is the use of codeine, which is permitted. Preparations containing hydrocodone are prohibited. Although morphine administration is prohibited by both the USOC and major league baseball, it is not included on the NCAA list.

E. Anabolic Agents

The USOC, NCAA, and the National Football League (NFL) prohibit use of these substances. As with all prohibited substances, related compounds are also prohibited. Because of its anabolic properties, the foreign β_2-agonist stimulant clenbuterol is included under this classification by the USOC.

F. Peptide and Glycoprotein Hormones and Analogues

This group includes corticotropin (ACTH), erythropoietin (EPO), human chorionic gonadotropin (HCG), human growth hormone (hGH), and any and all of their respective releasing factors (GnRF).

G. Glucocorticosteroids

Corticosteroids are allowed in all forms by the NCAA. The USOC permits topical (ear, eye, or skin) use, but prohibits rectal, oral, intramuscular, and intravenous routes of administration. However, inhaled administration is acceptable by the USOC, with certain restrictions. A physician-written letter of notification must be sent to the USOC before athlete competition.

H. Diuretics

Because of their ability to mask detection of other prohibited substances through urine dilution, diuretics are not allowed by either the USOC or NCAA. In sports where weight categories are a factor, diuretics have been known to be misused to decrease weight quickly and are prohibited for this reason as well.

I. β-Blockers

The β-blockers are tested for at the request of an international federation (IF) and at the discretion of the USOC in the following USOC sports: archery, biathlon, bobsled, curling, diving, equestrian, fencing, free-style skiing, gymnastics, luge, modern pentathlon, sailing, shooting, ski jumping, and synchronized swimming. The NCAA tests for these medications in rifle events only.

J. Sedatives

Any substance with a sedative action is prohibited by such international sport federations as archery and modern pentathlon or biathlon. They are not allowed for use in NCAA rifle events.

K. Alcohol

Alcohol is prohibited by the NCAA as well as by certain sport international federations. The USOC maintains the right to determine breath or blood alcohol levels and may conduct tests for ethanol.

L. Marijuana

Prohibited by both the NCAA and major league baseball, marijuana may be tested for at the request of a USOC National Governing Body (NGB) or an international federation as well as the International Olympic Committee.

M. Anesthetics

Although local or intra-articular administration of anesthetics is permitted by the NCAA, documentation is required by the USOC under the following conditions: bupivacaine, lidocaine, mepivacaine, and procaine, may be used, but not cocaine. Epinephrine (adrenaline) or other vasoconstrictor agents, may be administered concurrently. Intramuscular and intravascular injections are prohibited by both organizations.

N. Blood Doping

All forms of blood doping are prohibited by the USOC and NCAA. Erythropoietin, prohibited under the classification of peptide and glycoprotein hormones and analogues, is also included in this category.

O. Urine Manipulation

The USOC and NCAA prohibit all forms of pharmacological, chemical, and physical manipulation of the urine specimen. Epitestosterone, used to mask testosterone abuse, is prohibited in certain concentrations.

P. No Advance Notice Program

It is important to note that doping regulations included in this chapter pertain to the in-competition programs. As the various no advance notice programs continue to expand, education about their regulations is necessary. At the time of printing, the only substances tested for in the no advance notice program include anabolic agents, diuretics, peptide and glycoprotein hormones and their analogues, and urine manipulation.

Appendix A USOC Status of Medications Used for Treating Asthma

Medication	Status
Antihistamines	Prohibited by some international federations, (i.e., archery, modern pentathlon/biathlon)
Anticholinergic agents	
Atropine sulfate	Allowed
Ipratropium bromide	Allowed
Diluents	
Sodium chloride	Allowed
Glucocorticosteroids[a]	
Beclomethasone diproprionate, aerosol	Allowed[b]
Budesonide, aerosol	Allowed[b]
Dexamethasone sodium phosphate, aerosol	Allowed[b]
Flunisolide, aerosol	Allowed[b]
Hydrocortisone, IV	Prohibited
Prednisolone, oral	Prohibited
Prednisone, oral	Prohibited
Triamcinolone acetonide, aerosol	Allowed[b]
Miscellaneous	
Cromolyn	Allowed
Nedocromil sodium	Allowed
Mucolytics	
Acetylcysteine	Allowed
Nasal decongestants	
Desoxyephedrine	Prohibited
Ephedrine	Prohibited
Epinephrine	Prohibited
Naphazoline, topical	Allowed
Oxymetazoline, topical	Allowed
Phenylephrine	
Oral	Prohibited
Topical	Allowed (IOC 9/94)
Phenylpropanolamine	Prohibited
Propylhexadrine, topical	Prohibited
Pseudoephdrine	Prohibited
Tetrahydrozoline, topical	Allowed
Xylometazoline, topical	Allowed
Sympathomimetic bronchodilators	
Bitolterol mesylate[d,e]	Prohibited
Ephedrine sulfate	Prohibited
Epinephrine	Prohibited
Ethylnorepinephrine HCl	Prohibited
Fenoterol[e]	Prohibited

Appendix A Continued

Medication	Status
Isoetharine HCl[e]	Prohibited
Metaproterenol sulfate[e]	Prohibited
Orciprenaline[d,e]	Prohibited
Rimiterol hydrobromide[d,e]	Prohibited
Pirbuterol acetate[e]	Prohibited
Salbutamol (albuterol)[c,d,f]	
Aerosol	Allowed[b]
Rotocap	Allowed[b]
Oral	Prohibited
Salmeterol[g]	Allowed[b]
Terbutaline sulfate[c,d,f]	
Aerosol	Allowed[b]
Oral	Prohibited
Intramuscular	Prohibited
Isoproterenol	Prohibited
Xanthine drivatives	
Aminophylline	Allowed
Diphylline	Allowed
Oxtriphylline	Allowed
Theophylline	Allowed

[a] History of glucocorticosteroid regulations

1975 IOC attempted to restrict their use during the Olympic Games by requiring a declaration by the team doctors, because it was known that they were being used nontherapeutically by the oral, intramuscular, and even the intravenous route in some sports.

1984 Not prohibited

1986 The problem was not solved by previous restrictions and stronger measures designed not to interfere with the appropriate medical use became necessary. Prohibited except for topical use (aural, ophthalmological, and dermatological), inhalational therapy (asthma, allergic rhinitis), and local or intra-articular injections. Written notification required.

[b] Allowed with physician notification sent to USOC before competition.

History of β_2-agonist regulations

[c] 1984 Permitted with team doctor notifying head physican for the games in writing before competition.

[d] 7/1986 Aerosol use allowed. Oral use is prohibited.

[e] 3/1993 Permission to use in aerosol form withdrawn.

[f] 3/1993 Aerosol use allowed only with written notification from prescribing physician sent to USOC before competition.

[g] 3/1996 Aerosol use allowed only with written notification from prescribing physician sent to USOC before competition.

Appendix B Regulations
The following are, or have been reported in the past to be, prohibited. Additional substances may also be prohibited. Regulations constantly change, no list can be absolutely up-to-date and accurate. Contact the governing organizations for current regulations.

Prohibited Drug	USOC	MLB	NBA	NCAA	NFL	MTC
Stimulants						
Decongestants	B			#		
Amphetamines	B			B	B	B
Caffeine	C			C		
β-Agonists	B			A		
Aerosol	B			A		
Salbuterol, Inh	#			A		
Salmeterol, Inh	#			A		
Terbutaline Inh	#			A		
Street drugs						
Cocaine	B	B	B	B	B	B
Heroin	B	B	B	B	B	B
Narcotic analgesics	B			A		
Codeine	A			A		
Morphine	B	B		A		
Anabolic agents	B			B	B	
Peptide hormones	B			B		
Corticosteroids						
Systemic	B			A		
Inhaled	#			A		
Diuretics	B			B		
β-Blockers	B*			B*		
Drugs with sedative action	*			*		
Alcohol	*			*		
Marijuana	M	B		B		
Anesthetics						
Local	#			A		
IM, IV	B			B		
Blood doping	B			B		
Urine manipulation	B			B		

A Allowed
B Prohibited
B* Prohibited in some sports
* Prohibited by some international federations (IFs)
C Caffeine
USOC prohibits greater than 12 μg/mL in urine.
NCAA prohibits greater than 15 μg/mL in urine.
M Tested for at IOC/NGB request

App. B. continues

Appendix B Continued

#	Restricted use
NHL	In the process of forming a formal drug testing program as part of collective bargaining agreement.
PGA	Confidential drug testing policy.
USPF	Adheres to USOC guidelines.
USTA	Juniors follow USOC guidelines. Professionals follow MTC.

Appendix C Contacts for Complete, Up-to-Date Information

International Olympic Committee (IOC)
Prince Alexandre de Merode, Chairman
Medical Commission
Rue Vergote
26, 1200 Brussels, Belgium

Major League Baseball (MLB)
Office of the Commissioner
350 Park Avenue
New York, NY 10022

National Basketball Association (NBA)
645 5th Avenue
New York, NY 10022

National Collegiate Athletic Association (NCAA)
6201 College Boulevard
Overland, KS 66211-2422

National Federation of State High School Association
Target Program
11724 N.W. Plaza Circle
P.O. Box 20626
Kansas City, MO 64195-0626

National Football League (NFL)
410 Park Avenue
New York, NY 10022

National Hockey League (NHL)
1251 Avenue of the Americas
47th Floor
New York, NY 10020-1198

United States Olympic Committee (USOC)
Drug Control Administration
One Olympic Plaza
Colorado Springs, CO 80909

Appendix C Continued

United States Powerlifting Federation (USPF)
Box 18485
Pensacola, FL 32523

United States Tennis Association (USTA)
70 West Red Oak Lane
White Plains, NY 10604-3602

Available Publications

Glaxo Wellcome
Athletic Drug Reference '96
Clean Data, Inc.
P.O. Box 12795
Research Triangle Park, NC 27709-2795
(Also available on disk)

US Olympic Committee
Drug Education Handbook
USOC Drug Education Program
One Olympic Plaza
Colorado Springs, CO 80909

REFERENCES

1. Wadler GI, Hainline B. Drugs and the athlete. Philadelphia: FA Davis, 1989.
2. Mandell AJ, Stewart KD, Russo PV. The Sunday syndrome: from kinetics to altered consciousness. Fed Proc 1981; 40:2693.
3. Catlin DH. Detection of drug use by athletes. In: Stauss RH, ed. Drugs and performance in sports. Philadelphia; WB Saunders, 1987; 103.
4. Donohoe T, Johnson N. Foul play: drug abuse in sports. New York: Basil Blackwell, 1986.
5. International Olympic Charter Against Doping in Sport. Comite International Olympique. Ottawa, Canada, 1988.
6. de Merode A. IOC medical commission-doping in sport. Letter 27 January. Lausanne: Comite International Olympique, 1985.
7. Beresford H. Legal consideration. In: Wadler GI, Hainline B, eds. Drugs and the athlete. Philadelphia: FA Davis, 1989; 234–247.
8. Hanley DF. Drug and sex testing: regulations for international competition. Clin Sports Med, 1986.

9. Mahler DA. Exercise-induced asthma. Med Sci Sports Exer 1993; 25(5): 554–561.
10. Voy RO. The US Olympic Committee experience with exercise-induced bronchospasm, 1994. Med Sci Sports Exer 1986; 18:328–330.
11. Stamford B. Exercise-induced asthma: taking the wheeze out of your workout. Physician Sports Med 1991; 19:139–140.

24

Do Asthma Medications Enhance Sports Performance in Athletes Who Do Not Have Asthma?

William W. Storms
University of Colorado Health Sciences Center, Colorado Springs, Colorado

I. INTRODUCTION

Physicians who treat patients with exercise-induced asthma attempt to control the asthma so that the patient is able to be active physically, and even participate in competitive sports. This approach is based on the understanding that exercise will cause asthma to become worse if pretreatment is not provided. The preferred therapy is to pretreat with medications that will block exercise-induced asthma (EIA) to allow normal exercise. Use of a medication to give an asthmatic an even chance on the playing field seems a natural thing to do. But what if that same medication is shown to enhance the performance of a normal, nonasthmatic individual? A performance-enhancing drug must be banned for all competitors, asthmatic or otherwise. Drug control regulations have been formulated to prevent the use of drugs that enhance performance.

II. DRUG CONTROL REGULATIONS

The United States Olympic Committee (USOC) has a drug education and doping control program [1] to educate athletes about banned medications so that athletes are directed to take only the medications that are permitted, to avoid disqualification. The International Olympic Committee (IOC) has defined a list of substances that are considered "doping." *Doping* is defined as " . . . the administration of or use by a competing athlete of any substance foreign to the body or any physiological substance taken in abnormal quantity or taken by an abnormal route of entry into the body with the sole intention of increasing in an artificial and unfair manner his/her performance in competition." In addition, if treatment requires the use of any substance that because of the nature, dosage, or application is able to boost the athlete's performance in competition in an artificial and unfair manner, this too is considered by the IOC as doping.

The IOC has published a list of banned substances, and has instituted a drug-testing program at the Olympics to deter the use of these substances (see also Chap. 23). The USOC provides support to athletes with its drug control department, and it even provides a hotline for athletes and their physicians (1-800-233-0393) to make sure that athletes are treated only with drugs that comply with the IOC guidelines.

III. DRUGS THAT ENHANCE ATHLETIC PERFORMANCE

The IOC has identified five classes of doping, or drugs that enhance performance:

Stimulants
Narcotics
Anabolic agents
Diuretics
Peptide hormones and analogues

IV. STIMULANTS

Stimulants are drugs that increase alertness, reduce fatigue, and may increase competitiveness and hostility. Although these drugs produce both a psychological and physical stimulus to athletic performance, they also cause variable side effects that can be detrimental. They produce anxiety, tremor, and aggressiveness, which can lead to poor judgment, placing the individual and his or her fellow competitors at risk of injury. Heart rate and blood pressure can be increased. Other side effects include the risk of cerebral hemorrhage and cardiac arrhythmias.

Performance enhancement effects have been associated with certain β-adrenergic agonists, such as clenbuterol or oral albuterol. Clenbuterol is a veterinary drug, not approved for use in humans, which increases muscle mass when given orally to human subjects. This drug has been abused by some who have desired to build up their muscle mass; however, it is not as effective as anabolic steroids for this use. There are several stimulatory side effects from clenbuterol that may interfere with athletic performance, including insomnia, jitters, palpitations, nervousness, and headaches. Oral albtuerol is a recognized therapy for the treatment of asthma (albuterol syrup, Ventolin, Proventil; albuterol tablets, Volmax, Proventil Repetabs). This form of albuterol is banned because of the potential for increase in muscle mass. Volmax has increased muscle strength in lower leg muscles in volunteers. Whether or not this effect can be translated to enhanced performance is unclear, especially because tolerance to this effect appears to occur after even short-term use. In any event, the oral β-agonists are banned.

Amphetamines and related compounds have the most notorious reputation for producing problems in sports. There is no medical justification for the use of stimulants (i.e., amphetamines, cocaine, and related substances) in sports. Some examples of stimulants are listed in Table 1.

Table 1 Examples of Stimulant Drugs

Generic name	Example (trade name)
Desoxyephedrine	Vicks inhaler
Ephedrine	Tedral, Bronkotabs, Rynatuss, Primatene
Isoetharine HCl	Bronkosol, Bronkometer, Dilabron
Isoproterenol	Isuprel, Norisodrine, Medihaler-ISO
Metaproterenol (oral)	Alupent, Metaprel (oral)

A. Over the-Counter Medications Containing Stimulants

One group of stimulants is the sympathomimetic amines, including ephedrine, pseudoephedrine, phenylpropanolamine, and norpseudoephedrine. These are often present as decongestants in cold and hay fever preparations purchased without a prescription. Because of their availability and common use, athletes must be careful not to take these banned substances.

Thus, no product for use in colds, flu, or hay fever purchased by a competitor or given to him or her should be used without first checking with a doctor or pharmacist to ensure that the product does not contain a drug of the banned stimulants class. Please refer to the following few examples (Table 2).

Table 2 Over-the Counter Medications Containing Stimulants[a]

Generic name	Example
Desoxyephedrine	Vicks Inhaler
Pseudoephedrine	Actifed, Ambenyl, Anamine, Afrin tablets, Afrinol, Co-Tylenol, Deconamine, Dimacol, Emprazil, Fedahist, Fedrazil, Histalet, Isoclor, LoTussin, Nasalspan, Novafed, Nucofed, Poly-Histine, Pseudo-Bid, Pseudo-Hist, Rhinosym, Ryna, Sudafed, Triprolidine, Tussend, Chlorafed, Chlor-Trimetron-DC, Disphoral, Drixoral, Polaramine Expectorant, Rondec, and others
Phenylephrine	Coricidin, Dristan, NTZ, Neo-Synephrine, Sinex
Phenylpropanolamine	ARM, Allerest, Alka-Seltzer Plus, Contac, Dexatrim, Dietac, 4-Way Formula 44, Naldecon, Novahistine, Arnex, Sine-Aid, Sine-Off, Sinutab, Triaminic, Triaminicin, Sucrets Cold Decongestant, and related products
Propylhexedrine	Benzedrex Inhaler
Ephedrine	Bronkaid, Collyrium with Ephedrine, Pazo Suppository, Wyanoid Suppository, Vitronol Nose Drops, Nyquil Nighttime Cold Medicine, Herbal Teas and Medicines containing Ma Huang (Chinese Ephedra)
Ma Huang (herbal ephedrine)	Action Caps, Bishop's Tea, Breathe Easy Herbal Decongestant Tea, Brigham Tea, Chi Powder, Energy Rise, Ephedra, Excel, Free Herbal "Energy Tablets," Joint Fir, Mexican Tea, Miner's Tea Popotillo, Quick Shot Vitamin B_{12}, Squaw Tea, Super Charge and Teamster's Tea

[a] **Caution**: *This is not a complete list. There are new products on the market almost monthly, and all products carrying the name "decongestant" generally contain banned substances.*

B. Caffeine

An amount of caffeine greater than 12 μg/mL in the urine is considered doping. As an example, to reach this limit one would have to consume approximately 6–8 cups of coffee in one sitting and be tested within 2–3 h. However, there are other sources of caffeine. The examples listed in Table 3 indicate how excessive levels might be inadvertently accumulated.

The choice of medication in the treatment of asthma and respiratory ailments has posed many problems. Some years ago, ephedrine, and related substances, were administered quite frequently. However, these substances are prohibited because they are classed in the category of

Table 3 Amount of Caffeine in Some Common Products

Caffeine products	Amount/dose (mg)	Equivalent in urine within 2–3 h ($\mu g\ mL^{-1}$)
Decaffeinated coffee	2–3	0.03–0.04
1 cup of coffee	100.0	1.50
1 Coca-Cola/Diet Coke	45.6	0.65
1 Tab	44.0	0.70
1 Dr. Pepper	39.5	0.99
1 Diet Pepsi/Pepsi Light	36.0	0.34
1 NoDoz	200.0	1.50
1 Vivarin	200.0	3.00
1 Anacin, or aspirin	32.0	0.68
1 Excedrin	65.0	0.97
1 Midol	32.4	0.68

Note: These are only examples: Accurate equivalents are based on age, body size, weight, and metabolic rate.

"sympathomimetic amines" and, therefore, are considered to be stimulants. The use of the following β_2-agonists is permitted in the *aerosol* or *inhalant* form only.

Generic name	Example
Salbutamol	Albuterol; Ventolin, Proventil, Airet
Terbutaline	Brethaire
Salmeterol	Serevent

Any team doctor wishing to prescribe these drugs to an athlete must give written notification to the USOC.

Note. Other β_2-agonists have been permitted in the past, but are now considered *banned*.

V. MEDICATIONS FOR USE IN ASTHMA OR ALLERGIES

A. Stimulants

Permission to use inhaled-β_2-agonists, such as the following, has been withdrawn, and they are *banned*:

Bitolterol (Tornalate)
Fenoterol (Berotec)

Metaproterenol sulfate (Alupent and Metaprel)
Orciprenaline
Rimiterol hydrobromide
Pirbuterol (Maxair)

The following β_2-agonists are permitted by *inhalation only*, and *only* with written notification from the prescribing physician sent before competition:

Salbutamol (albuterol: Proventil, Ventolin, Airet)
Terbutaline (Brethaire)
Salmeterol (Serevent)

B. Corticosteroids

1. Oral, rectal, intramuscular, and intravenous use of corticosteroids is banned.
2. Topical use (aural, ophthalmological, and dermatological) is allowed.
3. Inhalation therapy (asthma, allergic rhinitis) and local or intra-articular injections are allowed *only* with written notification sent before competition.

Note that inhalation therapy is no longer allowed without written notification. The following inhaled corticosteroid preparations are examples of medications previously allowed that now require written notification:

Beclomethasone (Beclovent, Beconase, Vancenase, Vanceril)
Dexamethasone (Decadron Phosphate Respihaler and Turbinaire, Dexamethasone Aerosol and Respihaler)
Flunisolide (Aerobid, Nasalide)
Triamcinolone (Azmacort, Kenalog, Nasacort)
Fluticasone (Flovent)

In the past, rectal administration of corticosteroids was allowed with notification. This is no longer true, and rectal preparations are now *banned*.

VI. ASTHMA MEDICATIONS AND ATHLETES' PERFORMANCE

Asthma medications can be divided into two categories: (a) bronchodilators, and (b) anti-inflammatory drugs.

Bronchodilators include β-agonists (given orally and by inhalation), theophylline (oral), and anticholinergics (inhaled). Of these, the only category that might have a potential for enhancing performance would be the β-agonists. The primary drug of this category used in asthma is albuterol (Proventil, Ventolin); this is usually given by the inhaled route and is the treatment of choice for exercise-induced asthma. In this setting it is usually given as a pretreatment 15 mins before exercise.

Albuterol is a sympathomimetic amine compound that has a β-adrenergic stimulatory effect on smooth muscle, with preference for bronchial smooth muscle over cardiac smooth muscle, thus minimizing any cardiostimulatory side effects. Because this drug is related to ephedrine and epinephrine, it must be considered as having potential for enhancing performance.

In one study, albuterol was given to asthmatics performing cycle ergometry [2] and had no effect on $\dot{V}O_2max$ when compared with placebo aerosol; these authors felt that albuterol aerosol had no ergogenic effect. Another study [3] assessed the effect of nebulized albuterol on normal volunteers and found an increase in pulse rate, systolic blood pressure, and blood glucose, concluding that this drug might produce unwanted side effects. These results might also suggest that albuterol may impair performance, although these measurements were not done.

A study showing enhanced performance with albuterol was performed in nonasthmatic cyclists [4]. Fifteen subjects were exercised to exhaustion with and without albuterol pretreatment. The only parameters showing statistically significant changes were the 1-s forced expiratory volume (FEV_1) and the total ride time. The FEV_1 change was noted only after drug administration before exercise; there was no change after exercise. Thus, inhaled albuterol reversed the small amount of smooth-muscle bronchodilator tone found in normal persons, but there was no further change after exercise. The amount of improvement in FEV_1 was very small, about 2.9%. This study excluded asthma patients by a medical history and a pulmonary function test; no specific challenge for airway reactivity (such as histamine, methacholine, or cold air inhalation) was performed to definitively exclude subclinical cases of asthma from the subject population. If one or two of the subjects had airway reactivity, this might have influenced the results.

Another measure of performance is total power output, in which subjects exercise on a bicycle ergometer for a short time (15 s) at supramaximal effort. The effects of albuterol on performance in this test were studied in 15 nonasthmatic athletes [5]; the results showed improved performance, as shown by peak power output, fatigue, and pulmonary function values. The authors concluded that albuterol had an ergogenic effect; however, these subjects were also not screened for airway reactivity with challenge tests. Therefore, the comments raised with the previous study apply similarly to this one.

Treadmill testing is an accepted standardized measure of performance. Nineteen nonatopic athletes were exercised maximally on a treadmill, with and without albuterol pretreatment [6]. There was no effect of albuterol treatment on the $\dot{V}O_2max$, pulmonary function tests, or heart rate. The authors concluded that there was no evidence of an ergogenic effect of albuterol.

Another study of the effect of albuterol on performance [7] examined seven elite nonasthmatic athletes. Meeuwisse et al. evaluated both maximal power output and a sprint to exhaustion on a cycle ergometer. They found no difference in peak power, maximal heart rate, endurance sprint time, Wingate peak power, or total work. These authors concluded that there was no ergogenic effect of albuterol in this study.

Two other studies [8,9] were performed at the Sports Medicine Division of the US Olympic Committee in Colorado Springs. Both of these studies included prescreening of all athletes with methacholine inhalation to exclude airway reactivity.

In these two studies some elite cyclists failed the methacholine inhalation challenge despite a negative history of asthma or atopic disease, indicating the presence of undiagnosed airways reactivity. One of the studies evaluated the effects of albuterol on maximal power output and the other evaluated exercise to exhaustion. Both studies showed no ergogenic effects of albuterol on performance.

The level of athletic performance may have an effect on the level of symptoms of exercise-induced asthma experienced by a given athlete. If one athlete competes at a higher level than another and trains more intensely, it may be that this continued higher level of exercise stimulation may produce more problems with EIA than it would if less exercise was undertaken. Thus, the elite level athlete with EIA may require more medication to control the asthma than would a nonelite athlete.

To summarize the data on albuterol, it can be concluded that this drug has no ergogenic effects on the performance of nonasthmatic athletes.

The other bronchodilators in use for asthma, including theophylline and anticholinergics, have not been shown to have ergogenic effects in athletes. The same holds true for the inhaled anti-inflammatory drugs—cromolyn, nedrocromil, and steroids. Thus, these medications should be available to asthmatic athletes in competition.

Systemic steroids are occasionally needed for patients with asthma and may have the potential for enhancing performance.

VII. SUMMARY

The International Olympic Committee has attempted to restrict the use in athletes of any drug that may enhance performance. In so doing, this has led to the restriction of some of the drugs used to treat asthma and exercise-induced asthma in athletes. However, there remains a wide variety of medication of different classes that are still permitted for treatment. Physicians should not have difficulty in choosing adequate therapy from the list of permitted drugs. Because the list of permitted drugs changes occasionally, it is very important for the physician, the trainer, and the patient to call the USOC drug hotline (1-800-233-0393) for a review of the patient's therapy and suggestions for any changes that may need to be made. This notification should be made as early as possible, so that the patient may be stabilized on the new treatment before competition begins.

REFERENCES

1. United States Olympic Committee Drug Education and Doping Control Program. Guide to banned medications, 1993.
2. Neville A, Palmer JBD, Gaddie J, et al. Metabolic effects of salbutamol: comparison of aerosol and intravenous administration. Br Med J 1977; 1: 413–414.
3. Smith SR, Ryder C, Kendall MJ, et al. Cardiovascular and biochemical responses to nebulised salbutamol in normal subjects. Br J Clin Pharm 1984; 18:641–644.
4. Bedi JF, Gong H Jr, Horvath SM. Enhancement of exercise performance with inhaled albuterol. Can J Sport Sci 1988; 13:144–148.
5. Signorile JF, Kaplan TA, Appelegate B, et al. Effects of acute inhalation of the bronchodilator, albuterol, on power output. Med Sci Sports Exerc 1992; 24:638–642.
6. McKenzie DC, Rhodes EC, Stirling DR, et al. Salbutamol and treadmill performance in nonatopic athletes. Med Sci Sports Exerc 1983; 15:520–522.
7. Meeuwisse WH, McKenzie DC, Hopkins SR, et al. The effect of salbutamol on performance in elite nonasthmatic athletes. Med Sci Sports Exerc 1992; 24:1161–1166.
8. Fleck SJ, Lucia A, Storms WW, et al. Effects of acute inhalation of albuterol on submaximal and maximal $\dot{V}O_2$ and blood lactate. Int J Sports Med 1993; 14:239–243.

9. Lemmer JT, Fleck SJ, Wallach JM, et al. The effects of albuterol on power output in non-asthmatic athletes. Int J Sports Med 1995; 16:243–249.
10. Fitch KD. The use of anti-asthmatic drugs. Do they affect sports performance? Sports Med 1986; 3:136–150.
11. DiPasquale G. Clenbuterol: a new anabolic drug. Drugs Sports 1992; 1:8–10.
12. Martineau L, et al. Salbutimol, a beta-2 adrenoreceptor agonist, increases skeletal muscle strength in young men. Clin Sci 1992; 83:615–621.

25

Recognition and Management of Asthma and Related Diseases in Children Participating in School Sports and Physical Education Programs

Robert E. Coifman
Allergy & Asthma of South Jersey, Vineland, New Jersey

I. HYPOTHESES/PREMISES

A. Asthma has been identified as the most common chronic disorder in children attending school. Exercise as an asthma trigger may be additive to, or synergistic with, other asthma triggers that may be active in a patient at any time. If this premise is correct, then sports and physical education (PE) should present a problem for children attending school. The term, "school sports and PE asthma," in this chapter will be used to mean asthma in all school settings associated with increased physical exertion, including interscholastic sports, physical education, physically active recess for young children, and such activities as climbing stairs, in schools with stairs, to go from one class to another.

B. There are four possible combinations of trigger and response pattern in school sports and PE asthma.

1. Exercise as the only trigger of asthma.
2. Exercise as one of many triggers of mild to moderate symptoms in individuals whose asthma may or may not be recognized, and may or may not be partially controlled.

3. Exercise as a trigger that provokes a severe, acute exacerbation of asthma, which is either undiagnosed or else known but inadequately controlled.
4. Exercise-associated respiratory symptoms which are incorrectly labeled as asthma.

C. Asthma morbidity and mortality in general are higher in ethnic minority and socioeconomically disadvantaged populations than in mostly Caucasian and more affluent population groups. These differences may have genetic, socioeconomic and cultural causes.

1. The socioeconomic/cultural cause may result from perception of the principal role of the health care system as providing emergency treatment, rather than prevention. Often minorities have decreased access to appropriate preventive care, and fewer resources to implement such measures as environmental control of dust mite and cockroach allergens, and avoidance of combustion products of tobacco and kerosene heaters.
2. The effect of asthma, and the management burden it places on school districts, might correspondingly be different in schools serving students from these different groups.
3. It is generally recognized that school districts serving socioeconomically disadvantaged populations must cope, at significant cost if it is to be done effectively, with deficiencies in the physical, psycho-social, and educational backgrounds from which their students come. Frequent school sports and severe PE asthma in a school district may be no more than a barometer of unresolved socioeconomic problems in its community. Effective management may require specific interventions that are made necessary by poverty, and for which equity requires funding from budgets based on need rather than per capita funding for education.

D. Asthma might be expected to differ in its presentation by grade level and between physical education programs and interscholastic sports.

1. Young children are intuitive enough not to do things that hurt. As such, they are more likely to limit their level of exercise than to push to levels that provoke symptoms. Older children are more motivated by recognition of achievement; consequently, they are more likely to persevere, even when an activity results in discomfort.
2. Because of the greater premium on performance, a student with asthma who participates in interscholastic sports may perform

at a greater intensity of exercise and trigger more asthma than a student in a physical education class, at recess, or during physical activities such as walking up stairs between classes. For the balance of this chapter, these potentially different risk areas, will be distinguished as *school sports asthma* and *school PE asthma*.

E. Having asthma may be a source of secondary gain:

1. Secondary gain constitutes whatever recognition, preferential treatment, benefits, reduction in demands, or other entitlements that may be derived from the achievement of a particular status, either by formal declaration or by peer or community acceptance. The seeking of a status providing secondary gain is not necessarily dysfunctional. Most members of our society are happy to accept the entitlements of Social Security and Medicare eligibility.
2. Similarly, secondary gains from the status of having school PE asthma may include the "entitlements" and peer recognition of disability status, being excused from physical education, and being allowed to use the elevator while the rest of the student body climbs stairs. One might expect the seeking of secondary gain entitlements from the status of having asthma to be more common in students from disadvantaged socioeconomic groups in which there are both a rational basis and a societal role model for seeking entitlements based on disability status as a way to enhance one's position in life.

II. A TALE OF TWO CITIES

In 1991, we presented an educational program on school sports and PE asthma for school nurses, physical education teachers, and sports coaches. We were then invited to work with a large, urban school district, to implement and evaluate a program for improved management of school sports and PE asthma employing use of peak flow meters (PFM) by gym teachers and coaches. This program was designed to foster communication with students' families and physicians by the schools' nurses, nurse practitioners, and school physicians. In 1993 and 1994, the district had about 21,000 students in grades K–12, attending 24 elementary , two junior high, and two high schools. About 80% of students were black, and 15% were Hispanic. The median 1993 per capita and household income in the municipality served by this district were 7,726 and 17,386 dollars, respectively. Every school had at least one nurse on duty during school hours. Each of the two high schools had a student health clinic, with full-time staffing by nurse practitioners and part time availability of a consultant pediatrician who subspecialized in adolescent medicine. Asthma was second only to issues of reproductive health among problems presenting for care at the high school clinics. Care at the school clinics had previously been covered by Medicaid, but was jeopardized by the contracting of Medicaid in this county to managed care plans unwilling to pay for care by school pediatricians.

School sports and PE asthma was not viewed to be a significant problem for the school health service in the elementary schools. Similarly, PE asthma was a minor problem in the junior high and high school physical education programs, in which instructors were familiar with PE asthma and reasonably astute at recognizing symptomatic children and sending them to the health service.

This is a school district in which excellence in a major interscholastic sport is one of the most effective ways for a student to leapfrog from the poverty and violence of the local community to college, and for the most gifted, to a professional sports career. Its coaches stress toughness, and have little appreciation for either the potential seriousness of sports asthma or the degree to which athletic performance can be improved if asthma is controlled. Sports asthma has been a recurring problem in the district's junior high and high schools, generating an average of one ambulance call for status asthmaticus per month to one of the four schools. The district's school-nursing administrator, with whom we worked, believed that the recent publicized asthma death of a promising high school basketball player, in a nearby city, might make the coaches receptive to asthma management strategies, other than denial, as ways to maximize the achievement of asthmatic student athletes.

However, following a change in composition of the school board and the appointment of a new superintendent, the district abruptly withdrew its request for us to help improve its management of school sports and PE asthma. The new superintendent voiced his concern about outsiders exploiting his district's poverty for their own agendas. About a year later, the district changed its contractor for school physician services to the pediatric department of a local teaching institution whose staff included a full-time pediatric allergist. We offered to collaborate with the district and its new contract physicians if they wanted to continue the PFM project. We received no reply. As we began to prepare this manuscript, we requested a meeting to review and update our notes about the district's experience with sports and PE asthma. However, the new superintendent considered this confidential information, which could not be shared without his specific prior approval. Our efforts at further communication have been ignored. This experience suggests that personal feelings at the administrative level may complicate the management of school sports and PE asthma in high-risk schools. In this chapter we will identify this district only as District "U" (urban) in deference to the superintendent's concerns and to leave the door open for possible future cooperation.

Slightly more than a mile away from urban District "U" is suburban District "S" serving about 10,000 students; 5,300 in 12 elementary schools, 1,500 in two junior highs, and 3,200 in two high schools. Eighty one percent of its students are white, 12% Asian, 5% black, and 2% Hispanic. Slightly less than 3% of students in the district qualified for aid to dependent children. Median 1993 per capita and household income in this municipality were 24,453 and 54,432 dollars, respectively. Slightly more than 6% of the district's 10,000 students were listed on school records as having asthma.

District "S" required that for elementary school students, all medications given in school, including inhaled asthma medications, be given by school nurses. Junior high and high school students were permitted to carry their own asthma inhalers, but were asked to report to the school health service if they did so. Use of inhalers for asthma was believed to be underreported. School records listed 300 students as receiving daily medications in school, most of these were elementary students receiving medications for attention deficit disorder. Five hundred students were listed as receiving medications as-needed. The director of nursing believed most of these students used asthma inhalers. Participation in interscholastic sports required submission of an authorization form, listing illnesses and medications, signed by both a parent and a physician. Asthma of such severity that it required intervention by a school nurse was rare in this district. The director of nursing, who did not remember any cases of sufficient severity to require activation of the emergency medical response system, offered to enlist the support of her administration if we wished to follow our retrospective study of the asthma experience of the two districts with a prospective study. In both school asthma experience and in receptiveness to working on school asthma with outsiders, the two districts were distinctly different.

III. FATALITIES IN SCHOOL SPORTS AND PHYSICAL EDUCATION ASTHMA

A 17-year-old African-American male high school basketball player, with a skill level believed sufficient to anticipate a professional basketball career, reported a history of childhood asthma on his school sports permission form. After a light, noncontact workout early in the basketball season, he became short of breath and collapsed while standing in the gymnasium. Emergency medical service personnel found him pulseless, and he did not respond to resuscitative efforts in the field, in transit, or in the emergency room. Results of a toxicology screen were negative. Autopsy findings indicated hyperexpanded, "fluffy" lungs, moderate bronchial mucosal hyperplasia, inspissated mucus in several bronchi that contained inflammatory cells including eosinophils, smooth-muscle hyperplasia of small bronchi, and marked thickening of bronchial basement membranes. These are gross and microscopic findings characteristic of acute bronchial asthma. The heart was grossly normal and microscopic sections revealed no evidence of myocarditis, cardiomyopathy, or other myocardial lesion. Single sections of sinoatrial and atrioventricular nodes were histologically unremarkable. Death was attributed to acute bronchial asthma.

Although information available to his school indicated that he had long since "outgrown" his asthma, he had an albuterol asthma inhaler in his pocket when he died of this disease. While it was not so-stated in the medical examiner's report, individuals familiar with this case believe the physician's signature on his school sports permission form was forged. This boy had a cousin, also a gifted basketball player, who died while playing basketball of a documented cardiac arrhythmia.

Three of 19 asthma deaths in school-aged children (age 5–18) recorded from 1975 to 1987 in Wayne County (Detroit), Michigan, occurred in the course of vigorous physical activity [1]. Two 15-year-old boys collapsed and died of asthma during vigorous running not associated with school sports or PE, one while being chased by a dog and the other while running to beat curfew. A 17-year-old girl collapsed and died of asthma while playing soccer; the published report does not indicate whether this event was associated with school sports or PE. Most patients in this series were stated to be known chronic asthmatics, and many had histories of previous emergency room treatment. Historical data, when available, were reported by the authors as indicating that most patients appeared to have been subjectively unaffected by increasing asthma symptoms until very shortly before their death, whereas both histology and, when available, past history, indicated long-standing, chronic asthma.

The department of Pulmonary and Critical Care Medicine at Temple University, with support from the National Athletic Trainers Association (NATA) maintains a national registry for asthma fatalities and near-fatalities caused by exertional activity in sports.* In its first 10 months of opera-

---

* c/o Gilbert D'Alonzo, DO, Division of Pulmonary and Critical Care Medicine, 1-800-204-3303, 215-707-7208, fax 215-707-7209, Temple University Health Sciences Center, Broad and Ontario Streets, Philadelphia PA 19140.

tion the registry received 15 case reports in which it could confirm exercise-induced bronchospasm to have been an important element contributing to death. The age range of these individuals at death was 10–39 years, with median age 19 years. Eleven of the 15 were males, and 9 of the 15 were African-Americans residing in low-income areas. The primary source of case reporting for fatalities was a national newspaper clipping service. Case-finding from such a source might reflect a media-reporting bias favoring individuals, such as our aforementioned basketball player, whose skill in a high media interest sport gave greater than average news-worthiness to his death.

The registry also collects reports of life-threatening exercise-induced asthma requiring urgent or emergent medical care, with most cases reported by members of the NATA. Sixty cases of life-threatening sports-associated asthma were reported to the registry in the same 10 months. Most of the reports came from school sports activities or organized after-school sports activities in school-aged children. Near-fatalities were reported in sustained running sports (cross-country), repeated short aerobic burst sports (soccer), and also in the traditionally low–asthma-risk sport of swimming. The registry's analysis of its near-fatalities was insufficient to permit the reporting of demographic trends in time for inclusion in this chapter. The registry will probably be a valuable resource for information on the more severe presentations of sports-associated asthma in school-aged children in the future, although reporting of near-fatalities by members of the NATA will selectively favor the reporting of cases from those sports activities staffed by trainers.

IV. ASTHMA AT THE FINISH LINE

An otherwise healthy 16-year-old caucasian male had a positive family history of atopy and asthma, and a negative prior history except for spasms of cough, gagging, and choking "almost to the point of vomiting," beginning within a minute and lasting for 2 h after vigorous long-distance running. His problem began when he began serious competitive running, at age 14. He could complete a 4.8-km 3-mile cross-country run or run a 1.6-km (1 mile) in 4 min 30 s without symptoms, but would begin coughing and choking almost as soon as he stopped. His principal complaint was that his coach often wanted him to run in additional events after he completed the mile, and he could not do it because he was still coughing and choking. His only other sign of disease, elicited by careful questioning, was frequent throat clearing with body movement, but not when still, regardless of whether standing, sitting, or lying down. Chest x-ray films and baseline spirometry were normal.

An oral sustained-release theophylline with breakfast, supplemented by a gradual warm-up and two puffs from a pirbuterol inhaler before competing and a "cool-down" lap at the end of his race produced no improvement. He experienced no symptoms during his cool-down lap, but again began to cough within 30s after he stopped running. His coughing spasms gradually subsided over about 2 h, but recurred with movements including attempts to speak, during the 2-h period. He had no history suggesting gastroesophageal reflux.

In a free run exercise challenge test along the road outside our small town office, the need to slow down for traffic kept this young man from achieving a sufficient workload to reproduce his symptoms. Because his next races were only four days away, we empirically prescribed daily inhaled beclomethasone and nedocromil, plus pirbuterol and ipatropium before running. His race after four days' treatment was the first vigorous competitive mile he had ever run without post-exercise coughing and gagging. He subsequently determined that he could maintain complete symptom control with only beclomethasone, nedocromil, and ipatropium. Allergy evaluation indicated strong skin test reactivity to the dust mite, *D. pteronyssinus*, and a preference for sleeping in a sleeping bag on his carpeted bedroom floor as he found his mattress uncomfortably soft.

A 17-year-old black female had a similar history for the 3 years she has been running competitively, except that her coughing and choking spasms lasted for 3 days after competitive long-distance running, instead of 3 h. She could run a mile (1.6 km) in 5 min 20 s. She reported rhinorrhea as well as coughing, gagging, vomiting, and gasping for air after vigorous competitive running. She initially presented for care 4 days before her state sectional high school championships. A victory in this meet would qualify her for the state championship meet, 1 week later. Her spirogram suggested premature reflex glottic closure, limiting forced expiration (a pattern we have learned to identify as "bronchitic") both before and after bronchodilator administration, with significant improvement in PEFR and FEF25–75, but no change in FEV_1 or FVC following use of a bronchodilator.

She was treated in a manner similar to the preceding case but also instructed to use a 12-hr decongestant nose spray before each meet. Although she did not qualify for the state championships, her post-race symptoms were prevented. She subsequently found that she could maintain symptom control with only beclomethasone and nedocromil. She also had demonstrable allergy, with strong positive skin test reactions to ten of 26 molds tested, and moderate reactivity to *D. pteronyssinus*.

V. SCHOOL SPORTS AND PHYSICAL EDUCATION ASTHMA IN THE OFFICE OF THE PRIMARY CARE PHYSICIAN

We asked a large pediatric group and a large family practice group in our service area how school sports and PE asthma impinge on their practice. Both groups serve primarily middle-class, insured patients, often enrolled in managed care programs. The pediatric group did not find school sports and PE asthma to be a particular problem in their asthmatic patients attending school. The family practice group's only concern was the appropriateness of salmeterol as single-drug prophylaxis for exercise-induced asthma, as it was favored by some of their consultants but not by others.

VI. SCHOOL SPORTS AND PHYSICAL EDUCATION ASTHMA IN THE OFFICE OF THE SPECIALIST

We have a four-office, solo allergy practice which serves a mixed suburban–rural–small town population. We treat numerous hard-to-manage asthmatic children from low income families, on referral from other physicians. In this practice, sports-associated asthma or cough-variant asthma are unusual in the absence of other signs or symptoms of asthma. Most school-aged asthma patients report sports-associated respiratory symptoms when they enter our care, although their management does not always require taking medications at school. Among those children who appear physically fit, sports-associated respiratory symptoms typically appear following rather than during, maximal exertion. We usually confirm these to be exercise-induced exacerbations of asthma, and they usually respond to appropriate management of the asthma and associated allergies. Among the children who appear physically unfit, the most common exercise-associated respiratory complaints are shortness of breath and chest wall pain. These usually occur during, rather than after, maximal exertion, and reflect physical deconditioning even if the patient also has coexisting asthma.

Most patients we provide care for with asthma completely limited to school sports and PE are not like the two high school athletes described earlier, but fall into one of the following three groups.

1. Children formerly unable to participate in sports and PE because of their asthma, who continue to have exertional dyspnea after other manifestations of asthma have been controlled, Most such patients reproduce their dyspnea after a free-running exercise challenge, without a fall in pulmonary functions. These patients

are physically deconditioned as a result of their previous inability to exercise, and they respond to reassurance and graded exercise programs to get into better physical shape.

2. Children who may or may not have a diagnosis of asthma from their primary physicians, referred to us by their school nurses for evaluation of exertional dyspnea. Most patients in this group are obese and sedentary, and come from homes in which physical activity has not been encouraged. History and physical examination of these patients is usually negative for cardiopulmonary disease and suggests mild asthma or cough-variant asthma. These children almost invariably have normal or near-normal baseline spirometry and they experience dyspnea without a fall in pulmonary function on exercise challenge, suggesting that their problem, too, is physical deconditioning. These children usually respond to the same management as children in the preceding group. They have often been given gym excuses for asthma by other physicians, in the past.
3. Children almost exclusively from lower income families who seek certification of disability status, to be excused from physical education and to be permitted to ride the elevator instead of having to use the stairs at school. These patients are often already known to us, having been treated for medical care of asthma months or years earlier but not having returned as requested for follow-up. Remarkably, what they typically seek is not treatment for their reported symptoms, but certification of a disability status that will give them secondary gain. These patients typically report dyspnea during, rather than following exercise, again suggesting physical deconditioning, rather than asthma as the principal cause. If they return for exercise challenge, patients in this group rarely make more than a minimal gesture of exercising. Often, when offered treatment rather than disability certification, they terminate care and take their quest for disability certification elsewhere. These patients often file inappropriate claims for SSI disability certification because of asthma at about the same time that they seek disability certification for secondary gain at school. Many of these patients have been previously certified by other physicians as being disabled by asthma.

VII. DISCUSSION

Exercise-induced asthma occurs following the conclusion of exercise, rather than during the exercise itself [2]. McFadden and Gilbert noted also that, in general, "Exercise does not cause prolonged or intense airway obstruction that is dangerous or requires hospitalization" [2]. Cypcar and Lemanske, in another recent review, observed that, ". . such a situation almost invariably reflects advanced unattended disease or confounding trigger factors (i.e., concomitant allergen or irritant exposure), or both" [3]. Venge et al. [4] correlated severity of exercise-induced asthma with degree of underlying pulmonary eosinophilic inflammation, of which allergy is a common trigger. Knowledge of the pathophysiology of exercise-induced asthma and our observations support the following conclusions about school sports and PE asthma:

1. School sports and PE are common triggers of asthma, but sports and PE-associated symptoms do not commonly present significant management problems to either the school or the attending physician for children receiving appropriate medical care. School sports and PE may present significant problems for the individual in whom the association between atypical symptoms and asthma has not been recognized. School sports asthma appears to have been the trigger responsible for the death of the basketball player who did not seek medical care, but who forged the physician signature on his sports permission form and treated his symptoms with a borrowed albuterol inhaler.
2. There are probably children with all four of the trigger–response patterns listed in hypothesis B at the beginning of this chapter. However, despite our specific interest in school sports and PE asthma, we have never seen a patient in the first category with no complaints or demonstrable abnormalities other than postexertional asthma of the limited duration and severity meeting McFadden's definition of uncomplicated exercise-induced asthma. The majority of our physically active school-aged patients who report exercise as an asthma trigger represent the second category of school sports and PE asthma—mild to moderate asthma with exercise as one of multiple triggers. The male runner in Sec. IV falls into this category; we believe inflammation resulting from dust mite allergy contributed to both the severity and the duration of his symptoms. The female runner in Sec. IV and the basketball player whose death is described in Sec. III represent the third category, with allergic airway inflammation contributing to severe or prolonged post-exercise symptoms. The basketball player's airway was apparently sufficiently hyperreactive, as a result of other triggers at the time of his death, that a relatively modest level of exercise was able to provoke fatal airway obstruction. The fourth category comprises

children incorrectly classified as having school sports or PE asthma.

3. We have described the characteristics of two groups of children who may present with histories that falsely suggest or mimic school sports or PE asthma. Our experience suggests that such children are frequently mislabeled or misdiagnosed as having school sports or PE asthma. We believe it is a disservice to these children to label them as disabled or to restrict unnecessarily their physical activity because of a condition they do not have.
4. School sports and PE asthma may lead to an increase in morbidity and risk of mortality, similar to that of asthma in general, in socioeconomically disadvantaged, ethnic minority populations.
5. School sports and PE asthma is more severe in children of junior high and high school age than in younger children, and more severe in junior high and high school interscholastic sports than in PE, because of incentives to increase the level of aerobic exercise, to improve performance.
6. School sports and PE asthma of sufficient severity to come to medical attention almost always reflects activity of other asthma triggers, in addition to exercise. Allergies will almost invariably be contributory triggers in children of school age.

VIII. DIFFERENTIAL DIAGNOSIS AND ATYPICAL PRESENTATIONS

Exercise-induced asthma develops following rather than during, vigorous physical exercise. Shortness of breath from physical deconditioning presents during vigorous exercise. Cardiac events are uncommon in children and usually happen during, rather than following, vigorous physical exercise. A cardiac etiology should be suspected if there is a positive family history of similar events, of congenital cardiac arrhythmias, or of mitral valve prolapse or hypertrophic cardiomyopathy.

Pediatric cardiologists Nudel et al. found no cardiac pathology, but a 9.5% incidence of exercise-induced asthma in 147 children, ages 5–22 (mean 13.2) referred for evaluation of chest pain associated with exercise and studied with a standard cardiological progressive treadmill or bicycle ergometer progressive exercise challenge [5]. Wiens et al. reviewed the records of 88 children, ages 4–20 (mean 12.4) referred to their institution with similar histories. They performed a one step exercise challenge less likely to induce tolerance in exercise asthma than the progressive challenge used by Nudel et al., and found exercise-induced asthma in 72.7%

[6]. Neither group of authors discussed the temporal relation between the exercise and chest pain; specifically, whether the chest pain followed the time course defined by McFadden and others for exercise-induced asthma. Our own anecdotal clinical experience suggests that chest pain during, rather than following, maximal exertion in children and young adults with asthma, usually reflects either physical deconditioning or costosternal synovitis. In the latter case the pain can be reproduced by firm pressure on the affected costosternal joint or joints, and is sometimes accompanied by palpable synovial thickening.

Exercise-induced anaphylaxis is uncommon, particularly in children, and is usually associated with prominent itching and grossly visible urticaria and angioedema. Exercise-induced anaphylaxis is a syndrome of massive generalized histamine release, which should result in elevated levels of urinary histamine metabolites for several hours in survivors. Levels of other metabolic products of mast cell and basophil degranulation such as serum tryptase may be elevated in samples collected in a timely manner and appropriately preserved. Some cases are food-dependent, in which anaphylaxis is triggered by exercise, usually running, following ingestion of food [7]. We are not aware of these very uncommon cases being confused with school sports or PE asthma.

IX. EFFICIENT SURVEILLANCE

We believe surveillance for school sports and PE asthma should be simple, inexpensive, readily available, and reliable. Several investigators, including authors of other chapters in this book, have validated medically monitored exercise challenge protocols, either to screen entire school populations or to evaluate individual children for suspected school sports or PE asthma (see Chapter 26).

X. DEALING WITH EXERCISE-INDUCED ASTHMA IN SCHOOL CHILDREN

A. Goals and Steps to Achieve Them

Children with any chronic illness function best when the disruptive consequences of their illness are minimized, and they learn that their illness need not limit their ability to succeed. In school sports and PE asthma, this includes learning how to enjoy a healthy level of physical activity and the self esteem and peer recognition such participation can bring. The following steps will help school personnel facilitate the achievement of these goals:

1. Be alert for signs and symptoms of exercise-associated asthma and recognize suspicious cases.
2. Communicate observations and suspicions to parents or guardians, sharing in-school and out-of-school observations, to increase or decrease level of suspicion.
3. Remember the findings of McFadden [5] and Cypcar [6], that prolonged or intense post-exercise airflow obstruction indicates the presence of other triggering or aggravating factors, in addition to exercise.
4. Encourage appropriate medical evaluation and treatment.
5. Seek reports of physicians' findings and recommendations from parents or directly from physicians, when symptoms or illness impair a student's ability to function and develop healthy self confidence and self-sufficiency in school.

B. School Staffs and Administrators Should Recognize the Following

1. Children differ in access to appropriate medical care.
2. Children differ in parental oversight, ability, and resources to control other triggers that aggravate school sports and PE asthma.
3. Children and their families differ in ability to cope with the stress of this chronic disorder.
4. Deficiencies in the resources listed in this section are often socioeconomically based, and may reach epidemic proportions in schools serving socioeconomically disadvantaged communities.
5. Because high prevalences of these deficiencies are poverty-based rather than education-based, funding for costs of remediation may be most appropriately sought from poverty-based funds instead of siphoned from already limited educational budgets.

C. Modalities That May Facilitate Healthy, Rehabilitation at the Group Level

1. Support groups involving parents.
2. School-based support groups involving students.
3. Recruit participation of celebrities, particularly celebrity athletes, into health education curricular for all students (to facili-

tate peer acceptance) as role models who have overcome asthma.

In low-income, ethnic minority populations, in which the majority of asthmatics who have sports and PE-associated symptoms will not be gifted athletes, it would also be desirable to recruit other celebrity role models, such as the asthmatic rock musician who does not smoke, or the asthmatic pop singer who can sing only when her asthma is under control.

D. Policies and Practices to Facilitate Healthy Asthma Rehabilitation

Disability laws require that students have access to appropriate medications. This means teachers, particularly those supervising sports and other physical activities, must be trained and certified to administer simple medications normally given at home by parents, according to prescribed treatment schedules signed by both the child's physician and a legally responsible parent or guardian.

School asthma treatment schedules must permit dosing flexibility on an "as-needed" basis. Treatment may depend on the presence or absence of symptoms, or on readings on a child's own peak flow meter.

School asthma treatment schedules should be reviewed by a professional familiar with standards of asthma care. Usually, this will be a school nurse with specific training and experience in the management of asthma. This person must have the ability to seek informal consultation and review of questionable treatment schedules by appropriately qualified physicians, so that the school will not administer medically inappropriate treatments that could result in injury to a child and liability for the school.

Parents have asked to have drugs administered by nebulizer to their children at school. Is this appropriate? In none of these cases have we concluded that this was a medically appropriate use of school resources, even when a nebulizer has been available for this purpose. Young children sick enough to require nebulized medications during school hours are too sick to be at school.

Children need privacy for administration of medications. We cared for one child whose basketball coach interrupted practice, as soon as all children on the team had assembled, and grouped them into a circle in which he made derisive comments about one student who had delayed the start of practice because he had taken his asthma inhalers.

Students should be taught to self-administer asthma medication because metered-dose aerosols are the primary asthma drugs for which administration during school hours or at school activities is medically appropriate.

E. Off-the-Shelf Resources Available for Interested School Districts

The Allergy and Asthma Foundation of America (AAFA), Washington DC, (1-800-7-ASTHMA), is a source of asthma education programs and materials for lay individuals and groups of all ages. AAFA has regional chapters in several major metropolitan areas.

The American Lung Association (ALA) has offices nationwide, and is the lay arm of the American Thoracic Society (ATS), a medical specialty society of nonallergist specialists in pulmonary medicine. The ALA/ATS has literature describing exercise-induced asthma that may be obtained from state component organizations of the ALA/ATS.

Allergy and Asthma Network/Mothers of Asthmatics Inc. is a rapidly growing lay organization in Fairfax VA, (1-800-878-4403). It was founded by the mother of an asthmatic child who wanted answers to questions about her own child's disease and, on discovering the difficulty involved in finding them, sought the strength in numbers necessary to make them more accessible to others. The organization is consumer-oriented and does not reflect the biases of any individual medical discipline. Interested schools may become members of the network for a nominal fee.

The National Jewish Center for Immunology and Respiratory Medicine in Denver, Colorado, offers telephone access (1-800-222-LUNG) to its educational and information resources about asthma and other immunologic and respiratory diseases.

XI. SUMMARY

School sports and PE asthma is a barometer of the adequacy of asthma management in the communities. Its prevalence and severity can be minimized by recognition and appropriate management of the underlying asthma. Successful achievement of this goal requires accomplishment of an educational process strikingly similar to the educational process by which schools are charged with preparing children for other facets of life: Recognize differences in readiness. Adapt your program to meet prevailing readiness levels in your students. Encourage and recognize progress at every level of achievement, and make your target the learning of self-management skills and healthy adaptation patterns for life.

REFERENCES

1. Campbell S, Hood I, Ryan D, Biedrzycki L, Mirchandani H. Death as a result of asthma in Wayne County medical examiner cases, 1975–1987. J Forensic Sci 1990; 35:356–364.
2. McFadden FR, Gilbert IA. Exercise-induced asthma. N Engl J Med 1994; 330:1362–1367.
3. Cypcar D, Lemanske RF Jr. Asthma and exercise. Clin Chest Med 1994; 15: 351–368.
4. Venge P, Henricksen J, Dahl R. Eosinophils in exercise-induced asthma. J Allergy Clin Immunol 1991; 88:699–704.
5. Nudel DB, Diamant S, Brady T, Jarenwattananon M, Buckley BJ, Gootman N. Chest pain, dyspnea on exertion and exercise induced asthma in children and adolescents. Clin Pediatr 1987; 26:388–392.
6. Wiens L, Sabath R, Ewing L, Gowdamarajan R, Portnoy J, Scagliotti D. Chest pain in otherwise healthy children and adolescents is frequently caused by exercise-induced asthma. Pediatrics 1992; 90:350–353.
7. Kaplan AP. Urticaria and angioedema. In: Middleton E, Reed CE, Ellis EF, Adkinson NF, Yuninger JW, Busse W, eds. Allergy, principles and practice. St. Louis: CV Mosby, 1993; 1565.

26

Preparticipation Evaluation in the Athlete with Respiratory Disease

Christopher Randolph and Barbara Fraser
St. Mary's Hospital Regional Department of Pediatrics, Division of Yale University Medical Center, Waterbury, Connecticut

I. INTRODUCTION

Enthusiasm for organized sports activities is increasing for children and adults at all levels of competition [1]. This enthusiasm for sports participation is encouraging because it promotes cardiovascular fitness and general health and wellness, at the same time it demands increasing preparticipation evaluation surveillance, particularly for the previous nonathlete who is at highest risk of injury. The preparticipation evaluation requires an age-appropriate focused history and physical examination of the athlete. An evaluation is required for many athletic activities [2] and is recommended as a part of the overall health care for all student participants in organized sports [3]. The evaluation is usually performed by a physician using guidelines often established by medical societies or by other professional organizations to promote uniform standards for all such evaluations [3]. Decisions about sports participation are made by a qualified physician [3]. The focus of this chapter is to review the appropriate preparticipation history and physical examination for the athlete to identify respiratory disease, particularly of the lower respiratory system. Respiratory disease is a common disorder that has received relatively little attention compared with cardiovascular or orthopedic problems, which rightfully dominate the preparticipation examination [4].

II. THE DIMENSIONS AND DEMOGRAPHICS OF THE PROBLEM

About 3.5 million boys and 2 million girls competed in high school athletics during the years 1991–1992 [5]. As many as 46% of white, 52% of African–American and 46% of Hispanic boys participate in varsity sports at the high school level [6]. An estimated 22–39% of athletes are injured in sports, as defined by inability to complete a practice or game or absence from a subsequent practice or game [6]. Boys are injured at twice the rate of girls, particularly as a result of football and wrestling. In contrast gymnastics is the most injurious activity for girls.

The preparticipation athletic examination (PAE) is a paramount component of the general health care of the student participating in organized sports. Comprehensive health planning involves the coaches, trainers, parents, and adolescents; private and team physicians; and school administrators [7]. Each has designated responsibilities, such as addressing proper training and diet, education in injury recognition, mechanisms for appropriate rehabilitation, emergency preparation, record keeping, and systems for coordinating athletic and general health concerns [1].

There is a growing interest in exercise- and sports-related activities involving younger children, with many communities sponsoring organized sports, even at the preschool level. More than 20 million children are involved in community-sponsored sports programs.

More than 30 sports are now sanctioned for male participation and 27 for female participation. Increasing involvement of women, of disabled, the chronically ill, and of young children in adult sports, such as marathons, is creating the need for special knowledge on the part of the primary care provider. With young children participating in gymnastics or marathons, the "burned-out" child, who is expected to perform and win at early age is presenting a special challenge to the knowledgeable primary care provider [1]. These children risk injuries that may jeopardize their future. The role of the primary care provider is to identify those athletes whose medical condition may increase risk of injury or sudden death and to disqualify them or to provide appropriate medical treatment. Simultaneously, the provider should not disqualify athletes without a compelling medical reason. Objective medical criteria and guidelines should be employed to determine physical risks so that individual candidates are not arbitrarily penalized for being handicapped. Traditionally, the preparticipation athletic examination is a screening method to prevent life-threatening or disabling injuries, by identifying predisposing factors, recommending preparatory and rehabilitative measures, and assisting in matching the participant with an appropriate sport or position [8].

Table 1 Prevalence of Exercise-Induced Asthma

Author (xr)	Population
Kawabori (1976)	40% in allergic individuals, 90% in asthmatics
Weiler (1986)	50% by methacholine challenge in Iowa college football team
Randolph et al. (1991, 1992)	12% in unselected pediatric population
Rupp et al. (1992)	12% in preparticipation high school athletes
Rice et al. (1985)	2.8% in college athletes at University of Washington
Voy et al. (1984)	11% of Olympic athletes

However, 80–90% of adolescents report that the preparticipation athletic examination provides their only routine health evaluation, particularly among inner city youth. Therefore, there are proponents of a more extensive physical examination, including low-yield auscultation of the lungs and counseling for drugs, sex, and nutrition, instead of the more traditional examination focused on high-yield cardiovascular and musculoskeletal problems designed to determine physical risk for participating in a chosen sport. With the increasing numbers of youthful participants, the opponents of this broader approach argue that the examination must remain focused to be effective, because it is not a specific-screening test, particularly for rare cardiac diseases such as kinking of the coronary arteries or hypertrophic subaortic stenosis that predispose to sudden death [9]. The remaining focus of this chapter will be on the athlete with respiratory disease, which includes asthma, particularly exercise-induced asthma that affects at least 10% of the general population [10], 40% of allergic individuals, and up to 80–90% of asthmatics [11], as well as 11% of Olympic champions [12] (Table 1). The cost–benefit of screening for such a common disorder is indisputable. It is less clear what constitutes appropriate history, physical and exercise challenge as described in the following.

III. EXERCISE-RELATED PULMONARY SYNDROMES

Pulmonary disease that affects athletic performance includes various forms of chronic obstructive pulmonary disease, exercise-induced asthma (EIA), and rarely, exercise-induced anaphylaxis. These conditions must be differentiated from the far more common lack of conditioning. They must also be distinguished from causes of sudden death, such as hypertrophic cardiomyopathy, coronary artery disease, or anomalous kinking of the coronary vessels. Cardiac causes of exercise-related diseases are usually differentiated by dizziness, syncope, chest pain, or palpitations on exertion particularly in a child with known cardiac disease or with a family history of sudden death. This history demands a thorough cardiovascular evaluation. Unfortunately, even routine screening with 12-lead electrocardiogram (ECG) or with echocardiography are not cost-efficient in conjunction with history in differentiating the athlete with lack of conditioning from the athlete with compromising cardiac disease [13]. The preparticipation examination and history is not cost-efficient in screening for rare cardiac disease, which in Rhode Island afflicts 1:280,000 individuals, resulting in sudden death [14], or 1:7620 joggers in Rhode Island, age 30–65 years, who are afflicted with coronary artery disease [15]. However, examination and history may be more efficient in conjunction with exercise challenge in discriminating asthma, which afflicts up to 10% or more of exercising athletes [9]. Epstein and Maron [13] concluded that to identify a single athlete younger than 35 years who would die from sudden cardiac death, 200,000 competitive athletes would have to be screened and 1,000 would have to have cardiovascular disease. Even positive results on preparticipation history or physical examination are more often a variant of normal and a negative examination result does not rule out a catastrophic cardiac event [15].

Because athletic participation in all sports has increased dramatically during the 1980s the need for a simple and focused preparticipation history and physical examination has gained popularity as indicated by several editorials [16–19]. The original 1976 guidelines of the American Medical Association [20] were revised by American Academy of Pediatrics in 1988 [20], and the Academy of Family Physicians has a similar revision of an older 1984 guidelines [21]. The thrust of these guidelines and editorials is that a brief half-dozen or so historical questions and a focused preparticipation examination are essential to screen an estimated 14 million high school and an equal number of middle school students yearly [22].

The history and examination cannot be comprehensive, but can only focus on findings that would affect safe participation in sports. There are no universal guidelines for the performance of trials or focused examination for respiratory disease. However, the American Academy of Allergy Asthma, and Immunology, Sports Medicine Committee has attempted to develop a simplified questionnaire that is age-appropriate and concise to screen for exercise-related respiratory disorders, principally asthma and inhalant allergy (see Table 5). This questionnaire was derived after careful statistical analysis and trials from a more detailed Olympic questionnaire employed for the 1984 games [23]. This will be discussed in detail in a later section on exercise asthma.

The American Academy of Pediatrics, in its 1988 guidelines, and The Group on Science and Technology, designated by the American Medical Association, recommended the preparticipation athletic examination to identify adolescent athletes at risk for orthopedic disability, medical disorders, or sudden death from cardiac causes [3]. However, the same group could find no confirmation of the usefulness of the examination for previously unsuspected pulmonary disease.

Others have suggested that the most effective screening method for respiratory disease in the exercising athlete is appropriate challenge testing by cycling, running on a treadmill, or a free-running test, with monitoring of pulmonary functions by spirometry (1-S forced expiratory volume; FEV_1) or, less ideally, by peak flow meter readings [24,25]. Rupp and his colleagues demonstrated that when 1241 middle and high school student athletes were screened with questionnaire and resting spirometry as part of preparticipation screening, and then subsequently asked to run on a treadmill, if results of the questionnaire or screening were positive, 29% had previously unrecognized exercise-induced asthma [24].

If history alone was used as indication for challenge, only 28% had exercise-induced asthma, whereas when history was coupled with resting spirometry as an indication for challenge, 61% of the screened athletes had exercise-induced asthma and only 15% with positive spirometry alone had exercise-induced asthma based on treadmill testing [24]. Rupp's findings, which are consistent with earlier Olympic and collegiate studies [12,25,26], suggest that preparticipation history and examination are not sufficient to diagnose exercise-related syndromes, but may be used in conjunction with a challenge, such as treadmill and pulmonary function monitoring. We will now review the common exercise syndromes, including exercise-induced asthma, exercise in the athlete with chronic obstructive pulmonary disease, or allergic disease, as well as exercise-induced anaphylaxis [26].

IV. EXERCISE-INDUCED ASTHMA: PREPARTICIPATION EVALUATION

The significant differential diagnosis for the athletes with respiratory symptoms includes (a) lack of conditioning; (b) exercise-induced asthma, reflected by shortness of breath, cough or wheezing, or chest pain; (c) atopy, with typical eye or nasal itching, sneezing, or asthma on exposure to inhalant or ingested allergen; and (d) rarely, exercise-induced anaphylaxis, which may be dependent on ingestion of food in some individuals. The lung has the unique capacity to adapt to increased workloads, as evidenced by the ability to increase the pulmonary ventilation from 5–6 L/min at rest to 100–200 L/min during exercise. The limiting factors for the exercising athlete are the increases in cellular muscle metabolism and in the circulatory system that lead to the fatigued or "winded" state in the less well-conditioned athlete. However, the normal athlete, even at maximum cardiac output, consumes only 60% of maximum ventilatory capacity [26].

Lack of conditioning may be confused with exercise-induced asthma, but can be distinguished by the presence of cough or wheezing in association with exercise challenge in asthma. The poorly conditioned athlete may become winded, but rarely has any significant cough or wheezing [26]. This poorly conditioned person usually has a history indicating lack of appropriate exercise prescription to maintain sports activity or may have been previously injured and is at risk for orthopedic injuries, such as tendonitis, plantar fasciitis, or compartment syndromes.

These poorly conditioned individuals may be differentiated by a simple focused history, such as the 11-question form proposed by Fields [9]. The question "Has the athlete ever broken a bone, had to wear a cast, or had an injury to any joint?" will elicit previous injury, although not necessarily present condition. Knee and ankle injuries often recur. The most common injury is reinjury of a joint. Thus, a positive answer to this question places the athlete in a high-risk group. Counseling and rehabilitation may be indicated.

The patient with a rare cardiac syndrome, such as hypertrophic cardiomyopathy, an autosomal dominant condition that is the most common cause of sudden death in athletes younger than 15 years, can be screened by questions about sudden death in family members younger than 50 years. Other rare cardiac syndromes, such as arrhythmias or congenital anomalies of the coronary arteries may be differentiated by a question on exercise-related syncope, light-headedness, or dizziness [26]. Because sudden cardiac death in young athletes occurs only in 1:200,000, it is improbable that these questions will ever be verified as screening tools prospectively, but retrospective studies indicate that they identify the at-risk athlete [26]. The other questions in the 11-question history of Fields ask about of neurological injury (specifically concussion); heat-related illness; harmful health habits; general health related to chronic illness, medications, or injury to paired organs; and exercise-induced asthma and allergies [9]. The question for asthma or inhalant allergy is "Does the athlete have asthma (wheezing), hay fever, or coughing spells after exer-

Table 2 History of Notable Events

Aretaeus the Cappodochian (2nd century AD)
Sir John Floyer: Treatise (1698)
Heimlich et al.: The treadmill (1966)
Olympic swimmer deprived of medal (1972)
EIA incidence 11% in Olympic contenders (1984)

cise?'' This question exemplifies the presentation of exercise-induced asthma.

Table 2 provides a brief overview, from a historical perspectives of the recognition of exercise-induced asthma [27–49, 69].

V. SCREENING OF ATHLETES

The preparticipation or preseason examination and history provide an ideal setting to detect exercise-induced asthma and to develop a strategy for management of this disorder. The athlete should be asked about a history of environmental inhalant allergens (seasonal pollens such as grass, tree, or weed, or perennial allergies, such as mite, mold, or animal dander) or a history of cough or of wheezing at night, with respiratory infection, allergens or exertion. The athlete should also be asked about previous evaluations and medication use, such as antihistamines, decongestants, nasal sprays, and over-the-counter or prescriptions. Attention should be paid to use of cromolyn, nasal steroids, bronchodilators such as theophylline; or inhaled β-agonists or anti-inflammatory drugs.

Coach and trainer observations of ''locker room cough'' or an ''out-of-shape'' athlete in the middle of the season or repeated use of antibiotics for ''bronchitis'' should prompt further attention. A firm yes or no answer to cough, wheezing or shortness of breath with strenuous exercise should be sought in the evaluation questionnaire [26] Cough, wheezing, chest tightness, or shortness of breath with strenuous exercise, or respiratory infection resulting in missed school or work is particularly reliable historical information.

A. History

The focused preparticipation history is important [16] and required in at least 35 states [2] for junior and high school athletes [16]. The high-yield areas need to be addressed: (a) cardiovascular disease, (b) high blood pressure, and (c) orthopedic injury. A more detailed survey proposed as by Fields [9] should also address exercise-induced asthma, neurological disorders, and general health (including allergies to medications or bee venom, and health habits). The preparticipation examination should be a screening examination and not a comprehensive health maintenance examination.

Individual athletes with problems related to drug abuse or sexuality should be referred for further evaluation to the student's family physician, if one was identified or to a primary care physician [9]. Otherwise, the appropriate setting for the preparticipation physical (Table 3) examination and history depend on the resources, volume, and intentions of the examining physicians. The athlete's personal physician, if one is identified, may be able to perform the screening examination. Unfortunately, 78% of athletes have no primary care provider. However, a multistation approach as outlined by Smith [50] may also be used. In that case, vital signs, vision, height and weight, and sign-in are at one station run by nurses, coaches, or volunteer ancillary personnel, and a second station is used to perform orthepedic and general medicine examinations. Final clearance by a physician is ultimately required. Further stations, staffed by trainers, therapists, and physicians, may include specific orthopedic examination and evaluation of body composition, flexibility, strength, speed, endurance, agility, power, and balance. The personal physician approach clearly lacks the presence of personnel trained in specific orthopedic and medical subspecialties and has more time constraints and

Table 3 Preparticipation Format

Station examination: Efficient, multidisciplinary, but may be impersonal and superficial.

Personal physician: More thorough, allows counseling.

Objective: focused musculoskeletal and cardiovascular evaluation versus extended history to achieve counseling on drugs, sex, and conditioning.

Evaluation of athlete with respiratory disease:

- History: Focused on complaints of cough, wheezing, chest tightness or pain, dyspnea or syncopy, particularly with exertion.
- Spirometry before and after bronchodilator administration or treadmill, cycle or free-running athletic screening test (FRAST) with peak flow or spirometry monitoring as dictated by history or performance.
- Bodybox, blood gases, chest x-ray film, diffusing capacity for COPD or related cardiopulmonary disease.

inefficiency. The multistation approach is more efficient, but requires more personnel and organization and lacks privacy and familiarity with the athlete.

The purpose of the evaluation should be to detect limiting injuries and conditions to satisfy legal and insurance requirements and to determine the general health, maturity, fitness, and performance of the athlete. Secondarily, the evaluation may provide counseling on important health-related concerns, including drugs, sex, and conditioning. These secondary objectives are controversial [51]. The objective of the preparticipation examination is to provide a screening mechanism for conditions that preclude participation in sports, or those that may progress to disease or debilitating injury. The evaluation should also provide a mechanism for treatment and follow-up of medical or surgical conditions [52]. For example, the athlete might be referred to an allergist for follow-up and allergy skin testing or for pulmonary function testing.

The history remains the cornerstone of the preparticipation assessment detecting 63–74% of the conditions afflicting the athlete [53]. It may include as many as 20 questions [51,54] concerning general health, including recent physician visits, hospitalizations, or surgery in the last 12 months; family history of diabetes, allergies, migraine headaches, cardiac or blood pressure problems, and history of premature death (before age 50 years); neurological injuries, including concussions, skull injuries, convulsions, or neck injuries; emotional or psychiatric conditions; dental, vision, hearing, renal or gynecological problems; bone or joint injuries; anemia, diabetes, or dermatological conditions; allergies to medications or bee stings; inhalant allergy, asthma, or exercise-related symptoms, including asthma and anaphylaxis; or syncope. We will focus these on the athlete with respiratory symptoms (Tables 4 and 5).

For the athlete with respiratory symptoms, the three major concerns would be (a) asthma, particularly exercise-related, or bronchitis in the smoker; (b) allergic disease in the athlete with symptoms on exposure to allergens, such as inhalants, foods, medications, or stinging insects; and (c) rare conditions, such as exercise-induced anaphylaxis accompanied by hives and angioedema, or cardiac disease accompanied by exercise-related syncope [26]. The rare cardiac conditions have already been discussed and simple questions related to exercise syncopy and family history of sudden death or palpitations or chest pain will help identify these individuals and potentially avoid tragedy [54].

Standard questions include the following: Have you ever passed out, been dizzy, or experienced chest pain? Do you tire more easily than your friends during or after exercise? [53]. Further questions concerning blood pressure, murmurs, heart racing or skipped beats, or family history of

Table 4 Exercise Questionnaire: Answer Yes, No, or Unsure

1. Have you ever been told you have (had)
   a. Hay fever or allergic rhinitis (stuffy nose when you do not have a cold)
   b. Asthma
   c. Exercise-induced asthma
2. Do you *ever* have the following symptoms
   a. Chest tightness
   b. Cough
   c. Wheezing
   d. Prolonged shortness of breath
   e. Skin rash
3. When you exercise, do you often or occasionally have
   a. Chest tightness
   b. Cough
   c. Wheezing
   d. Prolonged shortness of breath
   e. Skin rash
   f. Chest pain
   g. Abdominal pain, nausea, or vomiting
   h. If yes, do you ever stop exercising because of any of these symptoms?
4. Do cold air, smoke, fumes (perfumes, paints), dust, or mold ever cause chest tightness, cough, or wheezing?
5. Does running ever cause chest tightness, cough or wheezing, or prolonged shortness of breath?
6. Do you frequently have ''head colds'' that end up with symptoms in your chest?
7. Have you had sinusitis?
8. Does anyone in your family have asthma, hayfever, or allergies?
   If yes, list who and describe briefly: ______________________
9. Do you get itchy eyes? If so, when? ______________________
10. Do you have a cold now or have you had a cold recently?
11. Have you ever had chest tightness, cough, wheezing, asthma, or other chest (lung) problems that made it difficult for you to perform in sports?
12. Have you ever missed school or work because of chest tightness, cough or wheezing, or prolonged shortness of breath?
13. Have you ever taken any medication for asthma or allergy? If yes, list below
    ____
14. Have you ever smoked? If yes, are you a current smoker?

Source: Courtesy John Weiler, M.D.

Table 5 Exercise Questionnaire (Short Form)

1. Have you ever been told you have (had) asthma or exercise-induced asthma?
   _____ No _____ Yes _____ Not sure
2. Do you ever have chest tightness?
   _____ No _____ Yes _____ Not sure
3. Do you ever have wheezing?
   _____ No _____ Yes _____ Not sure
4. Do you ever have itchy eyes?
   _____ No _____ Yes _____ Not sure
5. Do you ever have itching of the nose or throat or sneezing spells?
   _____ No _____ Yes _____ Not sure
6. Does running ever cause chest tightness, cough, wheezing, or prolonged shortness of breath?
   _____ No _____ Yes _____ Not sure
7. Have you ever had chest tightness, cough, wheezing, asthma, or other chest (lung) problems that made it difficult for you to perform in sports?
   _____ No _____ Yes _____ Not sure
8. Have you ever missed school or work because of chest tightness, cough, wheezing, or prolonged shortness of breath?
   _____ No _____ Yes _____ Not sure

Source: Courtesy John Weiler, M.D.

heart problems or sudden death, usually help identify these at-risk individuals. Unfortunately, the rarity of the cardiac causes of sudden death mandate a high level of suspicion because history, examination, and laboratory workup are often unrevealing [14]. Individuals with a suggestive history should be referred for cardiology evaluation, although the yield is low. It is imperative to ask about syncope, chest pains, palpitations, or shortness of breath with exercise or a family history of premature death, because this history may help discriminate the rare individual with Marfan's syndrome or hypertrophic cardiomyopathy, or more commonly, mitral valve prolapse, from the much more common lack of conditioning or from exercise-induced asthma [23]. Mitral valve prolapse is thought to be more common in female patients and may have a benign course if the athlete has no history of chest symptoms of syncope [55–57]. Chest pain is not always indicative of heart disease. As many as 70% of adolescents with chest pain and a negative cardiac workup in one series had exercise-induced asthma [49].

The question: Does the athlete have wheezing, suggestive of asthma, hay fever, or related symptoms with inhalants, or trouble breathing (shortness of breath), cough, or chest pain during or after exercise? [26,53] will help to discriminate exercise-related asthma from the out-of-shape athlete. The absence of hives, or angioedema, or hypotension after exercise (or exercise and food ingestion) helps rule out exercise-induced anaphylaxis [26,53]. Weiler has analyzed questionnaire histories for exercise-induced asthma for the Academy of Allergy, Asthma, and Immunology [unpublished]. He notes that certain questions seem to predict that an athlete will have a positive exercise challenge as described in the following. The more extensive Olympic questionnaire [12] and our own pediatric version demonstrate statistically significant correlation between a positive challenge and the presence of exercise-induced asthma only when all allergy and asthma-related questions were positive. Similarly, absence of allergy- and asthma-related symptoms correlates with a negative challenge [43,44]. Unfortunately our questionnaire is neither sensitive nor specific and a challenge by treadmill, cycle, or free-running is necessary to confirm exercise-induced asthma [24,36–38]. Questionnaires have been criticized for lack of sensitivity and specificity [35,58]. However, they have been used to identify 90% of Olympic [12] and 90% of high school athletes with asthma [35]. Weiler et al. [45] report that 37% of asymptomatic athletes had a positive methacholine bronchoprovocation test result, whereas 100% of athletes with symptoms had a positive challenge result. Overall, the higher the symptom score, the more likely the athlete had a positive result from methacholine bronchoprovocation ($p < 0.001$) [45]. In Weiler's analysis three questions predict a positive challenge result: (a) chest tightness, prolonged shortness of breath, cough, or wheezing, particularly with exercise; (b) chest tightness, prolonged shortness of breath, coughing or wheezing associated with missed school or work; and (c) the presence of itchy eyes (presumably suggesting allergy).

This information has allowed the development of more focused surveys (see Table 5) that may be more efficient than the longer Olympic-style questionnaire (see Table 4). One focused questionnaire is currently being used in a multicenter trial (see Table 5). Point scores can be developed to score wheezing, coughing, or shortness of breath with exercise or upper respiratory illness or history of asthma on exposure to cold air, smoke, or other irritants.

However, even the best questionnaire may be an unreliable predictor of exercise-induced asthma [24,47]. As demonstrated by the study of Kawabori [11] 78% of children with a history of exercise-induced asthma had positive exercise test result, but 54% of children who denied exercise-induced asthma also had a positive test result. A positive test was defined as a decrease in peak expiratory flow (PEF) by at least 15%, following 6 min of free-running. In the study of Bransford et al. [59] 201 school children in the age range of 12–13 years were challenged to a 6-min free-running test in a gymnasium, with peak flow monitoring before, immediately after, and 5 min after the run. Children were chosen based on a questionnaire about previous diagnosis of asthma, recent symptoms, and symptoms of allergic rhinitis. Of these children, 8.9% demonstrated exercise-induced asthma with 43% of those with symptomatic asthma and none of those with asymptomatic asthma demonstrating a positive challenge result. Only 7 (41%) of those with asthma, whose parents had reported exercise-related symptoms, could be demonstrated to have exercise-induced asthma. Parents of 20% of those asthmatic children who had exercise-induced asthma were unaware of the condition similar to later studies [24,36].

Only 39% of histories provided by athletes correspond to those their parents provided [60]. Thus, it is recommended that the athlete complete the history and have it reviewed and signed by parents before the examination [55,61]. The physician should further review the history with the athlete before the examination [50]. The highest yield on history is from orthopedics-related questions relevant to present conditioning and past injuries [9].

In summary, combinations of a challenge, such as the free-running test, that are easily adaptable to a track, hallway, or stair, or the treadmill or cycloergometer in conjunction with a questionnaire, are essential to diagnose exercise-induced asthma.

B. Timing of the Examination

The examination should be ideally scheduled 6 weeks before the onset of practice or competition to provide time to thoroughly assess and rehabilitate old injuries [3]. Recommendations for conditioning should be provided 6 weeks before the season. The multistation setting is favored for efficiency, with specialized medical personnel and fitness testing. Women may feel more comfortable discussing their gynecological concerns and personal questions with their own physician. A complete evaluation may be performed every 2 years with an interim history and examination during the other year.

C. Physical Examination

The preparticipation examination is focused on blood pressure, cardiovascular, and orthopedic components, particularly the knee and weight-bearing joints of the musculoskeletal system. The athlete with respiratory disease is a candidate for a focused ear, nose, and throat examination, as well as skin and pulmonary assessment, consisting of a chest examination.

Allergic stigmata, such as allergic shiners, creases, and the allergic "salute," pale boggy nasal mucosa, sinus tenderness, pruritic nasal discharge, or wheezing on chest examination, as well as hives or flexor or extensor eczema are hallmarks of the atopic athlete. The findings of hyperemic and pruritic conjunctiva with cobblestoning of the upper tarsal conjunctiva with serous, ropy ocular and nasal discharge suggest an allergic individual. In contrast, the athlete with clubbing, cyanosis, rales on chest examination, and nasal polyps may have cystic fibrosis or other malabsorptive disease. Further pulmonary function evaluation with spirometry before and after bronchodilator administration, and even evaluation of residual volume or diffusion capacity, may help differentiate the athlete with obstructive pulmonary disease. As with any complete examination, height and weight and nutritional status by skin-fold measurement and careful cardiovascular examination, including blood pressure, cardiac evaluation for murmurs, gallop, or tachycardia suggesting cardiac disease are mandatory. Further evaluation by a cardiologist is dictated if the examination suggests cardiac disease. As indicated earlier, the preparticipation evaluation is not a sensitive indicator of rare cardiac disease. Gynecological examination is indicated if the history is suggestive of menstrual irregularities, dyspareunia, dysmenorrhea or dysuria. Preventive counseling centering on drug abuse, proper nutrition and sexual issues such as birth control, and school and family issues including psychological issues should be either part of the evaluation or requires subsequent referral [3].

D. General Diagnostic Evaluation

General undirected laboratory testing such as complete blood count, urinalysis, serum ferritin, serum chemistries, or lipid determinations has no proven value. However, directed diagnostic studies, including exercise challenge, whether by treadmill, free-running, or cycle may establish the diagnosis of exercise-induced asthma. Similarly, pulmonary functions before and after bronchodilator administration are necessary to establish the diagnosis of chronic asthma. Epicutaneous skin tests may be performed and evaluated. Sexually active women of any age should have a Pap smear [54].

E. Directed Diagnostic Evaluation

Three diagnostic tests are available for exercise testing for suspected exercise-induced asthma; treadmill, cycle ergometry, and a free-running test (FRAST—free-running athletic screening test) (Table 6) [62]. Use of the methacholine bronchial provocation challenge or inhalation challenge with

Table 6 Methods of Screening

1. Questionnaire: insufficient and nonspecific.
2. Cycloergometer: least asthmogenic, but convenient for physiological measurements.
3. Treadmill: gold standard, expensive, but convenient for physiological measurements.
4. FRAST: convenient, familiar, inexpensive, most asthmogenic, but difficult to standardize for physiological measurements.
5. Challenge with consistent temperature, relative humidity and environment is essential to diagnosis.

cold, dry air or hyperosmolar saline are reserved for research settings [48] (see Table 5). Pulmonary function testing may be used to screen for individuals with less than 80% of predicted FEV_1. All exercise testing should be accompanied by cardiac monitoring, and individuals who develop arrhythmia or angina-like pain or evidence of circulatory insufficiency should have the exercise testing terminated promptly and should be evaluated by a cardiologist.

The exercise challenge consists of 6–8 min of strenuous exercise whether treadmill, FRAST, or cycloergometer at an intensity of 85–90% of the predicted maximal cardiac rate [48,59]. Most athletes achieve this heart rate by running on a 10% grade at a speed of 4–6 mph on a treadmill. An average of three resting spirometric measurements should be taken 2 min after exercise and then every 5 min for at least 15 min and preferably, for 30 min [24]. Monitoring for at least 8 h is controversial to detect the putative late phase. The maximal postexercise decline in spirometric measurements is compared with the resting baseline measurements to predict the percentage change. The diagnosis of exercise-induced asthma is based on documentation of a 10–15% or greater reduction in PER or FEV_1 in the postexercise period [48].

Environmental conditions should be controlled to provide a relative humidity of 40% or less, with an ambient temperature of 32.6°C (72°F). The challenge should be performed at least 4 h after the last dose of inhaler and 24 h after the last dose of sustained-release theophylline [26,48,56].

Athletes with a positive result by exercise challenge can be classified as having mild asthma with reduction of less than 25%, moderate with 25 35% reduction, and severe with greater than 35% reduction in FEV_1. Most competitive athletes fall in the mild-to-moderate range, including those with single or occasional medication use or those without a history of asthma or with only cough following rigorous exercise [26,63,64].

Whenever possible, a repeat exercise challenge should be performed under conditions identical with the initial challenge. Improvement in symptoms of cough, shortness of breath, or wheezing or chest pain in conjunction with a 50% or greater improvement in peak flow during challenge is indicative of successful therapy [26].

F. The Differential Diagnosis of Respiratory Disease in Athlete Preparticipation

The most common diagnosis in the young athlete with chronic lower respiratory disease is asthma. Less common diagnoses are exercise-induced anaphylaxis and cardiac disease, leading to sudden death (hypertrophic subaortic stenosis). In older athletes, coronary arteries disease and bronchitis should also be considered. More rarely, vocal cord dysfunction secondary to injury, abuse, or psychiatric syndromes, and cough-variant asthma must be considered.

G. Clearance for Participation

The critical issue for the athlete is whether it is safe to participate in a particular sport. The following questions must be answered for the athlete to receive clearance for medical or musculoskeletal condition [3]:

1. Does the condition predispose the athlete to increased risk of injury?
2. Does the condition expose another participant to increased risk of injury?
3. Can the athlete safely participate with therapy (i.e., rehabilitation, medication, padding, or other)?
4. Can limited participation be permitted while treatment is in progress?
5. If clearance is denied for some activities what activities are safe for the athlete to pursue?

The response to these questions may be in one of three categories: unrestricted, clearance after rehabilitation or evaluation, and not cleared [3]. Fortunately, few athletes fail to clear. In four studies [8,65–68] with preparticipation examinations on 17,500 male and female student athletes 85–94.8% passed, 5–13.5% passed conditionally and only 0.2–1.2% failed. Approval should be based on clinical assessment using American Academy of Pediatrics Recommendations for Participation in Competitive Sports [3]. Sports are classified by potential for injury as noncontact, limited contact, and collision. Noncontact activities are classified by their potential for exacerbating medical conditions: nonstrenuous, moderately strenuous, or strenuous. Recommendations for restriction are identical for males and females.

VI. SUMMARY

The preparticipation examination is a splendid opportunity for health care professionals to increase the safety for sports participation. Athletes may be provided education concerning conditioning, body composition, nutrition, musculoskeletal rehabilitation, and health maintenance. Athletes with respiratory disorders should be encouraged to participate. However, it is critical that the athletes be properly evaluated and that treatment be offered so that they may have a rewarding experience in their chosen sport.

REFERENCES

1. E Hulse, WB Strong. Preparticipation evaluation for athletics. Pediatr Rev 9:173, 1987.
2. JG Garrick. Orthopedic preparticipation screening examination. Pediatr Clin North Am 37:1047, 1990.
3. Athletic preparticipation examinations for adolescents. Report of Board of Trustees. Arch Pediatr Adolesc Med 148:93, 1994.
4. KB Fields. Clearing athletes for participation in sports. The North Carolina Medical Society Sports Medicine Committee's recommended examination. NC Med J 55:116, 1994.
5. National Federation of State High School Association. Sports Participation Survey. Kansas City MO. National Federation of State High School Associations, 1992.
6. EE Snyder, E Spreitzer. High school athletic participation as related to college attendance among black, Hispanic and white males. Youth Adolesc 21: 390, 1990.
7. SC Rice, JD Schlotfeldt, WE Foley. The Athletic Health Care and Training Program. A comprehensive approach to the prevention and management of athletic injuries in high school. West J Med 142:352, 1985.
8. CW Linder, RH DuRant, RM Seklecki, WB Strong. Preparticipation health screening of young athletes: results of 1268 examinations. Am J Sports Med 9:187, 1981.
9. KB Fields, M Delaney. Focusing the preparticipation sports examination. J Fam Pract 30:304, 1990.
10. M Nelson. Medical exclusion from sports. Pediatr Ann 21:149, 1992.

11. I Kawabori, WE Pierson, LL Conquest, CW Bierman. Incidence of exercise induced asthma in children. J Allergy Clin Immunol 58:447, 1976.
12. RO Voy. The U.S. Olympic Committee Experience with exercise-induced bronchospasm, 1984. Med Sci Sports Exerc 18:31, 1986.
13. JP Lewis, BJ Maron, JA Diggs, et al. Preparticipation echocardiographic screening for cardiovascular disease in large predominantly black population of intercollegiate athletes. Am J Cardiol 64:1029, 1989.
14. M Fahrenback, PD Thompson. The preparticipation sports exam and cardiovascular considerations for screening. Cardiol Clin 10:319, 1992.
15. M Ragos, J Crabtree, WQ Sturner, et al. Death during recreational exercise in the state of Rhode Island. Med Sci Sports Exerc 16:339, 1984.
16. JG Garrick, NJ Smith. Preparticipation sports assessment. Pediatrics 66:803, 1980.
17. PG Dyment. Another look at the sports preparticipation examination of the adolescent athlete. J Adolesc Health Care 7(suppl 16):130S, 1986.
18. DK Runyan. The preparticipation examination of young athlete: defining the essential. Clin Pediatr 22:674, 1983.
19. TR Thompson, JT Andrish, JA Bergfeld: A prospective study of preparticipation sports examinations of 2670 young athletes: Method and results. Cleve Clin O 49(4):225, 1982.
20. American Academy of Pediatrics—Committee on Sports Medicine: Recommendations for participation in competitive sports. Pediatrics 81:737, 1988.
21. Task Force on Sports Medicine: Athletic Competition Health Screening Form. Kansas City, MO, Academy of Family Physicians, 1984.
22. RA Feinstein, EJ Soileau, WA Daniel: A national survey of preparticipation physical examination requirements. Physician Sportsmed 16(5):51, 1989.
23. WE Pierson. Exercise induced bronchospasm in children and adolescents. Pediatric Allergic Disease Chapter of *Pediatric Clinics of North America Vol. 35 #5,* 1988.
24. NT Rupp, MF Guill, S. Brudno. Unrecognized exercise induced bronchospasm in adolescent athletes. American Journal Disease of Childhood 146: 941, 1992.
25. SC Rice, WW Bierman, GG Shapiro, et al. Identification of exercise-induced asthma among intercollegiate athletes. Ann Allergy 55:790, 1985.
26. JM Kyle. Exercise induced pulmonary syndromes. Med Clin North Am 78: 413, 1994.
27. Aretaeus the Cappadocian: The extant works of Aretaeus the Cappodocian. In: Samter M, ed. Excerpts from Classics of Allergy. Columbus OH: Ross Laboratories, 1969, p. 4.
28. JA Floyer, R Wilkin, W Innis. Treatise on Asthma, 1717.
29. RS McNeill, JR Nairn, RS Jill, et al. Exercise-induced asthma. Q J Med 35: 55, 1966.
30. S Godfrey. Symposium on special problems and management of allergic athletes. International Symposium on Special Problems and Management of Allergic Athletes Part 2. J Allergy Clin Immunol 73(suppl):630, 1984.

31. M Silverman, SD Anderson. Standardization of exercise tests in asthmatic children. Arch Dis Child 47:882, 1972.
32. ER McFadden Jr. Hypothesis: exercise-induced asthma as a vascular phenomenon. Lancet 335:880, 1990.
33. S Godfrey. Exercise induced asthma. In: Bierman CW, Pearlman DS, eds. Allergic Diseases from Infancy to Adulthood. 2nd ed. Philadelphia: WB Saunders, 1988, p. 597.
34. GJA Cropp. Grading, time course, and incidence of exercise induced airway obstruction and hyperinflation in asthmatic children. Pediatrics 56(suppl): 868, 1975.
35. BW Smith, JC Wong, JF Bremner, JC Puffer. The prevalence of exercise induced bronchospasm in high school athletes (submitted).
36. SD Williams, J Bruton, I Wilson. Screening a state middle school for asthma using a free running asthma screening test. Arch Dis Child 69:667, 1993.
37. JN Tsanakas, RDG Milner, OM Bannister, et al. Free running asthma screening test. Arch Dis Child 63:261, 1988.
38. S Bardagi, A Aguido, CA Gonzalez, DV Romero. Prevalence of exercise induced airway narrowing in school children in a Mediterranean town. Am Rev Respir Dis 47:1112, 1991.
39. DJ Keeley, P Neill, S Gallivan. Comparison of the prevalence of reversible airways obstruction in rural and urban Zimbabwean children. Thorax 46: 549, 1991.
40. RP Bransford, GM McNutt, JN Fink. Exercise induced asthma in adolescent gym class population. Int Arch Allergy Appl Immunol 94:272, 1991.
41. A Colin, E Said, WT Winter. Exercise induced asthma in school children. J Med Sci 21:40, 1985.
42. ML Burr, BA Eldridge, LK Borysiewicz. Peak expiratory flow rates before and after exercise in school children. Arch Dis Child 49:923, 1974.
43. CC Randolph, MF Randolph, B Fraser. Exercise-induced asthma in school children [abstract]. J Allergy Clin Immunol 87(part 2):341, 1991.
44. CC Randolph, MF Randolph, B Fraser. Ongoing evaluation of questionnaire (Q) for exercise asthma in children [abstract]. Ann Allergy 68:117, 1992.
45. JM Weiler, WJ Metzger, AL Donnelly, et al. Prevalence of bronchial hyperresponsiveness in highly trained athletes. Chest 90:23, 1986.
46. L Smith, R McFadden. Bronchial hyperreactivity revisited. Ann Allergy 74: 454, 1995.
47. S Shield, A Wang-Doulman. Incidence of exercise induced bronchospasm (EIB) in high school football players. J Allergy Clin Immunol 87:166, 1991.
48. S Anderson. Exercise-induced asthma. In: E. Middleton, CE Reed, EF Ellis, NF Adkinson, JF Yuninger, WW Busse eds. Allergy Principles and Practice, 4th ed. St Louis: Mosby Year Book, 1993.
49. L Weins, R Sabeth, L Ewing, R Goevdimarajan, J Portnoy, D Scagliotti. Chest pain in healthy children and adolescents is frequently caused by EIA. Pediatrics 90:350, 1992.
50. DM Smith, et al. The preparticipation evaluation. Primary Care 18:777, 1991.

51. RA Feinstein, EJ Soileau, WA Daniel. A national survey of physical exam requirements Physician Sportsmed 2:51, 1988.
52. Goldberg, et al. Children's sports injuries: are they unavoidable? Physician Sportsmed 7:9, 1979.
53. J Tanji. The preparticipation physical examination for sports. Am Fam Pract 42:397, 1990.
54. S Tanner. Preparticipation exam targeted for the female athlete. Clin Sports Med 23:337, 1994.
55. DC Warth, ME King, JM Cohen, et al. Prevalence of mitral valve prolapse in normal children. J Am Coll Cardiol 5:1173, 1985.
56. RL Washington. Mitral valve prolapse on active youth. Physician Sportsmed 21:136, 1993.
57. WW Briner, AL Sheffer. Exercise induced anaphylaxis. Med Sci Sports Exerc 24:849, 1992.
58. JF Frobase, JM Kyle, SD Hanna, JR Leaman, SL Hanshaw. Sensitivity of post exercise cough in predicting exercise induced bronchospasm in young athletes. Med Sci Sports Exerc 24:S143, 1992.
59. RP Bransford, GM McNutt, JN Fink. Exercise induced asthma in adolescent gym class population. Int Arch Allergy Appl Immunol 94:272, 1991.
60. WL Risser, EM Hoffman, GG Bellah. Frequency of preparticipation sports examinations in secondary school athletes. Are the university interscholastic league guidelines appropriate? Tex Med 81:35, 1985.
61. AS Lachman, P Schulman, CL Arfken, et al. Prevalence of mitral valve prolapse in non-care seeking adolescents. J Am Coll Cardiol 7:42A, 1986.
62. PA Eggleston, RR Rosenthal, SA Anderson, et al. Guidelines for the methodology of exercise challenge testing af asthmatics. J Allergy Clin Immunol 64: 642, 1979.
63. SD Anderson. EIA: new thinking and current management. J Respir Dis 7: 48, 1986.
64. W Bierman. Management of exercise induced asthma. Ann Allergy 68:119, 1992.
65. J Lewis, P Lieberman, G Treadwell, J Erffmeyer. Exercise-induced urticaria, angioedema, and anaphylactoid episodes. J Allergy Clin Immunol 68:432, 1981.
66. SA Magnes, JM Henderson, SC Hunter. What conditions limit sports participation? Experience with 10,540 athletes. Physician Sportsmed 20:143, 1992.
67. FS Tennant Jr, K Sorensen, CM Day. Benefits of preparticipation sports examination. J Fam Pract 13:287, 1981.
68. TR Thompson, JT Andrish, JA Bergfeld. A prospective study of preparticipation sports examinations of 2,670 young athletes: method and results. Cleve Clin Q 49:225, 1982.
69. EM Heimlich, L Strickl, RJ Busser. An exercise response test in childhood asthma. J Allergy 37:103(abstract), 1966.

Index

About the Editor

JOHN M. WEILER is a Professor of Internal Medicine in the College of Medicine at the University of Iowa, a Staff Physician at the Iowa City Veterans Affairs Medical Center, and a member of the Graduate College Interdisciplinary Program in Immunology. Since 1982, he has been an active participant in the Sports Medicine Services at the University of Iowa. He is coeditor of *Complement in Health and Disease*, Second Edition (1993). Dr. Weiler is a Fellow of the American College of Physicians, the American College of Rheumatology, and the American Academy of Allergy, Asthma and Immunology, and a member of the American Association of Immunologists, the American Society for Biochemistry and Molecular Biology, and the Central Society for Clinical Research. He received the B.S. degree (1967) from the University of Michigan, Ann Arbor, and the M.D. degree (1971) from Temple University School of Medicine, Philadelphia, Pennsylvania. He served for two years at the National Institutes of Health in the Blood Resources Branch of the National Heart, Lung and Blood Institute, and completed fellowship training at Harvard Medical School in the laboratory of Dr. K. Frank Austen at the Robert B. Brigham Hospital. He was a visiting investigator at Scripps Clinic and Research Foundation. He is certified by the American Board of Internal Medicine and by the American Board of Allergy and Immunology (for Allergy and Immunology and for Diagnostic Laboratory Immunology). His research has included studies of the complement system, especially of the interaction of complement proteins with highly charged substances such as heparin; investigations of heparin interactions with heparin-binding proteins and peptides; analyses of the prevalence of exercise-induced asthma; examinations of the role of nonsteroidal agents in sports medicine; and a variety of clinical trials, particularly in patients with hereditary angioedema. He has served as chair of the Sports Medicine Committee of the American Academy of Allergy, Asthma and Immunology, and as chair of the Publication Education Committee.